TECHNOLOGICAL INNOVATIONS IN TROPICAL LIVESTOCK DEVELOPMENT FOR ENVIRONMENTAL SUSTAINABILITY AND FOOD SECURITY

This book contains the proceedings of the fourth International Conference on Tropical Animal Production for Food Security (ITAPS) exploring **Technological Innovations in Tropical Livestock Development for Environmental Sustainability and Food Security**.

It discusses two interconnected issues: tropical livestock farming and environmental concerns, while addressing the adoption of innovative technologies and sustainable farming practices as a crucial step in addressing challenges related to tropical livestock farming. The contents of the proceedings include the latest research that can be applied in agricultural fields to improve the agriculture business, including topics such as:

- Leveraging environmentally friendly technologies to enhance production efficiency, manage waste effectively, and reduce carbon footprints
- Halal meat production in the modern era
- Availability of animal waste resources as alternative energy

The book will be valuable to students, researchers, and professionals in the agricultural fields and science.

PROCEEDINGS OF THE 4TH INTERNATIONAL CONFERENCE ON IMPROVING TROPICAL ANIMAL PRODUCTION FOR FOOD SECURITY (ITAPS 2023), 4–5 DECEMBER 2023, KENDARI, INDONESIA

Technological Innovations in Tropical Livestock Development for Environmental Sustainability and Food Security

Edited by

Purnaning Dhian Isnaeni
Halu Oleo University

Mashitah Shikh Maidin
University Putra Malaysia

Muh. Amrullah Pagala, Widhi Kurniawan and Asma Bio Kimestri
Halu Oleo University

CRC Press
Taylor & Francis Group
Boca Raton London New York Leiden

CRC Press is an imprint of the
Taylor & Francis Group, an **informa** business
A BALKEMA BOOK

First published 2024
by CRC Press/Balkema
4 Park Square, Milton Park, Abingdon, Oxon, OX14 4RN

and by CRC Press/Balkema
2385 NW Executive Center Drive, Suite 320, Boca Raton FL 33431

CRC Press/Balkema is an imprint of the Taylor & Francis Group, an informa business

British Library Cataloguing-in-Publication Data
A catalogue record for this book is available from the British Library

Library of Congress Cataloging-in-Publication Data
A catalog record has been requested for this book

ISBN: 978-1-032-74373-8 (hbk)
ISBN: 978-1-032-74376-9 (pbk)
ISBN: 978-1-003-46894-3 (ebk)

DOI: 10.1201/9781003468943

Typeset in Times New Roman
by MPS Limited, Chennai, India

Technological Innovations in Tropical Livestock Development for Environmental Sustainability and Food Security – P. Dhian Isnaeni et al. (eds)

Table of Contents

Technological Innovations in Tropical Livestock Development for Environmental Sustainability and Food Security – P. Dhian Isnaeni et al. (eds)
© 2025 The Editor(s), ISBN 978-1-032-74373-8
Open Access: www.taylorfrancis.com, CC BY-NC-ND 4.0 license

Committee of The 4th International Conference on Improving Tropical Animal Production for Food Security (ITAPS)

Host and Organizer:
Faculty of Animal Science, Universitas Halu Oleo, Kendari

Advisory Board:
1. Prof. Dr. Muhammad Zamrun F., S.Si., M.Si., M.Sc. (*Rector of Universitas Halu Oleo*)
2. Dr. Ir. Ali Bain, M.Si. (*Dean of Faculty of Animal Science*)

Scientific Board:
1. Prof. Dr. Ir Takdir Saili, M.Si.
2. Prof. Dr. Ir. Harapin Hafid H., M.Si, IPU
3. Prof. Dr. Ir. La Ode Nafiu, M.Si. IPU
4. Prof. Dr. Amrullah Pagala, S.Pt., M.Si, IPM
5. Mashitah Shikh Maidin, Ph.D.
6. Dr. Ir. Ali Bain, M.Si.
7. Dr. Ir. Andi Murlina Tasse, M.Si.
8. Dr. Muh. Rusdin, S.Pt., M.Si.
9. Dr. La Ode Arsad Sani, S.Pt., M.Sc.
10. Dr. Nur Santy Asminaya, S.Pt., M.Si.
11. Dr. Deki Zulkarnain, S.Pt., M.Sc.
12. Dr. La Malesi, S.Pt., M.Si
13. Dr. Ir. Syam Rahadi, S.Pt., M.P., M.M., IPM.
14. Sakinah Zubair, S.Pd., M.Pd
15. Muchammad Hifni, S.T., M.Sc.
16. Nur Hidayah, S.Pt., M.Si
17. Aditya Alqamal Alianta, S.Pt., M.Si.
18. Ir. Juni Sumarmono, M.Sc., Ph.D., IPU
19. Tutik Lusita Auliyani, S.Pt., M.Sc.
20. Dr. Bramanda Winiar Putra, S.Pt., M.Sc.
21. Aan Andriyanto, S.Pt., M.Sc.
22. Firman Nasiu, S.Pt., M.Sc.
23. Ulfiana Sara, S.Pt., M.Si.
24. Ima Malawati, S.Pt., M.Si.
25. Dr. Nadlirotun Lutfi, S.Pt., M.Si.
26. Dr. Nurul Chamidah, S.Sos.I., M.I.Kom
27. Lilil Krismiyanto, S.Pt., M.Si

Organizing Committee:

Chairman:	Dr. Ir. Rahman, S.Pt., M.T., IPM, ASEAN Eng.
Co-Chairman:	Dr. Fuji Astuty Auza, S.Pt., M.P.
Secretary:	drh. Purnaning Dhian Isnaeni, M.Pt
Treasurer:	Ashar, S.Sos., M.Si.

Program Coordinator:
1. Hamdan Has, S.Pt., M.Si.
2. Ir. Natsir Sandiah, MP.

3. Dr. ir. Andi Murlina tasse, M.Si.
4. drh. Yamin Yaddi, M.Si.
5. Andini Sulfitrana, S.Si., M.Kes.
6. Arby'in Pratiwi, S.Pt., M.Sc.
7. Dedem Sutopo, S.Pt., M.Sc.

Secretarial:
1. Dr. Ir. La Ode Arsad Sani, S.Pt., M.Sc., IPM
2. Astriana Napirah, S.Pt., M.Sc.
3. drh. Fadli Ma'mun Pancar, M.Si.
4. Nurhayu, S.Pt., M.Si.
5. Indriyani, S.Pt.
6. Muhammad Nur Afandy
7. Yumin

Proceedings and Publications:
1. Prof. Dr. Ir. Muh. Amrullah Pagala, S.Pt., M.Si., IPM, ASEAN. Eng.
2. Widhi Kurniawan, S.Pt., M.Si.
3. Asma Bio Kimestri, S.Pt., M.Sc.
4. Hairil A. Hadini, S.Pt., M.Sc.
5. drh. Restu Libriani, M.Si.
6. La Ode Munadi, S.Pt., M.P.
7. Rachmita Dewi S. Toba, S.Pt., M.Pt

Documentation:
1. drh. Putu Nara Kusuma Prasanjaya, M.Kes.
2. Andy Budi Novrianto, S.Pi
3. Eka Fitriani, S.Pt

Transportation:
1. Musram Abadi, S.Pt., M.P
2. Rahim Aka, S.Pt., M.P.
3. Amiluddin Indi, S.Pt., M.Si.
4. Samin, S.I.K.
5. Abustam Buduhami

Consumption:
1. Ardhayu, S.P.
2. Fitrianingsih, S.Pt., M.Sc.
3. Muharwasita, S.Pi.
4. Rina Hasmanah, S.M.

Technological Innovations in Tropical Livestock Development for Environmental Sustainability and Food Security – P. Dhian Isnaeni et al. (eds)
© 2025 The Author(s), ISBN 978-1-032-74373-8
Open Access: www.taylorfrancis.com, CC BY-NC-ND 4.0 license

Halal meat production in the modern era: Concepts and applications

Z.A. Jelan*
School of Veterinary Medicine, Faculty of Health and Medical Sciences, Taylor's University, Kuala Lumpur, Malaysia

A. Pratiwi & P.D. Isnaeni
Department of Animal Husbandry, Faculty of Animal Husbandry, Halu Oleo University, Indonesia

ABSTRACT: The recent decades have seen, an exponentially rising Moslem population worldwide have created increased demand for *halal* meat, particularly poultry. Conversely, Moslem consumers are often apprehensive of the *halal* status and the production processes of this meat in the market. Firstly, for meat to be *halal*, the animal is slaughtered according to Islamic regulations. The meat should be *tayyib* which implies the meat is wholesome, nutritious and good. *Tayyib* does not just involve post-slaughter processing, but the farming practices are obliged to provide good well-being to the animal and do not cause environmental degradation. The production processes of all meat are generally similar and there are possible poor or violation of the code of practice along the *halal* meat supply chain. Modern-day production of *halal* meat must still comply with the requirements of the Shariah law as prescribed in the Quran and Hadiths. Today, there are *halal* certification bodies in nearly all countries that are entirely responsible for managing the compliance of the *halalan* and *tayyiban* standards of the meat production chain from farming to distribution of *halal* meat. In recent years, research on *halal* meat production has received much emphasis and technologies have been developed to detect meat adulteration and contamination. Newer technologies and expertise are implemented for improved farming efficiency, product development and monitoring of *halal* meat that convinces Moslem consumers of acceptance and enhancing environment management.

Keywords: Halal Meat, Modern Era, Poultry, Moslem consumer

1 INTRODUCTION

Meat of livestock is a key source of protein food for the world's population. Global demand for meat is growing over the past 50 years and meat production has more than tripled to meet the fast-expanding population. In 2022, the *halal* meat market size was valued at USD 266 billion and is projected to be worth USD 724 billion by 2032 with a cumulative average growth rate of 9.7% (Statistical Report – March 2023). As a result, industrial farming commonly referred to as a factory production system evolved rapidly where livestock is reared intensively in a large population. Following a short farming duration, the finished animals are transported to the abattoir for slaughter. Industrial farming frequently denies animals favorable welfare, displays unethical practices and also has created substantial environmental degradation such as increasing greenhouse gas emissions, water contamination and land degradation. Therefore, one of the world's most critical challenges is to carry out animal farming responsibly and sustainably (Hannah *et al.* 2017).

*Corresponding Author: jelanzainal@yahoo.com

DOI: 10.1201/9781003468943-1

From the Islamic viewpoint, meat for the consumption of the Moslem population must be mandatorily produced following the *halalan* and *tayyiban* concepts throughout the entire supply chain. In addition, Islamic teachings have strongly reminded men of their responsibilities on the management and welfare of all animals including the farm animals and the care of the environment. Hence the production of meat as food for Muslims must adhere to the principles and practices mentioned in the Qur'an, the sacred guidebook of Islam and supported by the Hadiths, the sayings of the prophet Muhammad. The guidance was specified to all mankind more than 1400 years ago.

This article looks at the *halalan* and *tayyiban* concepts and their application in meat production and the recent challenges in producing meat that adhere to Islamic Law. It also highlights the Islamic perspectives on enhancing the management at various stages of the commercial meat production system from the processes of rearing the animals until the *halal* meat reaches the consumers.

2 DISCUSSION

2.1 *Farming of animals for meat*

The Quran mentioned in Surah 2: Verse 168: "O Mankind! Eat of what is permissible (*Halal*) and good (*Tayyib*) on earth and do not follow the footsteps of Satan; truly he is an open enemy to you". Similarly, God has prescribed even before Islam, Kosher food (proper and lawful under the Jewish law) as mentioned in the Torah, so proper food handling has always been a divine decree.

The production of livestock meat began with the rearing of animals in various systems of production with the aim of high animal productivity and profitability. The large-scale and intensive production of animals is a universal approach to maximize meat production while minimizing costs. Industrial farming is common in broiler, mutton/lamb and beef productions where animals with superior economic traits are reared to rapidly attain high finished body weight by feeding a high plane of nutrition in a short growth duration. The intensive farming system requires the provision of good animal welfare and management of the large number of wastes that potentially cause environmental deterioration. In global poultry production, the modern intensive farming method has been universally adopted, but it also causes a significant environmental footprint with enormous waste materials that can pose a severe threat to the environment and human health (Grzinic *et al.* 2023).

Irrespective of the kind of meat animals, the typical pathways of all commercial meat production systems are diagrammatically summarized in Figure 1. Each step has its

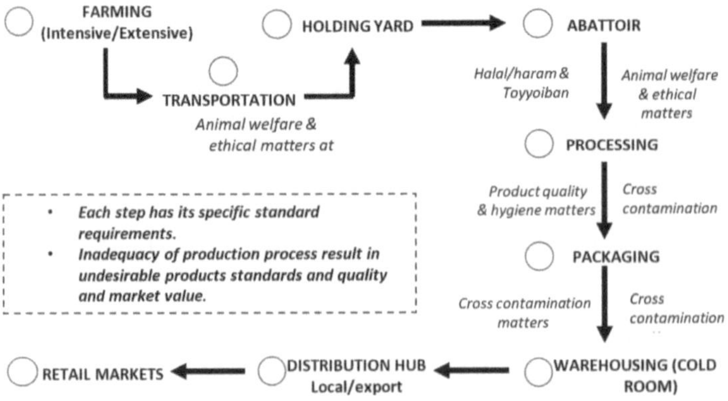

Figure 1. General pathways of the commercial production of meat of cattle, sheep and poultry along with the subjects of concern particularly among the Moslem consumers.

benchmark procedures to comply with and that the meat product is accountably produced and acceptable by the consumers. Unfavorable animal welfare and unethical issues of animal farming are likely to mainly occur at the farmland, the earliest step in meat production. Similar issues occur during gathering and transportation to the holding yard prior to slaughter and pre-slaughter handling of the animal at the abattoir.

Most apprehension about *halal* and *haram* meat production is associated with the management of animals at pre-slaughter, slaughter and post-slaughter procedures. Matters of animal welfare and cruelty are likely to occur during the handling of the animal at pre-slaughter, non-compliant procedures of slaughter and product quality and hygiene (*tayyib*) are prone to happen post-slaughter where processes of the carcass, meat de-boning and packaging engage direct human handling. Cross contamination and deterioration of meat can occur during storage at the warehouse, distribution/transportation and retailing of the meat products. The product packaging should be well-labelled and made traceable to the farm of origin, animal and abattoir/meat processing plant. These are the sections in the production pathways that require regular audits to ensure the meat is truly *halal* and *tayyiban*.

Islamic views on farming animals and conscientiousness of the operators' Islamic teachings clearly mentioned the importance and roles of animals to mankind. The Quran mentions "It is God who provided for you farm animals, that you may ride on some of them and from some you may derive your food. You also have other benefits from them for your use to satisfy your heart's desire. It is on them as on ships that you make your journeys." (The Quran, Surah 40 Ghafir: Verse 79–80). Islam is affirmative on the respect and compassion towards animals and the forbidden acts or attitudes of humans towards animals during their close association. The teaching clearly mentions that under any circumstances, it is not justifiable to cause unavoidable pain and suffering to His creations "There is not a moving (living) creature on earth, nor a bird that flies with its two wings, but are communities like you. We have neglected nothing in the Book, then unto their Lord they (all) shall be gathered" (The Quran, Surah 6 Al-An'am: Verse 38). The verse tells us that animals must not be treated as "lifeless things", but with care, compassion and respect.

Allah has created everything in its due proportion thus creating its balance for existence in accordance to the laws of nature as Allah has ordained. As long as this balance in nature is maintained, the earth has been designed to exist in a balanced state of harmony and the earth was created in accordance to His law of nature. Any unwarranted act of destruction or abuse can lead to the imbalance of nature's natural existence leading to grievous consequences (The Quran, Chapter 55 Ar-Rahman: Verse 5–10). Allah created this earth for humans and its contents to be used for man's benefit, but man is responsible for protecting it and preserving its balance. Nature is for man to use for his sustenance, so man can worship Allah. Proper management of resources as created by Allah is considered an act of worship, thus, the preservation (protection) of nature and animals is considered an act of worship. Good management of the environment is part of man's responsibility as vicegerents. These few verses of the Qur'an should competently remind and guide us to adopt and practice good animal farming methods and routine activities.

The producers or farm operators and the enforcing authorities should have a greater awareness and concerns about the welfare of the animals that are raised to produce food, non-food products or other purposes and the impact of the farming activities on the environment. Islam shows clear guidelines on the acceptable management of animals for whatever purpose, allowable food, preparation of food and even on how to eat your food.

2.2 *The halal concept*

The concepts of *halal*, *haram* and *tayyiban* in meat production *Halal* means lawful or permissible meaning compliance with the Islamic Law as defined in the Qur'an. Conversely, *haram* denotes not permissible or simply unlawful. Four verses in the Surah of the Quran comprehensively specify food that is lawful (*halal*) and prohibited which all Moslems must observe. These verses are (i) Al-Baqarah (The heifer), Surah 2: Verse 172, (ii) Surah Al-An'am (The cattle) Surah 6: Verse 145, (iii) Al-Ma'idah (Food dishes) Surah 5: Verse 3 and (iv) An-Nahl (The bees) Surah 16: Verse 115.

The word *halal* does not only refer to food products but includes Islamic financial services, media and recreations, Moslem-friendly travels, cosmetics, modest fashions, pharmaceuticals and human interactions following the principles and guidance of Islam (Aziz *et al.* 2013). In reality, *halal* is a universal term that refers to all aspects of life (Hafez *et al.* 2015). It is not restricted to the processes of slaughtering animals and meat products, freedom from porcine and its derivatives and alcohol, but it covers the whole process of production and services. *Halal* products have become a choice for both Moslems and non-Moslems (Nawai *et al.* 2007).

The term *tayyiban* means something that is good, beneficial, and useful for humans. Concerning meat, it means that the meat is *halal* and wholesome. Allah has called upon humans to eat and enjoy *halal* food that has been endowed on this earth. In Islam, the concepts of *halal* and *tayyib* are applied together as a package to affirm that the meat is consumable from lawful and wholesome aspects.

2.3 *Halal slaughter and stunning*

Slaughtering of an animal is a purposeful act to produce meat as food with ethical guidelines to conduct the act most conveniently. The action is a key clause in determining the *halal* status of the meat where the animal must be slaughtered in compliance with Islamic principles. The slaughtering act must be completed in the least painful manner as all the Islamic laws on the management of animals including the procedures of slaughter are based on compassion, respect and benevolence.

Many issues, arguments and requirements for *halal* certification of meat are largely centered on the procedures and practices at the abattoirs and processing plants. The processes of *halal* slaughtering of an animal involve restraining, stunning (if applied) and severing in a swift and single continuous action of making an incision with a sharp and clean knife across the neck of the animal to severe four anatomical structures namely the jugular veins, carotid arteries, trachea (windpipe) and oesophagus. Severing these structures ensures a rapid death with maximum drainage of blood from the body of the animal. Additionally, the animal must be alive and healthy at the point of slaughter, it is slaughtered in the name of Allah, slaughtering is conducted by a mentally sound Moslem slaughter man and as much blood is drained from the body. It is required that the slaughtering of animals and processing of the carcass and meat are conducted in a dedicated and accredited establishment meant for *halal* meat production.

The pre-slaughter stunning of an animal is a technical process that is now widely practised in abattoirs globally to induce unconsciousness and insensibility prior to slaughter. In some countries, pre-slaughter stunning is mandatory. The subject of pre-slaughter stunning has courted a great deal of concern and debate among Moslem scholars on the *halal* status of the meat from the stunned-slaughtered animal. From the animal welfare perspective, it is considered a humane method as stunning is viewed as a way of minimizing the fear, pain and discomfort experienced during the time of slaughter by the animal provided the stunning is correctly executed (Bergeaud-Blackler 2007; Nakyinsige *et al.* 2013). Different attitudes and solutions existed among authorities in Moslem-majority countries with regard to pre-slaughter stunning. Today, the Fatwa Council, a formal body on legal ruling on Islamic law and is binding on Moslems and Islamic Courts of most Moslem countries has accepted stunning as an act of compassion as stipulated in Islamic teaching. The acceptance of stunning is conditional that the procedure used shall be reversible and shall not kill or cause physical injury or death to the animal prior to the *halal* slaughter procedures (JAKIM, Malaysia 2003).

2.4 *Certification and authenticity of halal meat*

Halal certification is a guarantee that the meat is prepared in accordance with Islamic law and is unadulterated. *Halal* certification is one of the prerequisites for entering the global *halal* meat market. It does provide recognition of quality and safe products through the concept of *halalan tayyiban* for the entire supply chain, from farm to fork. In the *halal* meat industry, the system covers the practice of good animal husbandry on the farm until post-slaughter management in order to maintain the *halal* status. Animal welfare aspect and antemortem inspection are also highlighted in reducing the chances of slaughtering the injured or diseased animal which may not only affect the meat quality, but unhealthy for consumption. Maximum possible bleeding resulting from the slaughtering process ensures wholesomeness and will increase the shelf-life of the meat by reducing the risk of carcass contamination and product deterioration. As the concept of *tayyiban* is practised, the meat is free from any microbiological, physical and chemical hazards.

Every country has its own *halal* protocols designed by the national certification organization usually made up of experts from several related institutions including the Fatwa Council of each country. Their key role is in the certification and matters related to all *halal* products and production procedures. *Halal* certification bodies generally have common requirements with some minor differences among countries.

2.5 *Traceability of meat*

Product traceability is becoming normal across the agriculture food industry largely due to the demands for transparency within the food chain. Meat traceability is also a topic which is becoming increasingly discussed with the expansion of global trade, computerization and communications, food safety and disease surveillance. Moslem consumers in particular are constantly concerned about the *halal* status besides the safety of the meat they purchase. One solution to improve the guarantee of *halal* meat is to apply a more transparent and trustworthy *halal* meat supply chain system. With this supply chain system, all stakeholders, including consumers and suppliers could straightforwardly trace and obtain accurate information of the *halal* meat.

Traceability must create an effective link between all steps in the supply chain. In simplest words, meat traceability refers to the ability and the mechanism designed to track the movement of a meat item both upstream and downstream throughout the supply chain. A meat product in the market should be traceable to the abattoir where the animal is slaughtered, the farm where the animal is reared and the individual animal. The meat traceability system provides accurate information about the meat to the consumer. This is done by proper identification and recording of the animal and meat product at every stage of the production process beginning at the farm as indicated in Figure 1. There are many technologies developed for traceability systems especially in data management from the beginning of the supply chain until it reaches the destination. Such data can be quickly accessed and shared to provide assurance. The most integral part however is still the traceability system designed for the purposes of tracking the "journey" from a living animal to *halal* meat. This system can be incorporated with other tracking parameters such as temperature control to ensure proper handling at the product stage.

3 CONCLUSION

The *halal* meat industry is expected to grow significantly during the next decades as Moslem and non-Moslem consumers increasingly seek *halal*-certified meat and meat products that align with their values, emphasizing humane farming conditions and adherence to quality and safety standards. Islam is the fastest-growing religion in the world which will add to the increased demand for *halal* meat over and above the usual population growth in the existing Moslem population. The rising demand for convenience foods and value-added *halal* products reflects changes in consumer preferences for meat and meat products. *Halal* meat producers and the applicable authorities must ensure the integrity and authenticity of the *halal*an and *tayyiban* certification processes that will have a constructive influence on the *halal* meat market globally.

The global *halal* meat trade faces complexities due to the absence of universally recognized standards and regulations. Uncertainty surrounds *halal* standards because various entities, including government-affiliated organizations, private bodies and independent *halal* certification entities are involved in their formulation. Additionally, national, regional and international bodies contribute to the multifaceted landscape. Major meat producers and exporters are from non-Islamic countries. Different countries follow diverse regulatory frameworks in accordance with their laws and requirements, but numerous efforts have been organized to standardize and align rules governing *halal* meat exports and imports. There needs to be a clear understanding of *halal* meat requirements by exporting countries to ensure compliance with Islamic law.

As the standards and procedures are in place, ensuring the integrity of *halal* status throughout the chain until it reaches the consumers will be a very important task or it can nullify all the efforts taken. If the consumers are in doubt of the *halal* status, the meat can no longer be consumed. A tight traceability system is an important protocol that should be adopted in the modern-day *halal* meat production system. Many available technologies can be adopted to support the integrity of *halal* status, as the use of AI (artificial intelligence) is gaining popularity in supply chain management throughout the world. The use of mechanization in the distribution hub can avoid human error and cross-contamination.

REFERENCES

Aziz, Y.A., Chok, N.V. 2013. The role of *halal* awareness, *halal* certification, and marketing components in determining *halal* purchase intention among non-Moslems in Malaysia: A structural equation modelling approach. *J. Int. Food and Agribusiness Marketing*, 25 (1): 1–23.

Bergeaud-Blackler, F. 2007. New challenges for Islamic ritual slaughter: A European perspective. *J. Ethn. Migrat. Stud.* 33(6): 965–980.

Department of Islamic Development Malaysia (JAKIM). 2003. *The Malaysian Protocol for the Halal Meat and Poultry Productions*. Official Publication of JAKIM Malaysia.

Grzinic, G., Piotrowicz-Cieślak, A., Klimkowicz-Pawlas, A., Górny, R.L., Ławniczek-Wałczyk, A., Lidia Piechowicz, L., Olkowska, E., Potrykus, M., Tankiewicz, M., Krupka, M., Siebielec, G. and Wolska, L. 2023. Intensive poultry farming: A review of the impact on the environment and human health. *Sci. Total Environ.* 858: 160014.

Hafez, O.A., Zaiton, H., Nazmi, A.M.M. 2015. Effect of slaughtering methods on meat quality indicators, chemical changes and microbiological quality of broiler chicken meat during refrigerated storage. *IOSR Journal of Agriculture and Veterinary Science*, 8(9): 2319–2372.

Hannah, R., Pablo Rosado and Max Roser. 2017. *Meat and Dairy Production*. Published online at OurWorldInData.org. Retrieved from: 'https://ourworldindata.org/meat-production'.

Maheran, N.M.N. and C.F.F.M. I. Bidin. 2009. Positioning Malaysia as *halal*-hub: Integration role of supply chain strategy and *halal* assurance system. *Asian Social Science J.* 5(7): 44–52.

Nakyinsige, K., Man Y.B., Aghwan, Z.A., Zulkifli, I., Goh, Y.M., Abu Bakar, F., Al-Kahtani, H.A., and Sazili, A.Q. 2013. Stunning and animal welfare from Islamic and scientific perspectives. *Meat Sci.* 95: 352–361.

Nawai, N., M.N. Nooh, N. Ridzwan, S.M. Dali and H. Mohammad. 2007. An exploratory study on *halal* branding among consumers in Malaysia: Factor analysis technique," *J. of Muamalat and Islamic Finance Research*. 4(1): 19–44.

Statista Report – March 2023. *Global Halal Market- Statistics and Facts*. https://www.ststista.com.

Zakiah, S., Amal Hayati Ishak and Nurul Himmah Kassan. 2014. Understanding the development of *Halal food* standard: Suggestion for future research. *Int. J. of Social Science and Humanity*. 4(6): 482–486.

Technological Innovations in Tropical Livestock Development for Environmental Sustainability and Food Security – P. Dhian Isnaeni et al. (eds)
© 2025 The Author(s), ISBN 978-1-032-74373-8

Microbiological characteristics of beef in Kendari city market

H. Hafid*, A.M. Tasse & F.M. Pancar
Animal Science Faculty Animal Science at Halu Oleo University, Kendari, Indonesia

I.W. Kertanegara & S.H. Ananda
Program Study Nutrition at STIKES Karya Kesehatan, Kendari, Indonesia

E. Haryanto
Program Study Agribusiness at UPBJJ Terbuka University, Kendari, Indonesia

ABSTRACT: This study aims to determine the level of chemical contamination and contamination of microbial pathogens of beef in various markets in Kendari city. The study was prepared based on Completely Randomized Design (RAL) 3 × 2 and 3 replication factorial patterns. The first factor is the type of Market (Mandonga Market, Old Town Market and New Market Wua-Wua). The second factor is the sampling period (Morning and Day). The parameters measured were pathogenic microbial contamination (*Escherichia coli, Staphylococcus aureus* and *Salmonella sp*). The results of this study based on SNI 7387: 2009 showed that Salmonella sp and Staphylococcus aureus bacteria were not found in all samples of beef tested from Slaughterhouse and market in Kendari City. While the bacteria Escherichia coli found in beef since the Slaughterhouse and increasing after arriving in some markets in the city of Kendari, especially in the Old Town market. Increased bacteria are very dangerous, because it can affect human health. These results indicate that the quality of beef sold in some markets in Kendari City has not fully met the standards based on SNI 7387: 2009.

Keywords: beef, Escherichia coli, Staphylococcus aureus and Salmonella sp

1 INTRODUCTION

Beef as one of the main commodities of livestock products consumed by the community must be guaranteed its safety. The results showed the presence of heavy metal content and microbial contamination in beef originating from traditional farms in Kendari City (Hafid *et al.* 2015, 2016). Naturally beef is perishable because of the presence of endogenous enzymes (cathepsin) and contains many protein nutrients and water needed for the growth of spoilage bacteria (Hafid *et al.* 2018). This causes the possibility of animal food safety problems originating from beef in Kendari is quite high and alarming because there is no guarantee of beef health to consumers. The intended health insurance is free post-mortem beef from chemical (heavy metal) and microbiological (microbial) contamination from meat management in slaughterhouses, transportation, and in particular the process of marketing beef in the Kendari traditional market which does not meet the criteria Indonesian National Standard (SNI).

*Corresponding Author: harapin.hafid@uho.ac.id

DOI: 10.1201/9781003468943-2

The process of slaughtering cattle in the Kendari slaughterhouse is still traditional and handling of meat does not pay attention to hygiene so it is very easy for microbiological pollution. Meat management in slaughterhouses does not go through chilling process, after they are cut, they are directly transported to the market. Transporting beef from slaughterhouse to Kendari traditional market using open pickup vehicles and only covered with tarpaulin made of plastic. Such conditions facilitate the contamination of heavy metals and are also polluted by microbes resulting from pollution from hauling transport vehicles or other means of transport. In addition, the condition of traditional markets in Kendari City is prone to microbiological pollution because the meat sold is placed in open stalls without a cover and close to a place for selling fish and other products.

Handling of meat against bacterial contamination needs to be considered because it can interfere with consumer health. According to Hafid meat products must meet the requirements of safe, healthy, whole and halal so as to support the nutritional and health needs of consumers (Hafid 2017). Meat that contains certain heavy metals and bacteria that exceeds SNI limits and is even pathogenic can cause poisoning. Beef that is contaminated with heavy metals can cause health hazards to humans. The effect of heavy metal disruption on human health depends on which part of the heavy metal residue is bound in the body and the amount of heavy metal exposure dose. Some disorders of the body condition caused by heavy metal poisoning are anemia, disorders of various body organs and decreased intelligence.

Meat containing bacteria causes damage easily and decreases physical quality which in turn can interfere with consumer health. Some bacteria that can contaminate beef and cause health problems in humans can even cause death in humans such as *Escherichia coli*, *Staphylococcus aureus* and *Salmonella sp*. Verotoxin-producing *E. coli* generally results in bloody diarrhea and can cause hemolytic uremia, which is characterized by thrombocytopenia, hemolytic anemia, and acute kidney failure, especially in children. Salmonellosis is a disease caused by Salmonella contamination and can cause rheumatism, meningitis, splenic abscesses, pancreatitis, septicemia, and osteomyelitis. This encourages the need for research on the study of chemical and microbial residues in beef in the traditional markets of Kendari City.

2 MATERIALS AND METHODS

This research was conducted in March to April 2017 in Kendari Slaughterhouse, Traditional Markets such as Mandonga Market, Kota Lama Market and Pasar Baru. Sample testing was carried out at the Denpasar Veterinary Laboratory.

The study was arranged based on a completely randomized design (CRD) factorial pattern of 3×2 and 3 replications. The first factor is the Type of Market (P) with three levels, namely: Mandonga Market (P1), Old Market (P2), and New Market Wua-Wua (P3). The second factor is the sampling period (W) with two levels, namely: Morning (W1), and Afternoon (W2).

Parameters analyzed for chemical contamination include zinc (Zn), Lead (Pb) and Cadmium (Cd) residues. Whereas the microbial contamination was *E. coli*, *Staphylococcus aureus* and *Salmonella sp*.

Data from laboratory test results are statistically analyzed by testing average values, then each test value is compared with SNI (2008). Data analysis of heavy metal test results in the laboratory was carried out statistically descriptive by comparing the content of heavy metals (Zn, Cd, and Pb) in beef with applicable food safety standards. Variance of analysis is used to determine the influence of each factor and interaction between factors following the factorial completely randomized design, followed by the Least Significant Difference test to determine the extent of the difference between treatment factor levels (Rahmawati & Sahab 2002).

3 RESULTS AND DISCUSSION

3.1 *Microbial contamination*

3.1.1 *Salmonella contamination*

Salmonella sp is a pathogenic microbe that causes food borne disease which can cause death, which is called Salmonellosis. This can occur due to consuming food contaminated by these bacteria (Dominguez *et al.* 2002). Del Portillo states that the incidence of typhoid salmonellosis (enteric fever) is relatively stable with the lowest number occurring in developed countries, but the incidence of non-typhoid salmonellosis (gastroenteritis) is relatively increasing in all countries. Cases of acute gastroenteritis (diarrhea) are 1.3 billion cases with three million people died, while cases of enteric fever are 16 million cases with 600 thousand deaths (Moi *et al.* 2022).

Based on data from Table 1 it can be seen that the *Salmonella sp* bacteria in meat samples show negative results. This is thought to be due to the condition of the market environment that has a high level of humidity that inhibits bacterial growth. Gram-positive bacteria tend to live at higher air humidity compared to gram-negative bacteria associated with changes in the structure of cell membranes that contain lipid bilayers (Caldwell 2011).

Table 1. Average description of microbial pollution results based on the location and time of sampling on beef.

	Type of Microbes		
Source	*Salmonella sp*	*Staphylococcus aureus*	*Escherichia coli*
Slaughterhouse (Controlled)	negative	0	1,10
Mandonga Market	negative	0	5,30
Kota Lama Market	negative	0	32.52
Baru Market	negative	0	11,77
Average	negative	0	12,67

Research conducted in the Kendari City market shows that sanitation conditions are relatively good. In traditional markets, meat is sold by arranging it on a table without low temperature conditioning. While the detection results of *Salmonella sp* on the market in Kendari City on meat samples showed negative results, this was allegedly because the sampling was done in the morning and afternoon so the meat was still fresh and still very minimal contamination from contamination of other bacteria and from consumers (buyers), and the lack of flying flies.

Another factor that caused Salmonella bacteria was not found in the sample, which was thought to be caused by conditions that did not support the growth of Salmonella bacteria, namely the sampling was carried out in the rainy season where the room temperature conditions were relatively low so that it inhibited the growth of the bacteria. Salmonella bacteria thrive in warm temperatures. The development of Salmonella bacteria is quite fast and amazing, each cell is able to divide every 20 minutes at warm temperatures. Therefore, Salmonella infections are more common in the summer.

Indonesian National Standard SNI No. 01-6366-2000 concerning the maximum limit of bacterial contamination in fresh beef made by the government for the protection of consumers regarding the quality of animal products in circulation, for Salmonella is negative or beef does not contain *Salmonella sp* bacteria (BPOM RI 2022; SNI 2009).

Based on these standards, the fresh beef sold in several markets in Kendari City has met the set standards, because the results of this study indicate that the beef samples examined did not contain Salmonella sp. These results indicate the quality of beef sold in several markets in Kendari City is quite good.

3.1.2 *Staphylococcus aureus microbes contamination*

Based on the data in Table 1 it can be seen that the microbial contamination of *Staphylococcus aureus* shows 0 (zero) results, this is thought to be caused because the sampling is done on the condition of the meat is still fresh and still very minimal contamination from contamination of other bacteria and consumers (buyers), as well as the lack of flying flies.

Staphylococcus aureus contamination is one of the main causes of foodborne disease (FBD) because *Staphylococcus aureus* can contaminate food products during preparation and processing. This bacterium itself is found in the respiratory tract, the surface of the skin and hair are also commonly found in the environment around us such as land, water and air (Hafid & Patriani 2022).

This bacterium is often found in foods that contain high protein. This bacterium is able to survive well in freezing conditions. *Staphylococcus aureus* is easily removed by using heating to temperatures which are generally used to process meat and fish products. Microbial growth that exceeds 5.0 log CFU/g will produce heat-resistant enterotoxins (Hanum & Yurliasni 2022).

The environment around the place of selling meat such as a place of waste water, floors, walls, garbage disposal, as well as the block of selling beef in the market in the city of Kendari which is around the place of the sale of fish, which has a high level of humidity becomes a source of bacterial pollution. Market floor conditions that are dirty with soil are also contaminants of meat that are in the market. Anaerobic bacteria forming spores and gases, such as *Clostridium botulinum*, can be found in soil, water and fish (Soeparno 2015).

3.1.3 *Escherichia coli contamination*

The results of the Variance Analysis showed that the microbial contamination of *Escherichia coli* on the location and time of beef sampling was significantly affected (P <0.05). In Table 2 it can be seen that the average microbial contamination of *Escherichia coli* began to be seen in the Slaughterhouse which is 1.10 colonies/gram and in the market after distribution on the Mandonga market which is 5.30 colonies/gram and the highest in the Kota Lama market is 32.52 colonies/gram.

Table 2. Average *Escherichia coli* microbial contamination based on place and time of sampling on beef (5×10 MPN/gram).

	Sample Source				
Time Taken	Slaughterhouse	Mandonga Market	Kota Lama Market	Baru Market	Average
Morning	1,10	4,87	22,37	9,87	12,37
Noon		5,73	42,67	13,67	20,69
Average		$5{,}30^{a}$	$32{,}52^{b}$	$11{,}77^{ab}$	16,53

Note: Numbers followed by different letters in the same line indicate significant differences (P<0,05)

Microbial examination results from beef originating from slaughterhouses and from several markets in Kendari showed 100% positive results from samples infected with Escherichia coli, both those from slaughterhouses and those that had been distributed to the Mandonga market, Kota Lama market and Pasar Baru market. This situation shows that meat from slaughterhouses as well as those that have been distributed do not meet health requirements because they have been contaminated with *E. coli* according to SNI guidelines (SNI 2008, 2009).

Contamination can come from cow dung or human feces. The *E. coli* infection is likely to occur if workers after cleaning cages and animal dung (cows) then clean themselves and wash the tools used from water sources. Besides that, *E. coli* has a natural living habitat in the digestive tract of humans and animals that can directly contaminate the surrounding material including water, soil and meat.

The number of bacteria in meat will continue to increase depending on the handling and subsequent levels of pollution. The development of bacteria in meat can generally be known by the formation of mucus. Bacteria will look slimy, smell bad and damage if the number reaches 10 colonies/cm. It was also stated that the onset of odor was caused by the production of hydrogen sulfide produced by microorganisms (Hafid & Patriani 2022).

The results showed a high level of carcass/meat contamination in the Slaughterhouse Kendari due to several things including: (1) unavailability of hand washing facilities equipped with facilities and disposal water that can flow into the sewer, (2) the absence of clean and dirty room facilities clearly separated so cross-contamination is very likely to occur, (3) the condition of the Slaughterhouse main room and the equipment used are not clean and not disinfected after use, (4) most of the workers do not apply sanitation and hygiene, this is proven by absence of special and closed clothing, do not use boots, gloves, masks and head coverings, (5) the quality of water used for washing equipment, washing hands, washing carcasses/meat does not meet the requirements as clean water, (6) supporting equipment used uncleanly, (7) lack of supervision and employee awareness of the importance of importance sanitation conditions in Slaughterhouse and (8) the unavailability of adequate carcass/meat transport facilities. The results of the analysis indicate that the sanitation of the room, equipment and personnel that are not clean and hygienic in the implementation of the production process, resulting in the level of contamination of meat in Slaughterhouse increased.

The distribution of beef in Kendari does not meet the required SNI where shipments of meat from Slaughterhouse to traditional markets in Kendari City still use open cup vehicles. These conditions allow the possibility of heavy metal pollution through fuel emissions both from the car carrying the meat and from other vehicles.

During the process of distribution of beef from Slaughterhouse Kendari City, the quality decreased rapidly, this can be seen from the increasing microbial contamination in the market. Judging from the value of the number of *E. coli* bacteria, since the slaughterhouse produced beef has been in a bacterial contaminated condition and during the distribution process the condition has worsened. Bacterial contamination in the process of slaughtering cattle is very possible, because the process of slaughtering, especially the removal of viscera, is the most vulnerable point for contamination from the outside of the skin and contents of the digestive tract. Moreover, the level of cleanliness of Kendari slaughterhouse facilities and operators is low, so the allegation of bacterial contamination during the cutting process becomes even more convincing. As an illustration in the USA with a high level of hygiene of the Slaughterhouse alone Consumer Report states that contamination of *Escherichia coli* from the surface of the skin to the meat is still found in the beef market Kuntoro *et al.* 2013).

The increase in the number of bacteria in meat occurs when arriving at traditional markets as a place of distribution of meat from slaughterhouses. Market traders generally do not practice hygiene, the habit of washing their hands is still bad, do not use special aprons that are clean while selling. Bacteria that come from the hands of sellers and buyers in the market which alternately hold beef, increase bacterial contamination higher (Muchtadi 2015).

4 CONCLUSION

Based on the results of this study, it was concluded that *Escherichia coli* found in beef originated from Slaughterhouse and increased after arriving at several markets in Kendari, especially in the Kota Lama market. This increase in bacteria exceeds the threshold according to SNI 7387: 2009 and is very dangerous, because it can have an impact on human health. *Salmonella sp* and *Staphylococcus aureus* were not found in all beef samples from Slaughterhouse and Pasar in Kendari. Further research needs to be done about the origin and patterns of livestock raising to determine the presence of Escherichia coli contamination.

REFERENCES

BPOM RI. *Persyaratan Cemaran Logam Berat Dalam Pangan Olahan. Peraturan Badan Pengawas Obat Dan Makanan Nomor 9 Tahun 2022.*

Caldwell A. *The Effects of Ultraviolet Light on Bacterial Growth.* http://www.ehow.com/facts_5871403_effects-ultraviolet-lightbacterial-growth.html. 2011. Accessed on Juni, 24th 2017.

Dominguez, C.L. Gomez, and J. Zumalacarregui. Prevalence of salmonella and campylobacter in retail outlet in spain. *Int. J. Food Microbiol*, 2002, 72(1): 165168. https://doi.org/:10.1016/s0168-1605(01)00638-9

Hafid H, Rahman, Nuraini, Y Wati, Inderawati, S H Ananda and L Ba'a. Production of broiler chicken carcass fed on rice bran biomass in different marketed ages. *IOP Conf Series: Earth and Environmental Sci.*, 2018, pp. 1–9.

Hafid, H. *Pengantar Pengolahan Daging: Teori dan Praktik. Cetakan Pertama, Alfabeta, Bandung*, 2017.

Hafid, H., A.M. Tasse, Nuraini, Inderawati and M. Hasdar. Evaluation of heavy metal content in beef at slaughterhouse in kendari city. *Proceeding International Seminar Improving Tropical Animal Production.* Faculty of Animal Science Halu Oleo University, 2015, pp. 255.

Hafid, H., A.M. Tasse, Nuraini, Inderawati and M. Hasdar. Microbial contamination on slaughterhouse in kendari. *Proceeding International Conference 3th ADRI*, 2016, pp. 459–463.

Hafid, H., P. Patriani. *Teknologi Pasca Panen Peternakan, Penerbit Widina Bhakti Persada, Bandung*, 2022.

Hanum Z dan Yurliasni. *Mikrobiologi Pangan Hasil Peternakan*, Syiah Kuala University Press, 2022.

Ibrahim Musa Moi, Zuhairu Ibrahim, Bashir Mohammed Abubakar, Yahaya Mohammed Katagum, Auwal Abdullahi, Gandi Ajibji Yiga, Badamasi Abdullahi, Ibrahim Mustapha, Jallaba Ali, Zinat Mahmud, Hamisu Maimusa, Halima Oge Katagum, Aisha Muhammad Malami, Aminu Mustapha dan Istifanus Ayuba. *Sifat Patogen Bawaan Makanan dan Penyakitnya*. Penerbit Intechopen. 22 Agustus 2022.

Kuntoro B, R.R.A. Maheswari, dan H. Nuraini. Mutu fisik dan mikrobiologi daging sapi asal rumah potong hewan (RPH) kota pekanbaru, *Jurnal Peternakan* 10 (1): 1–8. 2013.

Muchtadi D. Pangan, Gizi dan Kesehatan, *Penerbit Alfabeta*, Bandung, 2015.

Rahmawati F and M. A. Sahab. *Modul Praktikum Perancangan Percobaan.* Prodi Statistika dan Sains Data Fakultas Matematika dan Ilmu Pengetahuan Alam Institut Pertanian Bogor, 2022.

SNI (Standar Nasional Indonesia). *Batas Maksimum Cemaran Logam Berat Dalam Pangan, SNI 7387:2009. ICS 67.220.20*, 2009

SNI. *Standar Nasional Indonesia 3932:2008 Mutu Karkas dan Daging Sapi.* Badan Standarisasi Nasional. Jakarta, 2008.

Soeparno. *Ilmu dan Teknologi Daging Edisi Revisi.* Gadjah Mada University Press, Yogyakarta, 2015.

Technological Innovations in Tropical Livestock Development for Environmental Sustainability and Food Security – P. Dhian Isnaeni et al. (eds)
© 2025 The Author(s), ISBN 978-1-032-74373-8

Follicle Stimulating Hormone (FSH) and Luteinizing Hormone (LH) concentrations of bovine pituitary extract extracted by different methods

I. Novita*
Graduate School of Mathematics and Applied Sciences, Universitas Syiah Kuala, Banda Aceh, Indonesia

T.N. Siregar
Laboratory of Reproduction, Faculty of Veterinary Medicine, Universitas Syiah Kuala, Banda Aceh, Indonesia

N.W.K. Karja
Department of Veterinary Clinic, Reproduction and Pathology, Faculty of Veterinary Medicine, IPB University, Bogor, Indonesia

K. Eriani
Department of Biology, Faculty of Mathematics and Natural Sciences, Syiah Kuala University, Banda Aceh, Indonesia

A.R. Aru, M. Delima, H. Latif, E. Mariana & Z.M. Gaznur
Department of Animal Husbandry, Faculty of Agriculture, Universitas Syiah Kuala, Banda Aceh, Indonesia

ABSTRACT: The utilization of pituitary extract as a source of natural gonadotropin hormones is expected to be an alternative to commercial gonadotropin hormones that can be used in reproductive manipulation to improve livestock reproductive performance. A study on the effect of different extraction methods was conducted to obtain bovine pituitary extract with the highest concentration of FSH and LH. T-test was conducted to determine the effect of extraction method on FSH and LH concentrations. The pituitary gland used in this study came from 20 local bulls slaughtered at the abattoir. The method used was based on Isnaini & Sayudi (2004) and Sutiyono *et al.* (2008). The results showed that the treatment of different extraction methods did not show a very significant difference (P<0,01) in the concentration of FSH and LH. The second method (Sutiyono *et al.* 2008) showed better results than the first method (Isnaini dan Sayudi 2004) (232,99 mIU/ml vs 40,35 mIU/ml).

In conclusion

Keywords: Bovine pituitary, Extraction, FSH, LH, technology reproduction

1 INTRODUCTION

Reproductive manipulation aims to improve reproductive capabilities in living things. One of the reproductive manipulation techniques that have been carried out to increase reproductive productivity is hormonal reproductive manipulation and has been proven to accelerate gonadal cell maturation, improve gonadal production ability and even increase gonadal productivity. The hormones commonly used in this hormonal reproduction

*Corresponding Author: cutintan@usk.ac.id

DOI: 10.1201/9781003468943-3

manipulation are commercial gonadotropin hormones. However, this hormone is relatively expensive and still difficult to obtain in the local market. Therefore, alternative sources of hormones that have the same effectiveness as the commercial hormones are needed.

Gonadotropin hormones are secreted by the anterior part of the pituitary gland (Amar & Weiss 2003). FSH and LH hormones are gonadotropins that function in gonadal maturation. In male animals, FSH and LH together with testosterone play an important role in spermatogenesis (Oduwole *et al.* 2018). In female animals FSH functions to stimulate the expansion of cumulus cells, and stimulates and regulates chromatin condensation for the process of meiotic division, while LH functions to complement the action of FSH in stimulating follicular development, theca cells and granulosa cells so that oestrogen secretion increases, which will also stimulate oocyte maturation. These hormones are necessary in the reproductive cycle (Howles 2000).

In abattoirs or other slaughterhouses, the pituitary gland is a waste that is usually discarded with the skull. Several studies on the utilisation of pituitary extracts in improving reproductive performance have been conducted and shown to show good results, including overcoming reproductive performance problems in postpartum sows (Outang *et al.* 2017) and balinese cows (Nalley *et al.* 2017). Other studies reported that the addition of pituitary extract can improve the early behaviour of kaligesing goats (Setiawan *et al.* 2019; Priatin *et al.* 2019), can improve the pregnancy and birth profile of kaligesing goats (Isnaeni *et al.* 2020), can improve the quality of lambing and the quantity of pregnant sheep (Sutiyono *et al.* 2008), and can increase the productivity of laying hens (Amiruddin *et al.* 2014). In addition, studies on the use of equine pituitary extract in superovulation in mares are continuous (Alvarenga *et al.* 2008; Blanco 2009; de sá *et al.* 2017; Machado *et al.* 2005; Scoggin *et al.* 2002; Squires and McCue 2007). This suggests that the hypophysis isolated from cattle after slaughter has considerable potential as an alternative source of gonadotropins. However, some of these reports recommend that studies be conducted on the concentration of gonadotropin hormone contained in the pituitary extract so that the dose given can be more precise so that the results obtained can be maximised,

FSH and LH are gonadotropin hormones composed of glycoproteins. Glycoproteins are complex compounds between proteins with covalently bound oligosaccharide chains (glycans). Glycoproteins can be damaged during extraction due to the use of solvents and stirring/centrifugation (Aziz *et al.* 2007), therefore the extraction method used determines the concentration of FSH and LH contained in the hypophyseal extract. Extraction of the hypophysis has been done with various methods, including extraction using distilled water (Isnaini & Sayudi 2004) and 0.9% Physiological NaCl (Sutiyono 2008) as solvents as well as the dialysis-lyophilisation method (Kang *et al.* 2012). So far, no studies have been found that report on the content of gonadotropin hormones in hypophyseal extracts extracted by these methods. Therefore, it is necessary to study the concentration of FSH and LH in the hypophysis extracted by different methods.

2 MATERIAL AND METHOD

2.1 *Materials*

The pituitary gland used in this study came from 20 aceh bulls slaughtered at the abattoir.

2.2 *Sample preparation*

The pituitary gland was isolated from local bulls immediately after slaughter, and immediately put into a thermos to be taken to the laboratory. Then the pituitary glands were cleaned of connective tissue and separated from the outer membrane. Subsequently, extraction was carried out. First method: This method was carried out based on Isnaini & Suyadi (2004), as follows, the pituitary was ground until smooth, then distilled water was added as much as 10 ml for each gram of hypophysis, then filtered using filter paper. The solution obtained was centrifuged at 3,000 rpm for 20 minutes, then the supernatant was taken. The centrifuged supernatant is the pituitary extract.

Second method: This method is based on Sutiyono *et al.* (2008), pituitary was soaked in 90% alcohol solution for 16 hours, changing the alcohol solution every 4 hours so that the water content of the pituitary evaporates. Furthermore, the pituitary gland soak was aerated so that the alcohol solution could evaporate and then mashed. The obtained pituitary powder was put into a centrifuge tube and 0.9% Physiological NaCl was added as much as 10 ml for every 1 gram of pituitary. The solution was then centrifuged at 3000 rpm for 30 minutes. The supernatant obtained was the pituitary extract.

2.3 *FSH and LH concentration analysis*

To determine the concentration of FSH and LH in the hypophyseal extract was done by ELISA method. The kit used is FSH and LH ELISA Kit (Bioassay, USA). The kit contains stand ard solution, enzyme conjugate, washing buffer, substrate A and B, and stop dilution. 50 μl of standard solution, samples were put into wells, then 100 μl of enzyme conjugate was added to the solution and mixed for 30 seconds. The suspension was incubated at 37°C for 1 hour. Microtiter wells were rinsed 3 times with 100 ml buffer. 100 μl of substrate A and B (1:1) was added. The suspension was incubated at 37°C for 15 min under dark conditions. The reaction was stopped by adding 50 μl HCl as stop dilution to each suspension. Optical Density was calculated at 450 nm wavelength with a microtiter reader. The data obtained from the standard readings were recorded and a standard curve was made, with the absorbance value placed on the vertical axis (Y) and the FSH concentration on the horizontal axis (X). Based on the standard curve, a linear equation formula was obtained which was used to calculate the con-centration of FSH in the samples. For testing LH concentration, the same thing was done as in testing FSH concentration.

2.4 *Data analysis*

The data obtained will be analyzed by two side tests.

3 RESULT AND DISCUSSION

3.1 *Morphology and morphology of the pituitary gland of Aceh cattle*

In biology, morphology is a branch of science that studies the shape and structure of living things. According to Takàcs *et al.* (2016), morphological characteristics are very important to study in biological disciplines. In this study, the shape and structure to be studied is the pituitary gland found in Aceh cattle. The pituitary gland is located inside the front lower skull just in front of the brain stem. The pituitary gland is located under the diaphragm sellae which is a sheet of dura mater that forms the roof of the pituitary fossa (Shah & Elsanafiry 2018). The diaphragm sellae and the pituitary gland obtained in this study can be seen in Figure 1.

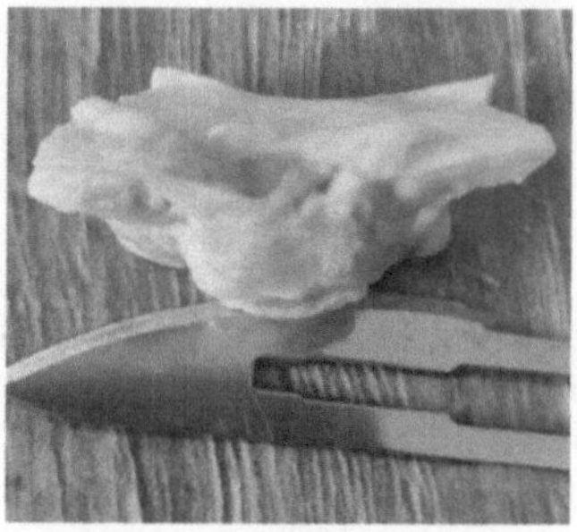

Figure 1. Diaphragm sellae (ds) and pituitary gland (pg).

The pituitary gland is protected by a thin membrane (Figure 2) and consists of 2 (two) parts, namely the anterior part (adenohypophysis) and the posterior part (neurohypophysis) (Figure 3).

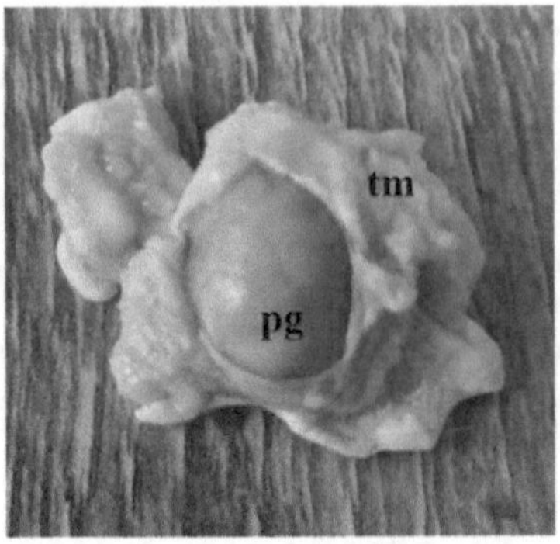

Figure 2. The pituitary gland (pg) and thin membrane (tm).

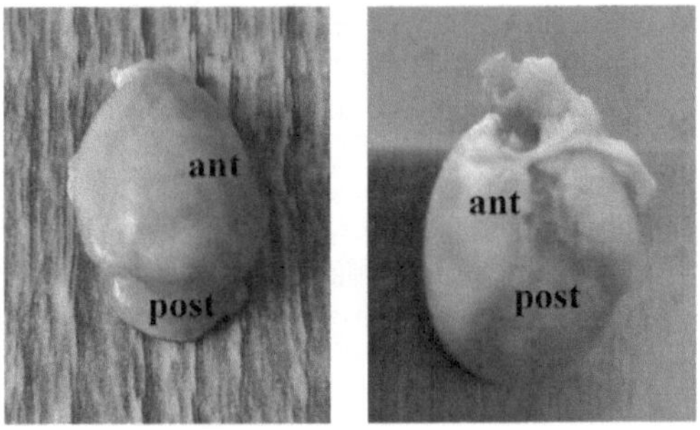

Figure 3. Anterior pituitary (ant) and posterior pituitary (post).

Morphometric data of the pituitary glands of Aceh cattle are presented in Table 1.

Table 1. Morphometry of the pituitary gland of aceh cattle

Parameters	Measurement
Weight (gram)	5,0 ± 0,3
Length (mm)	14,0 ± 1,2
Width (mm)	12,0 ± 0,9

3.2 *FSH and LH concentrations of bovine pituitary extracts with different extraction methods*

FSH and LH are gonadotropin hormones that are important in reproductive performance in both male and female livestock. Analysis of FSH and LH concentrations in pituitary extracts of aceh cattle extracted by different methods was conducted using Elisa test. The mean values of FSH and LH concentrations in pituitary extracts of Aceh cattle extracted by different methods are presented in Table 2.

The results of the analysis showed that the extraction method gave a very significant difference ($P<0.01$) to the FSH concentration of Aceh cow hypophysis extract, where the second

Table 2. Mean values of FSH and LH concentrations of bovine pituitary extracts with different extraction methods (mIU/mg).

	Average		Standard deviation			
types of hormones	Method I	Method II	Method I	Method II	t-table (P<0,01)	t-count
FSH	40,355	232,994	20,75241	47,93291	t<−2.878 atau t> 2.878	−11,6628
LH	10,257	32,082	5,744532	7,630957		−7,22575

method (Sutiyono *et al.* 2008) gave higher results than the first method (Isnaini & Sayudi 2004), namely 232.92 mIU/mg and 40.355 mIU/mg, as well as the concentration of LH (32.82 mIU/mg vs 10.26 mIU/mg), this is thought to be because in the extraction using the second method before dissolving the hypophysis was first dehydrated in alcohol for 16 hours. Dehydration in alcohol makes the sample lose water and become dry. This dry condition makes the sample denser so that the concentration of FSH and LH is also higher than the first method. The solvent used in this method is also different, in the first method the solvent used is distilled water while in the second method the solvent used is physiological 0.9% NaCl. Water-based solvents such as distilled water and 0.9% physiological NaCl have the same effectiveness. Distilled water is a universal solvent that can dissolve many chemicals including organic molecules, while 0.9% physiological sodium chloride (NaCl) solution is a standard physiological solution to maintain cell metabolic activity. Another difference is the length of centrifugation time, in the first method for 20 minutes, while in the second method for 30 minutes. However, in this study the use of both solvents and centrifugation time cannot be compared because each method has different procedures. Some studies using the first method in the extraction of the pituitary gland showed good results, as reported by Sayuti *et al.* (2022) that injection of bovine hypophysis glands can increase the concentration of estrogen, progesterone and the number of fetuses in rabbits. Similarly, Hanifah *et al.* (2023) where superovulation using a combination of prostaglandin F2α (PGFFα) and pituitary extract can increase estrus intensity and pregnancy rates compared to without the addition of pituitary extract. In the research of Siregar *et al.* (2020), giving bovine pituitary extract can increase folliculogenesis activity in white rats. Similarly, in studies using the second method, as reported by Outang *et al.* (2017) where the addition of pituitary extract can increase estrus intensity, estrus duration, number of services in heat, conception rate, litter size, litter weight and milk production. The concentrations of FSH and LH obtained in this study are different from those reported by Kang *et al.* (2012) which were 5.73 and 139.66 mIU/mg, respectively. The extraction method used is different from the two methods tested in this study. Where Kang *et al.* (2012) used ammonium acetate and alcohol as solvents. This study also tested commercial pituitary extract (bovine pituitary extract (BPE) (Gybsco, Germany), and showed FSH and LH concentrations of 586.5 and 87.72 mIU/mg, respectively. The concentration of FSH and LH in BPE is much higher, this is thought to be because the extraction method used is a protein isolation method, so the protein content, as the main element forming gonadotropin hormones, is much higher.

4 CONCLUSION

The best method of bovine pituitary extraction is the method of Sutiyono *et al.* (2008), because it produces the highest concentration of FSH and LH.

REFERENCES

Alvarenga, M. A., Carmo, M. T., & Landim-Alvarenga, F. C. (2008). Superovulation in mares: Limitations and perspectives. *Pferdeheilkunde*, 24(1), 88–91.

Amar, A. P., & Weiss, M. H. (2003). Pituitary anatomy and physiology. *Neurosurgery Clinics*, 14(1), 11–23.

Amiruddin, A., Siregar, T. N., Azhari, A., Jalaluddi, J., Zulkifli, Z., Rahman, A. A., & Hamdan, H. (2014). Pengaruh pemberian ekstrak hipofisa sapi terhadap peningkatan produktivitas ayam petelur pada fase akhir produksi. *Jurnal Kedokteran Hewan-Indonesian Journal of Veterinary Sciences*, 8(1), 80–84.

Aziz, Z., Thamrin Wikanta, & Tirta subagio. 2007. Analisis Glikoprotein dalam daging Mytilus viridis, Anadara granosa, dan Anadara maculosa. *Jurnal Ilmu Kefarmasian Indonesia*. 5(1), 1–6.

Blanco, I. D. P., Devito, L. G., Ferreira, H. N., Araujo, G. H. M., Fernandes, C.B., Alvarenga, M. A., & Landim-Alvarenga, F. D. C. (2009). Aspiration of equine oocytes from immature follicles after treatment with Equine Pituitary Extract (EPE) alone or in combination with hCG. *Animal Reproduction Science*, 114(1–3), 203–209.

de Sá, M. A. F., de Oliveira Santos, G., Bezerra, L. L., Moreno, M. P., Barbosa, C. G., Alvarenga, M. A., & Jacob, J. C. F. (2017). Use of Equine Pituitary Extract (EPE) in low doses to induce double ovulation in mares. *Brazilian Journal of Veterinary Medicine*, 39(2), 115–119.

Hafizuddin, Suryani, Yusmadi, Siregar, T. N., & Armansyah, T. (2010). Respons superovulasi mencit dengan ekstrak hipofisa: Suatu upaya menemukan agen superovulasi dengan biaya murah. *Prosiding Seminar Nasional Peternakan Berkelanjutan*. 2010.

Hanifah, D. M., Andanawari, S., Wibowo, H. T., Zulfikhar, R., Nawangsari, D. N., Sunardi, S., ... & Cahyani, A. P. (2023). The reproductive performance of local sheep following induced superovulation with cattle hypophisa extracts. *Formosa Journal of Applied Sciences*, 2(12), 3371–3378.

Howles, C. M. (2000). Role of LH and FSH in ovarian function. *Molecular and Cellular Endocrinology*, 161 (1–2), 25–30.

Isnaeni, I., Iskandar, F., & Wibawanti, J. M. W. (2020). Profil kebuntingan dan kelahiran kambing kaligesing (Capra Aegragus Hircus) betina yang diinjeksi ekstrak hipofisa dengan level yang berbeda. *Jurnal Ilmu Pertanian dan Peternakan*, 9(2), 98–108.

Isnaini, N., & Suyadi. (2004). Pengaruh sistem pemberian ekstrak hipofisa terhadap respon berahi dan respon ovari sapi perah anestrus postpartum. *Jurnal Ilmu-Ilmu Hayati*, 16(1), 33–40.

Kang, J. D., Lee, H. S., Liang, S., Li, S., Lu, Y., Kong, I. K., & Yin, X. J. (2012). Effect of crude canine pituitary extract (cCPE) on the in vitro production of progesterone and nuclear maturation of canine oocytes. *African Journal of Biotechnology*, 11(23), 6321–6316.

Machado, M. S., Carmo, M. T., Squires, E. L., Roser, J. F., & Alvarenga, M. A. (2005). Follicular dynamic, superovulatory response and embryo recovery rates in mares treated with constant and decreasing doses of Equine Pituitary Extract (EPE) and purified equine FSH. *Equine Embryo Transfer*, 1, 75–76.

Nalley, W. M., Hine, T. M., & Kune, P. (2021). Penyuntikan tiga kali ekstrak pituitari selama induk sapi bali bunting meningkatkan bobot lahir dan produksi air susu. *Jurnal Veteriner Juni*, 22(2), 271–277.

Oduwole, O. O., Peltoketo, H., & Huhtaniemi, I.T. 2018. Role of follicle-stimulating hormone in spermatogenesis. *Frontiers in Endocrinology*, 9, 763.

Outang, T. M. T., Nalley, W. M., & Hine, T. M. (2017). Pemanfaatan ekstrak hipofisis sapi untuk memperbaiki performans reproduksi induk babi post partum. *Jurnal Veteriner* September, 18(3), 383–392.

Priatin, T., Iskandar, F., & Arifin, H. D. (2019). Perubahan biologis awal berahi kambing kaligesing betina yang disuntik ekstrak hipofisa dengan level berbeda. *Jurnal Riset Agribisnis dan Peternakan*, 4(2), 30–38.

Sayuti, A., Hamdan, H., Jannah, M., Safriadi, S., Nasri, T., & Siregar, T. N. (2022). Superovulation induction with bovine pituitary extract in local rabbits. *Punjab Univ. J. Zool*, 37(1), 29–34.

Scoggin, C. F., Meira, C. D., McCue, P. M., Carnevale, E. M., Nett, T. M., & Squires, E. L. (2002). Strategies to improve the ovarian response to equine pituitary extract in cyclic mares. *Theriogenology*, 58(1), 151–164.

Setiawan, D., Iskandar, F., & Arifin, H. D. (2019). Tingkah laku awal berahi kambing kaligesing (Capra aegagrus Hircus) betina yang di injeksi ekstrak hipofisa dengan level Berbeda. *Jurnal Riset Agribisnis dan Peternakan*, 4(2), 48–55.

Shah, A., & Elsanafiry, M. S. M. (2018). Diaphragma sellae: Anatomical and surgical implication in surgery for pituitary adenomas–highlighting contributions by Goel. *Journal of Craniovertebral Junction & Spine*, 9(3), 135.

Siregar (2020).

Siregar, T. N., Siregar, I. K., Armansyah, T., & Sayuti, A. (2013). Ampilan reproduksi kambing lokal hasil induksi superovulasi dengan ekstrak pituitary sapi. *J. Vet*, 14, 91–98.

Squires, E. L., & McCue, P. M. (2007). Superovulation in mares. *Animal Reproduction Science*, 99(1–2), 1–8.

Sutiyono, S., Setiatin, E. T., Kuncara, S., & Mayasari, M. (2008). The influence of hypophysis exstracts on oestrous and fertility of ewes synchronized by progesterone. *Journal of the Indonesian Tropical Animal Agriculture*, 33(1), 20–26.

Takács, P., Vitál, Z., Ferincz, Á., & Staszny, Á. (2016). Repeatability, reproducibility, separative power and subjectivity of different fish morphometric analysis methods. *PLoS One*, 11(6), e0157890.

Technological Innovations in Tropical Livestock Development for Environmental Sustainability and Food Security – P. Dhian Isnaeni et al. (eds)

Environmental and genetic influences on milk composition of Sapera goat

A. Anggraeni*, A. Hafid & Asepriyadi
Research Center for Animal Husbandry, Research Organization for Agriculture and Food, BRIN, Cibinong, Bogor, West Java, Indonesia

E. Anggraini
Department of Animal Production and Technology, Faculty of Animal Science, IPB University, Bogor, Indonesia

ABSTRACT: Examination of the non-genetic and genetic factors was done on the milk composition of the 'Sapera' goat. Milk components (%) were analyzed from 220 daily milk yields. The General Linear Model was used to investigate non-genetic and sire effects. Heritability values were estimated using the Paternal Half Sib Correlation Method. The averages of fat, protein, lactose, and SNP contents were 4.38 ± 0.08%, 3.70 ± 0.05%, 3.52 ± 0.04%, and 7.67 ± 0.08%, respectively. Season- and year of kidding had very significant effects ($P<0.01$) on fat%, instead of the stage of lactation and period of lactation ($P>0.05$). Moreover, other milk components were not significantly ($P>0.05$) influenced by these environmental factors. Estimation of heritability values of fat%, protein%, lactose% and SNF% were 0.1355 ± 0.0906, 0.1841 ± 0.0914, 0.14311 ± 0.0909, and 0.1073 ± 0.0925 respectively. Improving the genetic quality of milk components through selection would be effective for local crossing dairy goats.

Keywords: Milk component, non-genetic, heritability, dairy goats

1 INTRODUCTION

Breeding programs to improve the performance of dairy goat farming depend on selecting livestock that have superior genetic lactation traits. Knowledge of non-genetic factors and estimation of genetic parameters that influence economically important traits is a basic consideration of selection programs. Heritability of the expression of the genetic diversity of a trait requires the elimination of the influence of environmental factors or non-genetic factors so that the heritability value (h2) can be estimated accurately in predicting breeding values and in developing efficient breeding schemes (Bagnicka *et al.* 2015). Milk quality and composition are important characteristics of dairy livestock. Quality is associated with health, nutritional value, cleanliness, and sensory aspects that satisfy the needs of consumers, while composition refers to the contents of the various elements contained in milk (Msalya *et al.* 2021).

Dairy goat milk composition can be influenced by many factors such as management, body weight, parity (age), stage of lactation, nutrition, the season of birth, and year of birth (Addass *et al.* 2013; El-Tarabany *et al.* 2018; Ibrahim & Jalil 2022; Idowu & Adewumi 2017; Msalya *et al.* 2021). Heritability value (h2) is required to calculate

*Corresponding Author: ria.anneke@yahoo.co.id

DOI: 10.1201/9781003468943-4

breeding values to determine the best parents for the next mating to make genetic improvements of the offspring for the desired trait (Anggraeni *et al.* 2020; El-den *et al.* 2020; Mucha *et al.* 2014). Heritability is essential to know selection responses of the considered trait and other correlated traits and to develop selection indexes on economically valuable traits (Bagnicka *et al.* 2015; Mucha *et al.* 2014). Several studies have found that goat's milk components such as protein, fat, lactose, solid non-fat (SNF), and total dry matter (DM) are controlled by genetic factors ranging from moderate to high. The h2 value for the component (%) of fat by 0.21–0.34; protein by 0.37–0.69; and lactose by 0.17–0.29 (Brito *et al.* 2011; El-den *et al.* 2020; Torres-Vázquez *et al.* 2010). Saanen goats kept at the government breeding station at BBPTU Baturraden at their first lactation resulted in the h2 values of the components (%) of fat, protein, lactose, and SNF were sequentially 0.11 ± 0.16; 0.12 ± 0.16; 0.10 ± 0.14; and 0.11 ± 0.16 (Irawati *et al.* 2020).

Dairy goats can be an alternative to supply the community's milk needs which are mainly sourced from Holstein Friesian dairy cattle in Indonesia. Local PE goats a local breed of dual-purpose goats, producing both milk and meat, were crossed with Saanen dairy goats at IRIAP (Indonesian Research Institute for Animal Production). This crossing program produced a local cross-dairy goat with a genetic composition of PE 50% x Saanen 50% commercially called the 'Sapera' goat. The crossing program aimed to obtain a combination of superiority and heterosis effects from the milk production and adaptation traits of both parental breeds (Anggraeni 2023; Anggraeni *et al.* 2020). Selection for Sapera in our research has been primarily conducted on milk production traits, but milk components are also an important consideration for genetic improvement.

This research was conducted to evaluate the influence of various non-genetic factors and estimate the genetic influence on milk quality in Sapera goats raised under an intensive IRIAP management system.

2 MATERIAL AND METHOD

2.1 *Location*

The study was carried out at the Indonesian Research Institute for Animal Production (IRIAP) Dairy Goat Station, which is situated in Ciawi Subdistrict, Bogor District, West Java. IRIAP was located between 450 and 500 m above sea level in Banjar Waru Village, Ciawi Subdistrict, Bogor Regency, with an annual precipitation range of 3,500 to 4,000 mm. The IRIAP Dairy Goat Station and Dairy Laboratory and Animal Product Technology of the Faculty of Animal Husbandry, Bogor Agriculture University, Bogor were the laboratories that conducted analyses on milk components.

2.2 *Material*

The research samples of this study used the Sapera goat, as the local crossing dairy goat with a genetic combination of 50% PE and 50% Saanen. The animal samples were 66 does in the status of month of lactation of 1–12 mo., lactation phase 1–6, and within the year of observation in 2020–2022. In addition, 8 bucks were used for possessing female offspring with milk component records between 14–49 records.

A lactoscan machine was used to analyse the components (%) of milk protein and other milk components. A basic procedure involved placing a milk sample into the machine's tiny tube and passing it via a sound wave beam to calculate the percentage of milk protein and other components. A number of 220 daily test milk yields were calculated as the sum of morning and midday productions to assess the daily milk components of the individual doe.

2.3 *Management*

Does were fed concentrate as sources of protein and energy with a protein content of 16–18% with a TDN of 70–80% for about 2% of live body weight around 0.8–1 kg/hd/d. Feeding forages consisted of elephant grass and calliandra legume. Additionally, the tofu waste was fed as a source of protein at a ratio of 1 kg of concentrate to approximately 4 kg of tofu waste. The tofu was fed for a doe by 0.8 kg/hd/d and for a young female by 0.5 kg/hd/d.

2.4 *Data analysis*

2.4.1 *General linear model*

Data of 220 milk components from 220 female offsprings (does) and eight sires were used to estimate heritability values (h2) by the paternal half-sib method. General Linear Model (GLM) analysis for unbalanced data was performed to investigate the effects of both genetic and non-genetic factors. The GLM was fitted by considering each of the milk components as independent variables. Whereas dependent variables were considered as fixed variables providing buck, stage of lactation, period of lactation, season-, year of kidding, or initial lactation. The statistical formula was followed:

$$\text{Yijklmn} = \mu + \text{Bi} + \text{SLj} + \text{LPk} + \text{SKl} + \text{YKm} + \text{ejklmn}$$

Yijklm: each of the mth milk components,
μ: overall average,
Bi: the ith sire effect (i = 1,2,3, ...10),
SLj: the jth stage of lactation effect (j = 1 & 2, 3, 4, 5, 6, $\geq$ 7);
LPk: the jth period of lactation effect (j = 1, 2, 3, $\geq$ 4);
KSl: the kth season of kidding effect (k = 1–3, 4–6, 7–9, 10–12 mo.);
KYm: the lth year of kidding effect (l = 2020, 2021, 2022).
Eijklmn: the mth random error NID (0, Iσ2e).

2.4.2 *Estimation of heritability value*

Heritability value (h2) was calculated using paternal half-sib correlation method with the following formula as used by Anggraeni (2023):

$$h_s^2 = \frac{4\sigma_s^2}{\sigma_s^2 + +\sigma_w^2}$$

Description:

h = heritability value,
σ_s^2 = variance components among sires,
σ_w^2 = variance components among individuals within sire.

The standard error of heritability value was calculated using the following formula:

$$S.E\ (h^2) = 4\sqrt{\frac{2(1-t)^2[1+(k-1)t]^2}{k(k-1)(s-1)}}$$

Description:

t = correlation within class,
s = number of sires,
k = coefficient of the number of offspring per sire.

3 RESULT AND DISCUSSION

3.1 *Non-genetic effects*

The results of the GLM analysis of the fixed effects of non-genetic factors and sire on individual milk components from Sapera goats are presented in Table 1. The mean and SE values of milk contents (%) of fat, protein, lactose, and SNP were 4.38 ± 0.08 %, 3.70 ± 0.05 %, 3.52 ± 0.04 %, and 7.67 ± 0.08 % respectively. The contents of the main milk components of this sapera were higher than those in Saanen goats aged 2–4 yr. kept at a farm in Malaysian tropical region, successively fat (2.77 ± 0.06% to 3.33 ± 0.06%), protein (2.77 ± 0.03% to 2.80 ± 0.00%) and lactose (4.1 ± 0.06% to 4.27 ± 0.03%); the exception for lower SNF (7.53 ± 0.11% to 7.80 ± 0.03% (Ibrahim & Jalil 2022). When compared with PE goat, in the treatment of feed supplements containing antioxidants, the milk components of this study were lower against those of fat (6,292–6,725%) and lactose (5,229–5,616%), but within the range for protein (3,427–3,783%) (Mardalena *et al.* 2011). Furthermore, pure Saanen and the local PE goat crosses (PExSaanen and PExEtawah) produced higher levels of fat (5.3 ± 0.50% to 6.6 ± 0.40%) and SNF (9.11 ± 0.04% to 9.25 ± 0.04%), but almost the same for protein content (3.70 ± 0.06% to 4.09 ± 0.03%) (Kabil *et al.* 2015). Meanwhile, Norwegian cross goats (blood composition 50% to >75%) yielded milk components for crude protein 3.47 ± 0.07% to 3.55 ± 0.11%, lactose 4.14 ± 0.19% to 4.19 ± 0.13%, SNF 7.82 ± 0.15% to 8.04 ± 0.17%, and total solid 11.81 ± 0.16% to 12.79 ± 0.14% (Msalya *et al.* 2021). The differences in milk components of Sapera goats from other studies could be caused by differences in animal genetics, feeding, management, environment, and tropical temperature.

Table 1. Non-genetic influences on milk components (%) of Sapera goat.

			Fat (%)	Protein (%)	Lactose (%)	SNF (%)
Non-genetic factor	Sub-factor	N	X ± SE	X ± SE	X ± SE	X ± SE
Stage of lactation	2	41	4.41 ± 0.03	3.60 ± 0.05	3.42 ± 0.03	7.45 ± 0.11
	3	45	4.36 ± 0.04	3.58 ± 0.09	3.41 ± 0.08	7.40 ± 0.05
	4	22	4.42 ± 0.09	3.66 ± 0.05	3.42 ± 0.06	7.41 ± 0.07
	5	30	4.18 ± 0.05	3.60 ± 0.04	3.43 ± 0.04	7.41 ± 0.06
	6	12	4.27 ± 0.11	3.89 ± 0.07	3.64 ± 0.11	7.91 ± 0.15
	7	70	4.34 ± 0.04	3.91 ± 0.05	3.74 ± 0.07	7.99 ± 0.09
Period of lactation	1	15	3.97 ± 0.12	3.64 ± 0.12	3.44 ± 0.06	7.51 ± 0.10
	2	95	4.76 ± 0.06	3.68 ± 0.06	3.49 ± 0.08	7.62 ± 0.13
	3	63	4.52 ± 0.04	3.81 ± 0.04	3.64 ± 0.04	7.79 ± 0.05
	4	47	4.65 ± 0.05	3.74 ± 0.05	3.55 ± 0.03	7.69 ± 0.04
Season of kidding	1	42	4.47 ± 0.03^{b}	3.57 ± 0.03	3.41 ± 0.02	7.48 ± 0.11
	2	80	3.98 ± 0.04^{a}	3.53 ± 0.05	3.33 ± 0.04	7.34 ± 0.05
	3	78	3.89 ± 0.06^{a}	3.80 ± 0.06	3.57 ± 0.05	7.81 ± 0.09
	4	20	4.67 ± 0.05^{b}	3.93 ± 0.05	3.73 ± 0.02	7.92 ± 0.07
Year of kidding	2020	103	4.41 ± 0.02^{ab}	3.74 ± 0.03	3.54 ± 0.03	7.66 ± 0.14
	2021	79	4.71 ± 0.04^{a}	3.67 ± 0.02	3.51 ± 0.05	7.71 ± 0.11
	2022	38	3.99 ± 0.03^{a}	3.71 ± 0.05	3.48 ± 0.02	7.52 ± 0.04
Total		220	4.38 ± 0.08	3.70 ± 0.05	3.52 ± 0.04	7.67 ± 0.08

Note: N: number of samples; SNF: solid non-fat.

Table 1 shows the influence of non-genetic factors including stage of lactation, period of lactation, season of kidding, and year of kidding on each milk component of the Sapera goat. Figures 1–4 also show the effects of these four non-genetic factors on each milk component of the Sapera goat, successive stage of lactation (Figure 1), period of lactation (Figure 2), season of kidding (Figure 3), and year of kidding (Figure 4). Season- and year of kidding statistically significant ($P<0.05$) affected on fat%, but stage of lactation and period of lactation had no significant ($P>0.05$) impact. Fat % was higher during lactation in the wet season (October to December) and January to March) compared to the dry season (April to September), with a difference of around 16.14%. Further, the highest milk fat % was during the year 2021 against 2020 and 2022, with the differences of 6.80% and 9.77%. Meanwhile, the levels (%) of protein, lactose, and SNF were not significantly influenced ($P>0.05$) by all non-genetic factors investigated. The availability of more forage during the rainy season was likely the cause of the increase in milk fat content from Sapera does. (Mlay *et al.* 2006) reported that the increasing feeding forage could increase acetate production in the rumen cause of increasing milk fat content, conversely, the increasing feeding concentrate could increase protein and total digestible nutrients. In line with this, Kabil *et al.* (2015) stated that milk fat content decreased by the reduced forage feeding. A previous study on three native Nigerian goat breeds found that lactation the period of lactation, parity, and kidding season influenced some milk components (Addass *et al.* 2013). During the colostrum stage, the highest levels of crude protein, fat, and milk lactose were achieved (i.e. 3.85 ± 0.04%, 5.35 ± 0.03%, and 5.02 ± 0.04%), whereas the lowest levels were during late lactation (3.20 ± 0.04%, 4.13 ± 0.03%, and 4.07 ± 0.04%). The highest percentages of fat and lactose occurred during the rainy season (i.e. 5.04 ± 0.02% and 4.85 ± 0.03%). Furthermore, milk fat and lactose percentages were highest at parities three and four (5.54 ± 0.03% and 5.30 ± 0.05%).

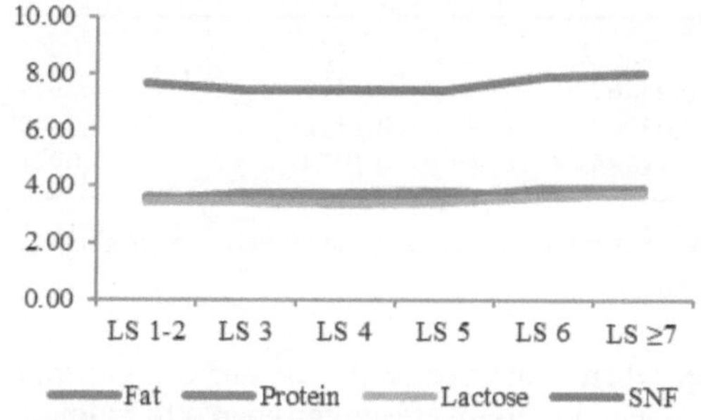

Figure 1. Effect of stage of lactation on milk components.

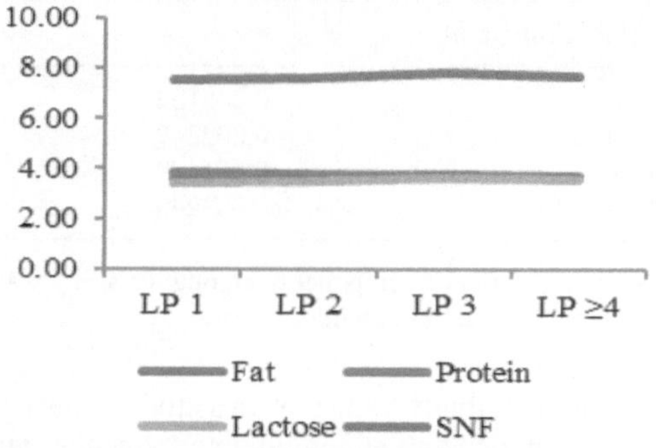

Figure 2. Effect of period of lactation on milk components.

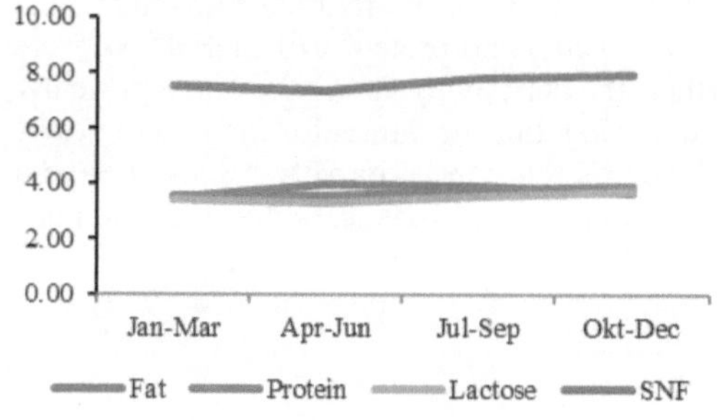

Figure 3. Effect of season of kidding on milk components.

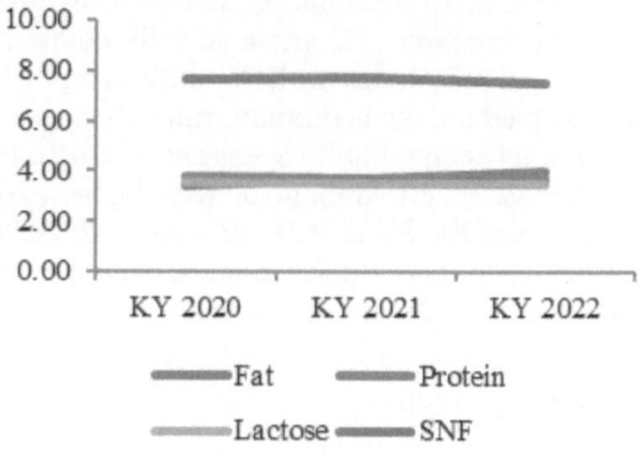

Figure 4. Effect of year of kidding on milk components.

Another study did not obtain significant differences (P>0.05) in the contents (%) of milk fat, lactose, and SNF by parity and stage of lactation, but these two factors had a significant effect (P>0.05) on milk crude protein level (Msalya *et al.* 2021). In a previous study at the first lactation the dairy goats resulted in the highest percentages of fat and protein, whilst the lowest yield (kg) of fat, protein, and milk (Bagnicka *et al.* 2015). In Damascus goats, the milk protein (%) during summer/spring was significantly higher ($P \leq 0.01$) than during Winter/Autumn, and the highest fat (%) ($P \leq 0.05$) was found in 2009, but no significant difference was between the type of birth for percentages (%) of protein and fat (El-den *et al.* 2020).

3.2 *Heritability values of milk components*

Heritability is essential to allow selection responses of the considered traits and other correlated traits and to develop index selection on economically valuable traits. The estimated heritability values for Sapera goat milk were for the components (%) fat by 0.1355 ± 0.0906, protein by 0.1841 ± 0.0914, lactose by 0.14311 ± 0.0909, and SNF by 0.1073 ± 0.0925. Based on the heritability criteria used to classify moderate values within a range of >0.10–0.30, the heritability values of milk components of Sapera goats from this study were at a moderate level (h2 = 0.158–0.228). The heritability value describes the contribution of additive gene influence to a particular trait. Thus, the presence of additive genetic variation of quite large value in milk components can be an indication of genetic improvement of the milk components through selection which will provide a fairly effective selection response in Sapera dairy goats.

Table 2. Heritability values (h^2) of milk components of Sapera goat.

Milk component	σ_s^2	σ_w^2	h^2	SE
Fat	0.006154	0.175488	0.1355	0.0906
Protein	0.002249	0.04662	0.1841	0.0914
Laktosa	0.001449	0.039051	0.14311	0.0909
SNF	0.003249	0.117867	0.1073	0.0925

Note: σ_s^2: variance components among sires, σ_w^2: variance components among individuals within sire; h^2: heritability value, SE: Standart error.

The heritability values of this study were lower when compared to those using a multi-trait animal model with animal and permanent environmental random effects considered to estimate genetic parameters in Saanen and Alpine goats. Heritability values of fat%, protein%, and lactose% were successively 0.21, 0.39, and 0.18; while the respective repeatability values were 0.34, 0.44, and 0.29 respectively (Brito *et al.* 2011). Likewise, the heritability values were lower for fat % (0.32 ± 0.06) and milk protein % (0.38 ± 0.07) in Saanen goat (Torres-Vázquez *et al.* 2010). Nevertheless, when Alpine goat milk components were examined using a single trait repeatability animal model, with variance components estimated using the residual maximum likelihood method, the heritability values for fat% (0.16 ± 0.003) and protein% (0.25 ± 0.004) were remarkably comparable (Špehar *et al.* 2019). Further, the heritability values for crude protein% in Damascus and Arabi goats were higher (0.69 and 0.37), but the values for fat% were nearly comparable (0.22 and 0.23) (El-den *et al.* 2020). The difference in heritability values of Sapera compared to other studies could be caused by differences in animal genetic, sample size, methods of analysis, and non-genetics factors considered in the model.

4 CONCLUSION

The milk quality of Sapera goat was fairly good as indicated by the quite high contents (%) of protein, fat, lactose, and SNF. The season- and year of kidding affected fat where doe lactation in the rainy season reached a higher fat than in the dry season. The season- and year of kidding affected significantly on fat%, where lactation during the rainy season reached a higher fat than in the dry season, but all non-genetic factors have minor effects on other milk components. The heritability values of milk components of Sapera goat were moderate (h2 = 0.1073 to 0.1841) indicating selection would be an effective way to improve the milk quality of cross-bred dairy goat.

REFERENCES

Addass, P. A., M. A. Tizhe, A. Midau, P. Alheri, and M. M. Yahya. 2013. Effect of genotype, stage of lactation, season and parity on milk composition of goat, in Mubi, Adamawa State, Nigeria. *Annals of Biological Research* 4(8):248–52.

Anggraeni, A. 2023. Estimated heritability values (h2) of milk yields of saanen goat. *AIP Conference Proceedings* 2628. doi: 10.1063/5.0144171.

Anggraeni, A., F. Saputra, A. Hafid, and A. B. L. Ishak. 2020. Non-genetic and genetic effects on growth traits from birth to 120 days of age of G2 sapera goat. 25:48–59. doi: http://dx.doi.org/10.14334/jitv.v25i2.2498 Information.

Bagnicka, E., H. Hamann, and O. Distl. 2015. Structure and the non-genetic and genetic effects on milk traits in polish dairy goat population. *Animal Science Papers and Reports* 33(1):59–69.

Brito, L. F., F. G. Silva, A. L. P. Melo, G. C. Caetano, R. A. Torres, M. T. Rodrigues, and G. R. O. Menezes. 2011. Genetic and environmental factors that influence production and quality of milk of alpine and saanen goats. *Genetics and Molecular Research* 10(4):3794–3802. doi: 10.4238/2011.December.14.9.

El-den, K. M., K. Mohammed, and A. Dahmoush. 2020. Genetic evaluation of milk yield and milk composition of Saudi Aradi and damascus goats. *Archives of Agriculture Sciences Journal* 3(2):118–26. doi: 10.21608/aasj.2020.41747.1031.

El-Tarabany, M. S., A. A. El-Tarabany, and E. M. Roushdy. 2018. Impact of lactation stage on milk composition and blood biochemical and hematological parameters of dairy baladi goats. *Saudi Journal of Biological Sciences* 25(8):1632–38. doi: 10.1016/j.sjbs.2016.08.003.

Ibrahim, N. S., and A. R. Jalil. 2022. The Effect of Age on Milk Yield and Milk Composition in Saanen Dairy Goats. *Journal of Agricultural Science and Technology A* 12(1):10–14. doi: 10.17265/2161-6256/2022.01.002.

Idowu, T. S., and O. O. Adewumi. 2017. Genetic and non-genetic factors affecting yield and milk composition in goats. *Advances in Dairy Research* 5(2):2–5. doi: 10.4172/2329-888x.1000175.

Irawati, N., D. Purwantini, and A. Sodiq. 2020. Estimating genetic parameter of saanen goat production characteristics using paternal half sib correlation. *Animal Production* 21(1):16. doi: 10.20884/1.jap.2019.21.1.710.

Kabil, O., M. Ali, E. Ibrahim, and H. El Barbary. 2015. Effect of seasonal variation on chemical composition of cow's milk. *Benha Veterinary Medical Journal* 28(1):150–54. doi: 10.21608/bvmj.2015.32728.

Mardalena, M., L. Warly, E. Nurdin, W. S. N. Rusmana, and F. Farizal. 2011. Milk quality of dairy goat by giving feed supplement as antioxidant source. *Journal of the Indonesian Tropical Animal Agriculture* 36 (3):205–12. doi: 10.14710/jitaa.36.3.205-212.

Mlay, P. S., A. Pereka, E. C. Phiri, Sakurani Balthazary, Jelantik Igusti, Torben Hvelplund, Martin Riis Weisbjerg, and Jørgen Madsen. 2006. Feed value of selected tropical grasses, legumes and concentrates. *Veterinarski Arhiv* 76(1):53–63.

Msalya, G. M., F. E. Urassa, and G. C. Kifaro. 2021. Quality of milk from Norwegian dairy goats bred and raised in mgeta division, Morogoro region, Tanzania. *Tanzania Journal of Agricultural Sciences* 20(1):54–62.

Mucha, S., R. Mrode, M. Coffey, and J. Conington. 2014. Estimation of genetic parameters for milk yield across lactations in mixed-breed dairy goats. *Journal of Dairy Science* 97(4):2455–61. doi: 10.3168/jds.2013-7319.

Špehar, Marija, D. Mulc, Z. Barać, B. Mioč, and A. Kasap. 2019. Estimation of genetic parameters for dairy traits using repeatability animal models based on test-day data for alpine goat in Croatia. *Mljekarstvo* 69 (4):215–21. doi: 10.15567/mljekarstvo.2019.0401.

Torres-Vázquez, J. Antonio, M. Valencia-Posadas, H. Castillo-Juárez, and H. H. Montaldo. 2010. Tendencias genéticas y fenotípicas para características de producción y composición de la leche en cabras saanen de México. *Tecnica Pecuaria En Mexico* 48(4):337–48.

Technological Innovations in Tropical Livestock Development for Environmental Sustainability and Food Security – P. Dhian Isnaeni et al. (eds)

Feeding elephant grass and *Gliricidia sepium* on performance of Bali calves during transitional diet

Nurmeiliasari*, A.H.K. Amrullah, H.D. Putranto, A. Riska & V.C. Hapsari
Department of Animal Science, Faculty of Agriculture, University of Bengkulu, Kandang Limun, Bengkulu, Indonesia

E. Yunita
Medical Study Program, Faculty of Medicine and Health Sciences, University of Bengkulu, Kandang Limun, Bengkulu, Indonesia

J. Firison
Research Center for Animal Husbandry, National Research and Innovation Agency, Bogor, Indonesia

ABSTRACT: A study investigated the effect of feeding elephant grass cv. Taiwan and a combination of elephant grass cv. Taiwan and *Gliricidia sepium* on the performance and body dimensions of Bali calves. This research was conducted for two months using eight pre-weaning Bali calves aged eight weeks, which were divided into 2 treatments (T1: 60% concentrate and 40% elephant grass cv. Taiwan, and T2: 60% concentrate + 20% elephant grass cv. Taiwan + 20% *Gliricidia sepium*). Different fiber sources did not affect dry matter consumption and weight gain (P>0.05). Various dietary fiber sources did not influence the body dimension of pre-weaning calves (P>0.05). To sum up, the transitional phase from a liquid to a solid diet in Bali's calves using elephant grass and a combination of elephant grass and *Gliricidia sepium* did not have negative effects on the production performance and body dimensions of Bali calves.

Keywords: Bali calves, elephant grass, Gliricidia sepium, performance, body dimension

1 INTRODUCTION

Newborn calves have underdeveloped rumen, and liquid feed is the main source of protein and energy. Changes in the feeding regime from a liquid to a solid diet are critical to stimulate rumen development as the main digestive system of ruminants. A successful dietary transition will enable a smooth shift from the pre-ruminant to the ruminant phase. Optimum growth of the rumen at a young age facilitates the utilization of energy from a solid diet for efficient growth when calves mature. The growth and development of the rumen are influenced by mechanical stimulation that occurs due to the supply of nutrients and the presence of fiber (physically adequate fiber) in the rumen. The triggers increase the number of rumen papillae, which are areas for absorbing feed nutrients (Nurmeiliasari *et al.* 2017).

Fiber feed is reported to alter the composition and content of VFA in the rumen, stimulating rumen growth and development. The epithelial papillae lining the rumen increase the surface area for VFA absorption (Gleason *et al.* 2022). The chemical composition of the feed and physical properties are the main factors that influence the morphological structure of rumen epithelial papillae (Liu *et al.* 2013; Steele *et al.* 2011).

*Corresponding Author: sari_nurmeiliasari@unib.ac.id

 DOI: 10.1201/9781003468943-5

Elephant grass is a popular source of feed in many beef cattle farms. However, feeding solely elephant grass is reported to have drawbacks in cattle performance due to its low crude protein content (Tibayungwa *et al.* 2011). Therefore, the utilization of elephant grass is supplemented with high-quality forages to meet the nutrient requirements of cattle. Elephant grass (Pennisetum purpureum) and *Gliricidia sepium* function as an energy source and protein source to complement the nutritional elements for basic living needs and growth (Rusdy 2016). This research aims to determine the effect of feeding forage elephant grass cv. Taiwan (Pennisetum purpureum cv. Taiwan) and *Gliricidia sepium* on the performance and body dimensions of Bali calves.

2 MATERIALS AND METHODS

2.1 *Research procedure*

This research used 8 pre-weaning Bali calves aged eight weeks to 14 weeks old distributed into an elephant grass-fed group and a combination of elephant grass and *Gliricidia sepium*. The concentrate consisted of dried cassava waste, corn meal, palm kernel cake, soybean meal, coffee husk, pollard, mineral, and salt. This research used a milk replacer (Nutri white) during the transition and adaptation to a solid diet. Milk replacers were given twice daily, and the amount of milk given was gradually reduced until none of the milk replacers were given; then, the research started. This transition continued to a solid diet. The treatments of the research were as follows:

T1: 60% Concentrate + Elephant Grass cv. Taiwan (*Pennisetum purpureum cv. Taiwan*) 40%
T2: 60% Concentrate + Elephant Grass cv. Taiwan (*Pennisetum purpureum cv. Taiwan*) 20% + *Gliricidia sepium* 20%.

The rations provision followed 3% body weight dry matter. The calves had free access to drinking water. Both treatment groups have 16% crude protein; however, the crude fiber in T1 was 17.18%; in contrast, T2 contained 8,41% crude fiber. The calves were fed twice daily at 08 AM and 15 PM. Feed refusal was collected and weighed every morning to calculate feed consumption. Body weight and dimensional measurements were carried out on day 1 of the study, day 30 of the study, and day 60 of the study. Research data was analyzed using an *independent t-test.* The level of significance in this study was 5% (0.05).

3 RESULTS AND DISCUSSION

3.1 *Dry matter consumption*

Table 1 showed that various dietary fiber sources did not influence dry matter intake in the 1st or the 2nd month or total dry matter consumption during the experiment ($P>0.05$). The nature of solid feed (forage and concentrate) promotes the initiation of solid feed consumption, all of which could affect the microbiome in developing calves (Khan *et al.* 2016).

Table 1. Average dry matter consumption of Bali calves.

Feed consumption (Kg)	T1	T2	P value
the 1st month	1.15 ± 0.03	0.93 ± 0,04	0.50
the 2nd month	1.38 ± 0.04	1.12 ± 0,06	0.54
2 months of the experiment	1.26 ± 0,04	1.03 ± 0,05	0.52

The calves in our research consumed 3% to 3.5% body weight dry matter. The amount of forage or non-forage NDF required to develop and stimulate rumination, saliva production, and stabilizing rumen pH is not clearly defined for calf diets (Khan *et al.* 2016). Similar feed intake in our research might not be influenced by dietary fiber treatment.

3.2 *Body weight gain*

The average daily gain was statistically the same between grass and a mixture of grass and legume treatment groups (P>0.05). Differences in crude fiber levels of grass and legume did not affect performance. Coverdale *et al.* (2004) reported that feeding higher levels of forage and a textured starter diet improved rumen development and growth in calves. Protein supplementation in ruminants fed low-quality grass feed such as elephant grass can increase the growth of rumen fibrolytic bacteria and increase feed degradation in the rumen (Rusdy *et al.* 2021). This is in accordance with that stated by Fitasari *et al.* (2018) that one of the important food substances for livestock growth is protein, because if the livestock lacks protein, then growth is disrupted

Marsetyo *et al.* (2012) reported that the daily gain was 0.174 g when Bali cattle fed sole elephant grass ad libitum, but increased to 0.311 g/day when elephant grass supplemented with legume at 10 g DM/kg body weight/day. In this study, the lowest daily weight gain occurred when calves were fed a mixture of elephant grass and nuts and reached the highest when single elephant grass was given to Bali cattle calves. Optimal legume levels are below 100%, because feeding Bali cattle with 100% legume results in lower daily body weight gain compared to feeding a mixture of elephant grass and legume feed (Marsetyo *et al.* 2012). Providing quality feed will be able to provide performance production such as postnatal body weight, milk production during the month of lactation and calf growth, as well as reducing Pastor's death in Bali cattle (Bamualim & Wirdahayati 2003).

Table 2. Average daily gain of Bali calves.

Average Daily Gain (Kg)	T1	T2	P value
the 1st month	0.17 ± 0.12	0.08 ± 0.06	0.24
the 2nd month	0.13 ± 0,08	0.15 ± 0,13	0.83
2 months of the experiment	9.25 ± 5,64	7.13 ± 5.76	0.62

3.3 *Body dimensions*

Measuring the body dimensions of livestock can be used as an effort to indicate that the livestock is experiencing growth. According to Sampurna (2014), one of the indicators for assessing growth and development is measuring the increase in body dimensions. Body dimensions are also measured to determine the appearance of livestock. Measuring tools commonly used are measuring tape and measuring sticks for the exterior of cattle. Average body dimensions of Bali calves for 2 months fed elephant grass cv. Taiwan and gliricidia are presented in Table 3.

Table 3. Average body dimensions of Bali calves for 2 months fed with elephant grass and *Gliricidia sepium.*

	Treatment		
Parameter (cm)	T1	T2	Probability
Heart girth	86,87 ± 9,06	78,50 ± 9,12	0,24
Body Length	58,79 ± 3,30	56,62 ± 5,61	0,53
Hip width	25,25 ± 2,47	23,75 ± 4,42	0,57
Withers height	74,29 ± 2,84	74,25 ± 7,24	0,99

An *independent t-test* showed that the treatment had no significant effect (P>0.05) on body dimensions, including chest circumference, body length, hip width, and withers height. It is assumed that calves experience the same rumen growth and development so that consuming the same feed will increase the same body dimensions in each treatment. Consumption that comes in first is intended for basic living needs. With sufficient basic living needs, the fulfillment of nutrition in the animal's body can help optimal growth, so that during the calf's pre-adult period, the body's bone and skeletal grow well.

Calves in the same age category have the same amount of feed consumption so that rumen growth and development are at the same stage. The growth and development of the rumen is stimulated by providing fibrous feed in the form of cv. Taiwan elephant grass. This cv. Taiwan elephant grass is a good source of energy for livestock. Elephant grass contains 30–40% cellulose and 25–30% hemicellulose; it is a potential energy source (Rusdy 2017).

The nutritional needs of the calf's body are of great concern because the feed given in the form of legumes contains good degradable protein. According to Wahiduddin (2008), gliricidia forage contains crude protein 20–30% BK, crude fiber 15%, and in *vitro* digestibility of dry matter 60–65 %. *Gliricidia sepium* contains 18–24% crude protein during the rainy season and 17–22% during the dry season.

Providing forage in the form of cv. Taiwan elephant grass and *Gliricidia sepium* is the first step to stimulate the growth and development of the rumen with the aim of optimal growth in the calf. An increase in body dimensions in calves characterizes growth. By making efforts to stimulate the rumen from an early age in calves mechanically, it has been reported that it can improve rumen motility, feeding behavior, rumination, and rumen proliferation by increasing the number of papillae and surface area of rumen absorption, which leads to increased performance (Nurmeiliasari 2018).

The growth and development of the rumen in the transition phase from pre-weaning to post-weaning is significant to pay attention to because it is the key to success in achieving production targets in ruminant livestock because most of the inefficiency in ruminant productivity occurs in the rumen (Ghozo and Mutsvangwa 2008; Koenig 2003). So, giving the calf fiber feed from an early age can stimulate the growth and development of the rumen for optimal growth in the calf, which is characterized by an increase in the calf's body dimensions.

4 CONCLUSION

Based on the research results, it can be concluded that feeding elephant grass cv. Taiwan (*Pennisetum purple cv. Taiwan*) and *Gliricidia sepium* do not have adverse effects on the performance and body dimensions of Bali's calves.

REFERENCES

Bamualim, A., & Wirdahayati, R. B. (2003). Nutrition and management strategies to improve Bali cattle productivity in Nusa Tenggara. In *Aciar Proceedings* (pp. 17–22). ACIAR; 1998.

Fitasari, E., Reo, K., & Niswi, N. (2016). The use of different levels of protein in free-range chickens affects the performance of protein production and digestibility. *Journal of Animal Science (Indonesian Journal of Animal Science)*, 26(2), 73–83.

Gleason, C. B., Beckett, L. M., & White, R. R. (2022). Rumen fermentation and epithelial gene expression responses to diet ingredients designed to differ in ruminally degradable protein and fiber supplies. *Scientific Reports*, 12(1), 2933. https://doi.org/10.1038/s41598-022-06890-5.

Liu, J. H., T. T. Xu, Y. J Liu, W. Y. Zhu, & S. Y. Mao. (2013). A high-grain diet causes massive disruption of ruminal epithelial tight junctions in goats. *American Journal of Physiology Regulatory Integrative and Comparative Physiology*. 305: R232–R241.

Marsetyo., Damry, S., Quigley, S. P., McLennan, S. R., & Poppy, P. (2012). Liveweight gain and feed intake of weaned Bali cattle fed a range of diets in Central Sulawesi, Indonesia. *Animal Production. Science*, 52: 630–635.

Nurmeiliasari, N. (2018). *Aplikasi Stimulator Mekanis Rumen Terhadap Performa Sapi brahman Cross Pada Penggemukan Tiga Bulan*. Animal Production and Technology. Bogor, Bogor Agricultural University. Doctoral: 102.

Nurmeiliasari, N., R. Priyanto, D.A. Astuti, Salundik, J. Takahashi, M. Okamoto, T. Okamoto & A. Jayanegara. (2017). Blood parameters and rumen wall histology of brahman crossbred steers in response to the administration of rumen mechanical stimulating brushes. *Pakistan Journal of Nutrition*. 16(12): 921–27.

Rusdy M. (2016). Elephant grass as forage for ruminant animals. *Livestock Research for Rural Development*. Volume 28, Article #49. Retrieved October 12, 2023, from http://www.lrrd.org/lrrd28/4/rusd28049.html

Rusdy, M., Hatta, M., & Rinduwati, S. Effect of supplementing elephant grass with Gliricidia sepium, Lannea coromandelica and concentrate feed on Bali cattle performance. *Livestock Research for Rural Development* 33 (8) 2021.

Sampurna I.P., I.K. Saka, I.G.L. Oka, & P. Sentana. (2014). Pattern of growth of Bali cattle body dimensions. *ARPN Journal of Science and Technology*. Vol 4, No 1, January 2014. ISSN: 2225-7217.

Sanderson, M.A. & R.A. Paul. (2008). Perennial forages as second-generation bioenergy crops. *International Journal of Molecular Sciences*, 9, 768–788.

Steele, M.A., J. Croom, M. Kahler, O. Alzahal, S.E. Hook, K. Plai-zier, & B.W. McBride. (2011). Bovine rumen epithelium under-goes rapid structural adaptations during grain-induced subacute ruminal acidosis. *American Journal of Physiology Regulatory Integrative and Comparative Physiology*. 300: R1515–R1523.

Sudardjat, D., & Sofjan. (2003). *National Report on Animal Genetic Resources Indonesia*. Directorate Generale of Livestock Services (DGLS), Directorate of Livestock Breeding. Indonesia.

Technological Innovations in Tropical Livestock Development for Environmental Sustainability and Food Security – P. Dhian Isnaeni et al. (eds)
© 2025 The Author(s), ISBN 978-1-032-74373-8
Open Access: www.taylorfrancis.com, CC BY-NC-ND 4.0 license

Estimated heritability value of egg weight and egg index of Tolaki chickens

R. Badaruddin*, L.O. Nafiu, M.A. Pagala & T. Saili
Animal Husbandry Department, Animal Husbandry Faculty, Halu Oleo University, Indonesia

ABSTRACT: Tolaki chicken is a breed of chicken native to Southeast Sulawesi and scattered in a few areas like Konawe, South Konawe and East Kolaka Regencies. Study This aim for analyze mark heritability egg weight, egg index and hatch weight of tolaki chicken. Breeding group was done with 10 roosters and 50 hens and each group contains of 1 rooster and 5 hens that produces 221 eggs of tolaki chicken. Research data analyzed by CRD (Completed Randomized Design) variance with pattern nested design (structure heararchy) for get component variety. Results study show that mark heritability weight eggs obtained is 0.52, index eggs 0.49 mark heritability in study This including category tall Because is at in above 0.30.

Keywords: Heritability, egg weight, egg index, Tolaki chicken

1 INTRODUCTION

Local chickens are the result of crosses or introductions from abroad that have been bred in Indonesia until the fifth generation or more. Local chickens have several families with distinctive morphological characteristics. One of Indonesia's local chickens is the Tolaki chicken, which is native germplasm of Southeast Sulawesi. Like other free-range chickens, the phenotypic and genotypic diversity of Tolaki chickens is still very high. This is reflected in the diverse egg weights. Selection programs in an effort to improve the genetic quality of livestock basically cannot be measured directly, but can be done through the calculation of the estimated breeding value based on the phenotype (Biscarini *et al.* 2010; Prihandini *et al.* 2012). The calculation of breeding value estimation in selection programs always involves genetic parameters. One of the genetic parameters used in estimating the breeding value of quantitative traits in livestock is heritability. Research on the calculation of heritability value has been conducted on Tolaki chickens with parameters including body weight during the growth period (Badaruddin *et al.* 2013). Heritability is the amount of influence of genetic diversity on phenotypic in a biological population. This value illustrates the ability of offspring to repeat the production achievements of their parents. The estimated value of heritability indicates whether a character is controlled by genetic factors or environmental factors, so that it can be known to what extent the character can be passed on to the next offspring (Lestari *et al.* 2006). Furthermore, it is said that heritability is the ratio between genetic variance to phenotypic variance (Dewi & Wahyuni 2020). The range of heritability value calculation is 0 to 1 (Widyawati *et al.* 2014). The high heritability value of a trait indicates a high correlation of phenotypic variance and genetic variance (Ciptadi *et al.* 2019). The value of genetic parameters of a trait in a particular population can be used as a guide to the direction of genetic quality improvement (Masili *et al.* 2018). Estimating genetic parameters, especially estimating the heritability of internal and external egg quality traits of

*Corresponding Author: rbadaruddin79@gmail.com

DOI: 10.1201/9781003468943-6

local chickens is very important to do because it can improve egg quality, increase egg size and increase production value which has an impact on increasing animal protein. Based on this description, research was conducted on estimating the heritability value of egg weight, egg index and hatching weight of Tolaki chickens, so that it can be the basis for the next selection process.

2 MATERIALS AND METHODS

This study used a digital scale with an accuracy of 0.1 g to weigh the weight of eggs. A calliper was used to measure the width and length of the egg to obtain the egg index value. The material used in this study was 400 tolaki chicken eggs obtained from the mating of 10 males with 50 hens, of which 1 male married 5 hens each, chicken mating was carried out using the Artificial Insemination (IB) method which was carried out 3 times a week. Eggs produced from mating were identified and coded according to the parents (male and female).

2.1 *Data collection*

Egg collection is done every day, by giving the code according to the parents (male and mother). Furthermore, the eggs that have been collected are weighed and measured egg length and egg width. The variables observed in this study were:

Egg weight (g), obtained by weighing eggs with digital scales sensitivity 0.01

Egg index (%), obtained by measuring the length and width of the egg Then calculated by the formula = (Egg width (%))

Egg shape index = Egg width (mm) Egg Length (mm) × 100% (Yuwanta 2010).

2.2 *Data analysis*

The research data were analysed using completely random design and analysis of variance nested design pattern (hierarchical structure) to obtain variance components of males and females. The mathematical model is as follows:

$$Yijk = \mu + Ji + \beta ij + \varepsilon ijk$$

Description:

Yijk = Observed values of offspring = I, feed = k, female = j and male
μ = General average of observations
Ji = Male effect (i = 1,2,...5)
βij = Effect of female (j = 1,2,...10) in male (i = 1,2,...5)
εijk = Effect of Ith offspring for each Ith male and jth female (individual error).

Through statistical analysis based on a hierarchical structure (nested design), variance components among males, among females within males and among offspring within females and males were calculated. The estimated genetic estimates based on the variance components are listed in Table 1.

The estimated heritability value is calculated based on the male variance component (ĥ2s), the female variance component (ĥ2d) and the combined male and female variance components (ĥ2s + d) (Becker 1992), which can be formulated as follows:

(1) Based on the male component (ĥ2s):

$$\hat{h}^2{}_s = 4s^2s^2 + d^2 + \sigma^2\epsilon$$

Table 1. Structure of analysis of variance nested design (hierarchical structure).

Source of Variance	Free degree	Sum of squares	Mean square	Group mean square
Among males	v – 1	$\sum X^2 i.. - C$	SSjtn/(v-1)	$\sigma^2\epsilon + k1\sigma^2♀ +$
Among females	v(m-1)	$\sum X^2 ij. - \sum X^2 i..$	SSbtn/v(m – 1)	$k2\sigma^2♂$
Among Offspring	vm(n-1)	$\sum X^2 ijk - \sum X^2 ij$	SSket/vm(n – 1)	$\sigma^2\epsilon + k3\sigma^2♀\ \sigma^2\epsilon$
TOTAL	Vmn-1		–	$\sigma^2T = \sigma^2\epsilon + \sigma^2♀ + \sigma^2♂^2$

σs^2: male variance component $\sigma^2\epsilon$: offspring/individual variance component error σd^2: female variance component

(2) Based on the female component ($\hat{h}2d$):

$$\hat{h}^2{}_d = 4d2s2 + d2 + 2\epsilon$$

(3) Based on male and female components ($\hat{h}2s + d$):

$$\hat{h}^2{}_{s+d} = 2s + d2s2 + d2 + 2\epsilon$$

Description:

$\hat{h}2s$: Heritability estimate based on male component
$\hat{h}2d$: Estimated heritability based on the female component
$\hat{h}2(s+d)$: Estimated heritability based on male and female components

3 RESULT AND DISCUSSION

3.1 *Tolaki chicken egg weight variance components*

Table 2 presents the distribution of variance components of egg weight based on the variance component of the male ($\sigma 2s$), the variance component of the mother ($\sigma 2d$), the variance component of the offspring (individual error) ($\sigma 2\epsilon$) and the total variance component ($\sigma 2total$) of Tolaki chicken. Based on the results of the hierarchical structure variance analysis used for estimating heritability values. The stud variance component ($\sigma 2s$) describes the relationship between half-siblings that does not give rise to the parent effect. The stud variance component is a component of genetic variance determined by the ability of the male as an additive gene estimation of the genetic variance component of weight and egg shape index of Tolaki chicken is presented in Table 2.

Table 2. Genetic variance components of egg weight and egg index of Tolaki chicken.

	Genetic Variance Component			
Parameters	σ^2_s	σ^2_d	σ^2_ϵ	σ^2_{total}
Egg weight	2.10	0.39	7.16	9.65
Egg index	5.40	2.65	24.70	32.75

Description:
$\sigma s2$: Male variance component $\sigma 2\epsilon$: Offspring variance component (individual error)
$\sigma 2$ total : Total variance component $\sigma 2d$: Female variance component

The parent variance component ($\sigma 2d$) describes the relationship between half-siblings based on the parent group, the resulting appearance in addition to being influenced by genetic factors, additives will also be determined by non-additive genetic factors (dominant, epistasis, interaction) and non-genetic (maternal effect). The offspring variance component ($\sigma 2\epsilon$) describes the combined genetic influence of males and parents together (additive, dominant and epistasis genes). The distribution of variance components based on the appearance of egg weight and egg shape index of Tolaki chickens shows that the variance component of males ($\sigma 2s$) is all positive both egg weight and egg index. The spread of the parent variance component ($\sigma 2d$) is all positive both egg weight and egg index. The distribution of the offspring/individual variance component ($\sigma 2\epsilon$) has no negative values which means it can be displayed on egg weight and egg index. The parent variance component is positive, indicating the ability of the parent in estimating additive genes can be displayed, this is due to a larger component of male variation. This is clearly seen from the distribution of the male variation component ($\sigma 2s$) which is much higher than the female variance component ($\sigma 2d$). As is known that the parent variance component is determined by additive, non-additive genetic factors (dominant, epistasis and interaction) and non-genetic (maternal effect) Pirchner cited by (Sidadolog & Sasongko 1990). The spread of the offspring variance component is shown in the stud and parent variance component ($\sigma 2\epsilon$) which is the appearance between siblings, can be displayed every egg weight and egg index with a relatively better estimation of the value of the spread of the variance component than the stud variance component or the parent variation component. Pirchner cited by Kismiati (1997), reported that the variance component of stud and parent is the combined genetic influence of stud and parent together (additive, dominant and epistasis genes).

3.2 *Estimation of heritability value of egg weight and egg index of Tolaki chicken*

Based on statistical analysis using hierarchical analysis of variance, the heritability value of egg weight based on the male component ($\hat{h}2s$), the parent variation component ($\hat{h}2d$), and the combined male and parent component $\hat{h}2s + d$ as presented in Table 3.

Table 3. Estimated heritability values of egg weight and egg index of Tolaki chicken.

	Heritability		
Parameters	$\hat{h}^2_s$	$\hat{h}^2_d$	$\hat{h}^2_{(s+d)}$
Egg weight	0.87 ± 0.54	0.16 ± 0.14	0.52 ± 0.42
Egg index	0.66 ± 0.41	0.32 ± 0.31	0.49 ± 0.38

$\hat{h}2s$: male component
$\hat{h}2d$: female component
$\hat{h}2s+d$: combined male and female components

Based on Table 3, it shows that the estimated heritability value of egg weight and egg index based on the male component ($\hat{h}2s$) which describes the half-sister relationship is positive. The heritability value based on the male component is heritability in the narrow sense which is the ability of the male in estimating additive genes. Kismiati (1997) stated that the estimation of this method is the purest for additive genetic variation among existing methods, if done properly. It is further explained that the estimated heritability of half-sisters does not include the dominant influence, but only includes 1/4 or less of the epistasy influence and no influence of the parent. The estimated heritability value of egg weight based on the male component ($\hat{h}2s$) is 0.87 and the estimated heritability of egg index based on the male component is 0.66. The values of the variance components will affect the heritability value, so changes in one of the components will affect the amount of heritability value. If there are differences in heritability values, this is natural, because heritability values are not absolute values but specific to certain populations at certain times, differences can occur due to differences in the materials used and environmental diversity. According to Falconer (1981) and Warwick *et al.* (1990), the estimation of the heritability value is theoretically between 0 and 1 but for estimating the heritability value of quantitative traits there is often a negative value, even greater than 1. The estimated heritability value of egg weight and egg index based on the parent component (ĥ2d) is positive. This positive value indicates that the genetic appearance of additive genes appears. The estimated heritability value of egg weight based on parent component (ĥ2d) was 0.16 and the estimated heritability of egg index based on parent component was 0.32. Estimation of heritability value based on the combined variance component of male and parent which is the estimation of individual heritability value is positive, where the heritability value displayed shows the heritability value that has been defined to be between 0 and 1. Kismiati (1997), the variance component of male and parent is a genetic influence that is a combination of male and parent together (additive, dominant and epistasis genes). Estimated heritability values of egg weight and egg index based on stud and parent components (ĥ2s + d) were 0.52 and 0.49. This indicates that 52% of the egg weight component is influenced by genetic and the rest is influenced by environmental factors, and 49% of the mother component is influenced by genetic and the rest is influenced by environmental factors. The heritability value of the combined variance component of males and parents (ĥ2s + d) in egg weight and egg index is a heritability value with a high category. The category of the size of the heritability value, namely: h2 smaller than 0.20 in the low category; 0.20–0.40 in the medium category; greater than 0.40 in the high category. The estimated heritability value in this study is higher than the heritability value of egg weight (0.08) and egg index (0.08) in kedu chicken (Kurnianto 2010). The heritability value in this study is almost the same as the research on the heritability of egg weight of crossbred chickens is 0.54. (Masili 2018). The same thing was also reported by (Pratiwi & Sidadolog 2015) the heritability value of egg weight of legund chickens is 0.94 while for egg index is 0.39 while the heritability of egg weight and egg index of normal chickens is 0.14 and 0.43. The same thing was reported (Anggraeni 2020) which stated that the heritability value of alabio duck egg weight was 0.52 ± 0.38.

4 CONCLUSION

The estimated heritability values of egg weight and egg index obtained were 0.52, and 0.49, and the estimated heritability values obtained were in the high category.

REFERENCES

Anggraeni R. (2020). Enhancing the revisit intention of nature-based tourism in Indonesia: The management and business research quarterly enhancing the revisit intention of nature-based tourism in Indonesia: *The Role of Memorable Tourism Experience and Satisfaction*. (January). https://doi.org/10.32038/mbrq.2019.11.02

Badaruddin R., J. H. Sidadolog and Y. Yuwanta. 2013. Phenotyping and genetic analysis of Tolaki chicken during growth period. *Livestock Bulletin*. 37 (2): 79–86.

Becker A. 1992. *Manual of Quantitative Genetics 4th edition*. Washington State University. Washington

Biscarini, F., H. Bovenh uis, E. D. Ellen, S. Addo, and J. A. M. van Arendonk. 2010. Estimation of heritability and breeding values for early egg production in laying hens from pooled data. *Poultry Science*, 89: 1842–1849.

Ciptadi, G., Aulanni'am., A. Budiarto., and Y. Oktanella. 2019. *Genetics and Breeding: Animal Husbandry-Veterinary. UB* Press. Malang.

Dewi, R. K. and Wahyuni. 2020. *Basic Livestock Breeding*. Unisla Research and Development Center. East Java.
Falconer D. S. and T. F. C. Mackay. 1996. *Introduction to Quantitative Genetics. 4 th Edition*, Addison Wesley Longman, Harlow.
Kismiati S. 1997. *Effect of Insemination Interval on Reproductive Performance and Growth Heritability of Black Kedu Chicken*. [Thesis] Master of Agriculture. Postgraduate Program, Gajah Mada University, Yogyakarta.
Kurnianto, E., S. Johari, and Y. Fadliyah. 2010. Appearance and heritability values of some quantitative traits in Kedu chicken. *Agromedia*, 28(1), 54–59
Lestari A. D. W., W. A. Dewi, M. Qosim, N. Rahardja, Rostini, and R. Setiamihardja. 2006. Genetic variability and heritability of yield and yield component characters of fifteen red chili genotypes. *Zuriat*. 17 (1): 97–98.
Masili, S., S. Dako, F. Ilham, and S. I. Gubali. 2018. Heritability of egg weight, hatching weight and body weight of 1-week-old crossbred chickens (DOC). *Jambura Jounal of Animal Science*, 1(1): 1–5.
Pratiwi A. C. and Sidadolog J. H. P. P. 2015 Estimation of heritability and ripitability values of egg weight, egg index and day-old chick (DOC) weight in mating legund and normal chickens.
Prihandini, P. W., L. Hakim, and V. A. Nurgiartiningsih. 2012. Male selection based on breeding value in Peranakan Ongole (PO) cattle at Grati-Pasuruan beef cattle research center. *Journal of Tropical Animal Production*,13(1): 9–18
Sidadolog J. H. P. and H. Sasongko. 1990. *Genetics of Egg Production and Growth in Native Chickens*. Research Report. No.232/P4M/DPPM/BD-XXI/ 1989, Faculty of Animal Science UGM.
Warwick E. J., J. M. Astuti and M. Hardjosubroto. 1990. *Livestock Breeding*. UGM Press. Yogyakarta
Widyawati, W., Y. Izmi, and Respatijarti. 2014. Heritability and genetic progress of f2 population expectations in large chili (*Capsicum annuum* L.). *Journal of Crop Production*, 2(3): 247–252.
Yuwanta, T. 2004. *Basic Poultry Farming*. Kanisius, Yogyakarta.

Technological Innovations in Tropical Livestock Development for Environmental Sustainability and Food Security – P. Dhian Isnaeni et al. (eds)
© 2025 The Author(s), ISBN 978-1-032-74373-8
Open Access: www.taylorfrancis.com, CC BY-NC-ND 4.0 license

Nutrient utilization and milk yield of dairy goats fed with diet containing garlic meal (*Allium sativum*) and organic minerals at a transition period

C.H. Prayitno*, Munasik & N. Hidayat
Faculty of Animal Science, Jenderal Soedirman University, Purwokerto, Central Java, Indonesia

ABSTRACT: The objective of this research was to determine nutrients utilization (intake and digestibility) and milk yield of dairy goats that consumed feed supplemented with garlic meal (*Allium sativum*) and organic minerals. The research was conducted corresponding to four treatments including basal feed (12.12% CP, 31.30% CF, 60.53% TDN). The feed given was 70% of corn forage silage and 30% of tofu with 3% of body weight. The research method used was experimental using the Latin Square Design. The treatments tested were T0: 70% forage corn silage + 30% tofu; T1: T0 + Rumensin 30 mg/body weight); T2: T0 + 250 ppm garlic meal (1.7% allicin); and T3: T0 + Organic Minerals (0.3 ppmSe + 1.5ppm Cr + 40 ppmZn-lysinate). Four heads of SAPERA dairy goats at a transition period at second lactation were used in this study. The results showed that supplemented rumensin, garlic meal, and organic mineral did not significantly affect (P>0.05) nutrient intake (DM, OM, CF), nutrient digestibility (DM, OM, CF, CP). However, treatment significantly (P<0.01) increased milk yield and production of total solid, solid non-fat and lactose and nutient intake of crude protein. The conclusion is supplementation of garlic meal can replace rumensin in the feed of dairy goat.

Keywords: dairy goat, garlic, methane inhibitor

1 INTRODUCTION

Ruminal methanogenesis is considered an inefficient process as it can result in the loss of 4 to 12% of the total energy consumed by the ruminant (Arif & Pazla 2023). During ruminal fermentation, a part of consumed energy and protein are excreted (as methane and ammonia nitrogen respectively) without being utilized by rumen microflora or host animal (Afdalla *et al.* 2021). For this reason, ruminant nutritionists have suggested optimising diet formulation and using feed additives (Banakar *et al.* 2021). However, the use of antibiotics as feed additives has been banned in many countries due to the risk of the appearance of antibiotic residues in milk and meat. Several plant extracts can be used as feed additives which can reduce methane gas emissions in ruminants and improve the rumen fermentation system. In vitro, garlic extract is effective in reducing methane (CH4) compared to onions and ginger. Garlic also reduces the ratio between acetate and propionate (A:P). Methane emissions in rumen fermentation have a close relationship with the A:P ratio (Kim *et al.* 2012). Reducing methane emissions will increase the concentration of propionate, so that the A:P ratio becomes low (Mitsumori *et al.* 2008; Prayitno and Hidayat 2013; Prayitno *et al.* 2013) and increase the efficiency of fermentation in the rumen on the ammoniated-rice straw-based feed of beef cattle (Prayitno *et al.* 2015). Garlic flour has dry matter, 93%, crude protein 19.2%, NDF 6.5% and ADF 5.1% (Wanapat *et al.* 2011). The introductory study

*Corresponding Author: caribuunsoed@gmail.com

DOI: 10.1201/9781003468943-7

showed that supplementations of Cr, Se, and Zn minerals combined with Sapindus arak and garlic extract were able to increase rumen efficiency in dairy cattle (Busquet *et al.* 2006). The purpose of this study was to evaluate the effects of supplementation of Garlic powder in feed and Cr, Se, and Zn minerals on feed digestibility and milk production.

2 MATERIAL AND METHODS

Four Saanen x Ettawa crossbred goats (SAPERA) at four-month gestation were allotted to individual cages, offered with feed (3% of body weight) composed of 70% whole corn crop silage, 30% concentrate, 0.3ppm Se, 1.5ppm Cr, 40 ppm *Zn-Lysinate*, 250 ppm garlic and rumensin. This experimental method used Lathin square design with four treatments, i.e., T_0: Basal feed (70% whole corn crop silage + 30% tofu dregs, 31.31% CF, 12.12 CP, 60.53% TDN); T_1: T_0 + 30 mg/kg BW rumensin; T_2: T_0 + 250 ppm garlic powder (1.7% allicin); dan T_3: T_0 + organic mineral (0.3 ppm Se, 1.5 ppm Cr, 40 ppm Zn-lysinate). Each treatment was replicated four times. Treatment feeds were given 4 weeks before parturition (transition period) Feed was offered two times a day at 08.00 am. and 04:00 pm (Total Mixed Ration) and treatment feed was offered at 7.30 pm. Data on feed intake and digestibility were gathered during the last five days of the feeding trial by collecting 5% of the feed residues and faeces (Afdala *et al.* 2021). A milk sample (50 ml) was collected during the last three days of the feeding trial for chemical composition analysis in which the milk was homogenized and preserved using *potassium dichromate*, then thawed before being subjected to lacto-scan analysis. This research was conducted in Pegumas Dairy Goat Farm, Gumelar Subdistrict, Banyumas District. The analysis of feed intake and digestibility was performed in the Feedstuff Laboratory, Faculty of Animal Science, Jenderal Soedirman University, Purwokerto.

3 RESULTS AND DISCUSSION

3.1 *Effect of treatment on feed intake*

The result of supplementing garlic (*Allium sativum*) powder and organic minerals into dairy goat feed did not significantly affect ($P>0.05$) the intake of dry matter, organic matter and crude fiber, but significantly affected crude protein. It shows that supplementing garlic powder and organic minerals into dairy goat feed did not contribute to the speed of feed particle movement in the digestive tract. Accordingly, goats may consume similar feed, but it impacts the structure of the ruminal microbe differently because it evidently increases crude protein intake, particularly in treatment feed supplemented with organic minerals. This outcome is contrary to previous findings which offered treatment feed in the post-partum period. Saanen goats supplemented with Moringa flour, Sauropus flour and Coleus flour obtained dry matter intake data between 1350 to 1473 g/day, crude protein of 217.35–254.82 g/day, crude fiber: 283.88–308.43 g/day (Novianti *et al.* 2021). Mahmoud (2022), who conducted research on dairy goats given broccoli products, obtained dry matter intake data of 1026–1086 g/day. Meanwhile, the Saanen crossbred that received a combination of *Gliricidia sepium* and *Indigofera zoolingeria* in its feed obtained crude fat intake and crude fibre intake data of 0.067 and 0.328 kg respectively, while those that received only Indigofera crude fat intake and crude fibre intake were 0.076 and 0.454 respectively. kg (Arief and Pazla 2023). Other researchers on Etawa crossbred goats fed swamp forage produced a dry matter intake of 428 – 536 g/day (Jaelani *et al.* 2021).

3.2 *Effect of treatment on feed digestibility*

The result of supplementing garlic powder (*Allium sativum*) and organic minerals into dairy goat feed did not significantly affect ($P>0.05$) the digestibility of dry matter, organic matter, crude fiber and crude protein. Garlic can improve ruminant digestibility, and a high digestibility is the result of high feed efficiency. Digestibility level is partly affected by the quality of ration offered to the goat. Feed digestibility in the present study is relatively high because the feed offered was suitable for the goat preference and ruminal microbe activities. Supplementation of garlic flour with coconut oil significantly increased dry matter digestibility by 9.8% higher than control feed (Kongmun *et al.* 2011). Alpine goats with limited access to feed obtained dry matter digestibility between 63.1–72.2%, organic matter digestibility, 64.6–71.2%, PK: 72.7–79.6%, NDF: 47.9–61.1% (Silva *et al.* 2018). Other researchers found that crude fat and crude fiber digestibility were 87.32 and 78.06% respectively in Saanen crossbred goats that received a combination of *Glirisidia sepium* and *Indigofera zoolingeria* (Arif & Pazla 2023).

Table 1. Effect of treatment on dry matter intake (DMI), organic matter intake (OMI), crude fiber intake (CFI), crude protein intake (CPI).

	Treatments				
Parameter	T_0	T_1	T_2	T_3	p-Value
DMI (g/d)	1334.03 ± 228.54	1317.81 ± 238.31	1264.23 ± 231.51	1275.95 ± 132.24	0.401
OMI (g/d)	530.66 ± 79.92	534.70 ± 99.06	519.08 ± 70.08	521.61 ± 48.49	0.850
CFI (g/d)	557.15 ± 1.09	557.13 ± 0.53	557.07 ± 1.0	557.52 ± 0.83	0.908
CPI (g/d)	111.68 ± 1.25^c	97.08 ± 0.45^a	102.63 ± 1.65^b	118.0 ± 0.73^d	0.058

Note: (T_0): basal feed (70% whole corn crop silage + 30% tofu, 12.12%CP, 31.30%CF, 60.53 %TDN (T_1): T_0 + rumensin 30 mg/kg BW), (T_2): T_0 + 250 ppm garlic powder (1.7% allicin), (T_3): T_0 + organic mineral (0.3 ppm Se + 1.5 ppm Cr + 40 ppm Zn-lysinate).

Table 2. Effect treatment on digestibility of dry matter (DMD), organic matter (OMD), crude fiber (CFD) and crude protein (CPD)

	Treatments				
Parameter	T_0	T_1	T_2	T_3	p-Value
DMD (%)	93.16 ± 2.59	91.83 ± 1.94	92.75 ± 2.56	92.54 ± 2.50	0.282
OMD (%)	82.83 ± 2.47	81.76 ± 2.26	82.71 ± 2.27	82.17 ± 2.53	0.532
CFD (%)	93.07 ± 0.65	93.36 ± 0.53	93.54 ± 0.58	93.54 ± 0.41	0.784
CPD (%)	88.51 ± 4.84	87.01 ± 2.33	87.94 ± 3.04	83.91 ± 4.82	0.380

Note: (T_0): basal feed (70% whole corn crop silage + 30% tofu, 12.12%CP, 31.30%CF, 60.53 %TDN (T_1): T_0 + rumensin 30 mg/kg BW), (T_2): T_0 + 250 ppm garlic powder (1.7% allicin), (T_3): T_0 + organic mineral (0.3 ppm Se + 1.5 ppm Cr + 40 ppm Zn-lysinate).

3.3 *Effect treatment on milk production and milk composition*

Supplementing garlic powder (*Allium sativum*) and organic minerals into dairy goat feed has improved milk production ($P<0.05$) without significant effect ($P>0.05$) on fat content, density, and casein, but significantly affected the produced total solid, SNF, and lactose. This result shows that either rumensin or garlic powder supplemented into goat feed has the capacity to affect secretory cells in milk synthesis. The results of this study show that garlic supplementation in goat feed can increase milk production. This condition is thought to result in energy savings that were originally used for methane synthesis being diverted to milk production.

This result shows that garlic is an effective anti-methanogenesis agent to reduce methanogen that synthesizes methane gas, thus conserving energy to convert to milk production. This is reflected in the increasing production of lactose and non-fat solid. Supplementing garlic powder in feed dairy goats may result in better feed efficiency compared to rumens in organic mineral supplementation. Efficiency relates to how much milk production quantities are able to be produced from the total feed intake. The supplementations of garlic powder increase significantly milk efficiency by 32.52 % relative to the control diet. Alpine goats with limited access to feed obtain milk production ranging from 1710 to 1845 g/day, with fat production between 51–73 g/day, protein, 41–52 g/day, lactose, 62–80 g/day (Silva *et al.* 2018). Saanen goats given Moringa, Sauropus and Coleus leaf flour obtained milk production data between 854.42 and 1152.42 ml/day (Novianti *et al.* 2021). The average production of Saanen goat milk is 2.15 + −0.13 with a maximum production of 2.80 + −0.1 kg, with a dry matter composition of 12.48, fat: 4.02, protein 3.55, lactose: 4.34%, SCC: 883.33 thousand/cm3 (Shuvarikov *et al.* 2021). Milk production of dairy goats really depends on their age: 2 years old: 571.1 + −89.7, 3 years old: 850.0 + −155, 4 years old 943.9 + −168 with fat composition respectively: 2.87, 2.77, and 3.33%, while SNF: 7.78, 7.80, 7.53% and lactose: 4.23, 4.27, 4.1% (Ibrahim and Jalil 2022). DMI/FCM conversion in dairy goats is 0.97–1.07 (Mahmoud 2022).

Table 3. Effect treatment on milk production, milk composition and milk efficiency.

	Treatments				
Parameter	T_0	T_1	T_2	T_3	p-Value
Milk yield (g/d)	901 ± 193.25^a	1140 ± 139.91^b	1194 ± 164.29^b	1059 ± 178.09^a	0.013
Total Solid (%)	11.49 ± 0.05	11.23 ± 0.35	11.68 ± 0.58	11.40 ± 0.25	0.355
Fat (%)	3.24 ± 0.19	3.58 ± 0.31	3.47 ± 0.46	3.39 ± 0.42	0.677
SNF (%)	8.34 ± 0.18	7.65 ± 0.47	8.21 ± 0.29	8.02 ± 0.34	0.114
Lactose (%)	3.82 ± 0.07	3.45 ± 0.22	3.76 ± 0.19	3.69 ± 0.23	0.827
Casein (%)	3.16 ± 0.04	2.91 ± 0.17	3.09 ± 0.09	2.98 ± 0.09	0.779
Relative density (g/ml)	1.030 ± 0.00058	1.030 ± 0.0005	1.030 ± 0.00082	1.030 ± 0.0005	0.758
Production of Total Solid (g/d)	103.51 ± 21.76^a	127.87 ± 15.23^b	140.14 ± 25.36^b	120.97 ± 22.03^b	0.018
Production of fat (g/d)	29.17 ± 6.34	40.51 ± 3.43	41.77 ± 9.68	36.40 ± 10.58	0.386
Production of SNF (g/d)	74.33 ± 15.7^a	87.36 ± 13.38^a	98.38 ± 16.58^b	84.57 ± 11.84^a	0.016
Production of Lactose (g/d)	34.4 ± 7.47^a	39.44 ± 6.15^a	45.12 ± 8.26^b	38.89 ± 5.56^a	0.015
Production of casein (g/d	28.55 ± 6.00	33.22 ± 4.95	37.02 ± 5.98	31.42 ± 4.42	0.727
Milk efficiency: DMI : milk yield	1.48 ± 0.12^c	1.16 ± 0.17^b	1.06 ± 0.01^a	1.20 ± 0.07^b	0.018

Note: (T_0): basal feed (70% whole corn crop silage + 30% tofu, 12.12%CP, 31.30%CF, 60.53%TDN (T_1): T_0 + rumensin 30 mg/kg BW), (T_2): T_0 + 250 ppm garlic powder (1.7% allicin), (T_3): T_0 + organic mineral (0.3 ppm Se + 1.5 ppm Cr + 40 ppm Zn-lysinate).

4 CONCLUSION

Supplementing garlic powder in feed dairy goats may result in better feed efficiency and milk yield compared to rumensin or organic mineral supplementation.

ACKNOWLEDGEMENT

The author would like to thank LPPM of Jenderal Soedirman University for funding this research through Scheme BLU.

REFERENCES

Afdala, M, D. Darlisa D., Adriania A. (2021). Digestibility, milk yields, and milk quality of Ettawa Crossbred goats fed *Coleus amboinicus* L. leaf extract. *Tropical Animal Science Journal.* 44(4): 441–450. https://doi.org/10.5398/tasj.2021.44.4.441

Arif and R. Pazla. 2023. Milk production and quality of Etawa crossbred goats with non-conventional forages and palm concentrates. *American Journal of Animal and Veterinary Sciences.* 18 (1): 9–18. DOI: https://doi.org/10.3844/ajavsp.2023.9.18

Banakar P., S., Kumar S., V. V. Vinay V.V., Dixit S., Tyagi N., & Tyagi A.K. (2021). Supplementation of *Aloe vera* extract in lactating goats' diet: Effects on rumen fermentation efficiency, nutrient utilization, lactation performance, and antioxidant status. *Tropical Anim.Health and Prod.* 53. DOI:10.1007/s11250-021-02894-x

Busquet, M., Calsamiglia S., Ferret A., & Kamel C. 2006. Plant extracts affect in vitro rumen microbial fermentation. *J. Dairy Sci.* 89:761–771. https://doi.org/10.3168/jds.S0022-0302(06)72137-3

Ibrahim, N. S., and Jalil A.R. (2022). The effect of age on milk yield and milk composition in Saanen dairy goats. *Journal of Agricultural Science and Technology* 12 (1): 10–14. doi: 10.17265/2161-6256/2022.01.002

Jaelani, A., Malik A., & Ni'mah Gk. (2021). The potential of Swamp forage-based feeding to on the qualities of digestibility and milk production in goat Etawa crossbreed. *Advances in Animal and Vet. Sci.* 9(4): 544–548. DOI: | http://dx.doi.org/10.17582/journal.aavs/2021/9.4.544.548

Kim S. H., Jung E.Y., Kang D.H., Un Jae Chang U. J., Hong Y., & Suh H. J. (2012). Physical stability, antioxidative properties, and photoprotective effects of a functionalized formulation containing black garlic extract. *J Photochem Photobiol B.* 117: 104–10. doi: 10.1016/j.jphotobiol.2012.08.01

Kongmun P., Wanapat M., Pakdee P., Navanukraw C. & Yu Z. (2011). Manipulation of rumen fermentation and ecology of swamp buffalo by coconut oil and garlic powder supplementation. *Livestock Science.* 135 (1): 84–92. https://doi.org/10.1016/j.livsci.2010.06.131

Kongmun, P., Wanapat M., Pakdee P., & Navanykraw C. (2010). Effect of coconut oil and garlic powder on in vitro fermentation using gas production technique. *J. Livestock Sci.* 127: 38–44. DOI 10.1016/j.livsci.2009.08.008

Mahmoud, Y. M. M. (2022). Improving performance of lactating goats fed rations containing boroccoli by product (*Brassica oleracea*). *Advances in Animal and Veterinary Science.* 10(7): 1623–1632.

Miranda, S. G., Purdie N.G., Osbome V.R., Coomber B.I., & Cant J.P. (2011). Selenomethionine increase proliferation and reduce apoptosis in bovine mammary epithellal cells under oxidative stress. *J. Dairy Sci,* 94: 165–173. DOI: 10.3168/jds.2010-3366

Mitsumori, M. & W. Sun. (2008). Control of rumen microbial fermentation for mitigrating methane emissions from the rumen. *Asian-Aust. J. Anim Sci.* 21:144–154. https://www.animbiosci.org/upload/pdf/21-22.pdf

Novianti, J., Purwanto B.P., Astuti D.A., & Atabany A. (2021). Milk production and metabolite profile of saanen goat fed with *Moringa oleifera, Saudopus androgynous* L. Merr and *Coleus amboinicus* lour leaves. *Livestock Research for Rural Development.* 33(9): 1–7. https://lrrd.org/lrrd33/9/33111jodi.html

O'Rourke, D. 2009. Nutrition and udder health in dairy cows. A review. *Irish Veterinary Journal.* 62:15–20. file:///C:/Users/Dell/Downloads/2046-0481-62-S4-S15.pdf

Prayitno, C.H. & Hidayat N. 2013. The Efficacy of methanol extract of garlic (*Allium sativum*) to improve rumen fermentation product. *Anim. Prod.* 15(1):69–75. http://animalproduction.net/index.php/JAP/article/view/412

Prayitno, C.H. and Suwarno. (2017). The effectively of garlic cake extract as an antimethanogenic agent in the feed of beef cattle. *Proceeding ICTA.* Nature-Springer.

Prayitno, C.H., Subagyo Y., and Suwarno. 2013. Effect of *Sapindus rarak* extract alone or its combination with garlic extract on in vitro ruminal fermentation. *Media Peternakan.*

Prayitno, C.H., Suwarno and Susanto A. 2015. In vitro assessment of digestibility and rumen fermentation of ammoniated rice straw-based beef cattle, supplemented with extract garlic and Sapindus rarak. *Livestock Res. Rur. Dev.* 27(5):1–7. https://www.lrrd.org/lrrd27/5/pray27094.htm

Shuvarikov, A.S., Pastukh. O.N., Zhukova E.V. & Zheltova O.A. 2021. The quality of milk of goats of Saanen, Alpine and Nubian breeds. *IOP: Conference Series: Earth and Environmental Science.* 640: 1–6. doi:10.1088/1755-1315/640/3/032031

Silva, Nhayandra C. D., Puchala R., Gipson T.A., Sahlu T., and C. Goetsch A.L. 2018. Effects of restricted periods of feed access on feed intake, digestions, behaviour, heat energy, and performance of Alpine goats. *Journal of Applied Animal Research.* 46(1): 994–1003. https://doi.org/10.1080/09712119.2018.1450259

Steel R. G. D., and Torrie J. H. 1995 *Principles and Procedures of Statistics.* Alih Bahasa Sumantri, B. Prinsip dan Prosedur Statistika. Edisi 4 (Jakarta: Penerbit PT Gramedia Pustaka Utama).

Wanapat M., Khejornsart P. & Pakdee P. 2008. Effect of supplementation of garlic powder on rumen ecology and digestibility of nutrients in ruminants. *J. The Science of Food and Agric.* 88 (13): 2231–2237. DOI:10.1002/jsfa.3333

Yang W. Z., Benchaar C., Ametaj B. N., Chaves A.V., He M.L. & McAllister T.A. (2007). Effects of garlic and juniper berry essential oils on ruminal fermentation and on the site and extent of digestion in lactating cows. *J. Dairy Sci.* 90. DOI: 10.3168/jds.2007-0369

Technological Innovations in Tropical Livestock Development for Environmental Sustainability and Food Security – P. Dhian Isnaeni et al. (eds)
© 2025 The Author(s), ISBN 978-1-032-74373-8
Open Access: www.taylorfrancis.com, CC BY-NC-ND 4.0 license

Blood profile of broiler chickens given boiled papaya leaves (*Carica papaya* L) through drinking water

M.A. Pagala*, R. Badaruddin & Nurhaida
Department of Animal Science, Faculty of Animal Science, Universitas Halu Oleo, Kendari, Southeast Sulawesi, Indonesia

ABSTRACT: Papaya leaves have benefits for the health of broiler chickens, such as improving the immune system by increasing antioxidant levels in the blood and stimulating the production of white blood cells. Papaya leaves also have natural antimicrobial and natural antibiotic. This study aims to analyze the blood profile of broiler chickens given papaya leaves in drinking water. The research was carried out on Jalan. Haji Lamuse, Lorong Semeru, Lepo-lepo Village, Baruga District, Kendari City from March to April 2023. The design used in this research was a completely randomized design (RAL) with 4 treatments and 5 replications, so there were 20 experimental units and each experimental unit consisted of 2 chickens. The experimental units used were 40 broiler chickens. The research treatments carried out were P1 = Use of plain water without additions, P2 = 2.5 ml of papaya leaf boiled liquid per liter of water, P3 = 5 ml of papaya leaf boiled liquid per liter of water, P4 = Use of 7.5 papaya leaf boiled liquid per liter of water. The variables observed include hemoglobin levels, hematocrit values, hematocrit values and leukocyte differential. The results showed that administering boiled papaya leaves through drinking water had a significant effect ($P<0.05$) on hemoglobin levels, hematocrit values, lymphocytes and monocytes.

Keywords: Papaya leaf decoction, broiler chickens, blood profiles

1 INTRODUCTION

Broiler chickens are known to have high productivity in producing meat. The ability to achieve fairly high body weight growth and low feed conversion can be achieved with a relatively short rearing time, namely 4 to 5 weeks of age. The meat produced contains high levels of animal protein which is provided by the quality of the feed provided during rearing, including the use of feed additives.

One of the traditional medicinal plants that can be used as a feed additive is papaya leaves. The papaya plant is a plant that contains natural phytochemical compounds such as alkaloids and proteolytic enzymes, papain, khimopapain and lysozyme. This compound works to make the intestines work easier in the digestive process and helps regulate amino acids and helps remove toxins from the body. Papaya leaves are also able to eradicate amoebas. can be used as an anthelmintic and to increase appetite (Rasbawati *et al.* 2022).

Papaya leaves contribute to supporting the health of broiler chickens. One of them comes from the vitamin C content of papaya leaves (165–205 mg/100g). Vitamin C is a powerful

*Corresponding Author: amrullah.pagala@uho.ac.id

 DOI: 10.1201/9781003468943-8

antioxidant that can improve the immune system by increasing antioxidant levels in the blood and stimulating the production of white blood cells. Likewise, red blood cells are needed to transport nutrients, as well as an indicator of livestock health. Papaya leaves contain phytochemical compounds that are antimicrobial such as flavonoids, saponins, tannins. Papaya leaves with low levels of 1–2% in the ration can replace antibiotics as a growth promoter (Antibiotic Growth Promoter) (Setyawan *et al.* 2014).

One indicator of livestock health is looking at the blood picture or blood profile. Blood profile is one of the physiological and pathological parameters of the body that reflects the health condition of livestock (Satyaningtijas *et al.* 2010). Blood is also one of the parameters of animal health status where the health condition of livestock can be observed through blood tests (Malik *et al.* 2022).

2 MATERIAL AND METHOD

The research was carried out from March to April 2023 on Jalan Haji Lamuse, Lorong Semeru, Lepo-lepo Village, Baruga District, Kendari City. The main material used was chicken blood obtained from 40 broiler chickens (4 weeks old). The equipment used is an Accupro tool and HB strips to determine hemoglobin levels. Apart from that, alcohol, cotton and Giemsa dye, papaya leaves, BP-11 feed, 3 ml syringe and needle, and EDTA tube are also used for blood collection and a microscope to determine leukocyte differential. Meanwhile, crestal cell hematocrit pipettes, centrifuges and hematocrit scales are used to determine hematocrit values in percent (%).

The cage used is a litter cage with the size of each cage plot being 40 × 35 cm which is equipped with a feeder and drinking water. Before the chicken is put into the cage it needs to be washed using disinfectant for 1 day to prevent microorganisms or pathogenic bacteria. After the cage is cleaned using disinfectant, the cage is left for 7 days. The experimental cages were carried out randomly, each cage plot consisted of 2 broiler chickens. The placement of broiler chickens in each cage plot is adjusted to the research.

The research design used was a Completely Randomized Design (CRD) with 4 treatments and 5 replications. Treatment consists of:

P1: Use ordinary water without additions
P2: Use 2.5 ml of papaya leaf boiled liquid per liter of water
P3: Use 5 ml of papaya leaf boiled liquid per liter of water
P4: Use 7.5 ml of papaya leaf boiled liquid per liter of water

The mathematical model in this research is:

$$Yij = \mu + \acute{\alpha}i + \varepsilon ij$$

With:

Yij = Observation results of administering the i-th and j-th repetition of papaya leaf decoction
μ = Average of observations
$\acute{\alpha}i$ = Effect of giving boiled papaya leaves i
εij = Effect of experimental error
i = 1,2,3,4, (giving boiled papaya leaves)
j = 1,2,3,4,5, (repetition)

The data obtained will be tabulated and then analyzed using variance to determine whether there is an effect of treatment. If the treatment has an effect, then further tests will be carried out using the Duncan Multiple Range Test (DMRT).

3 RESULTS AND DISCUSSION

3.1 *Hemoglobin*

Hemoglobin is a protein in red blood cells that plays an important role in transporting oxygen throughout the body. The results of the analysis of variance showed that giving boiled papaya leaves had a significant effect (P<0.05) on the blood hemoglobin levels of broiler chickens. Duncan's test results showed that the hemoglobin level of broiler chickens in treatment P4 was significantly higher than the hemoglobin level in treatment P1 (11.97 g/dl) but was not significantly different from treatment P3 (13.60 g/dl) and P2 (12.99 g /dl). This is because the vitamin C and flavonoid compounds contained in papaya leaves can increase hemoglobin levels. The average hemoglobin level from this study was 11.97 g/dl–14.89 g/dl, which is still within the normal range. The amount of hemoglobin varies depending on the type of animal and gender (Sherwood 2011). The hemoglobin value from this study is almost the same as the study reported by Melia *et al.* (2021) that the hemoglobin levels treated with betel leaves were 13.24–14.98 g/dl.

Table 1. Hemoglobin levels (g/dL) in the blood of broiler chickens given boiled papaya leaves in drinking water.

	Treatment			
Repetition	P1	P2	P3	P4
1	12.45	15.26	14.35	15.6
2	14.56	12.37	14.89	15.48
3	10.67	13.58	13.65	13.62
4	11.83	12.12	12.34	16.2
5	10.34	11.64	12.76	13.56
Average	$11.97^{a} \pm 1.68$	$12.99^{ab} \pm 1.45$	$13.60^{ab} \pm 1.06$	$14.89^{b} \pm 1.22$

Note: Different superscripts on the same line indicate significant differences (P<0.05).

3.2 *Hematocrit*

The results of research on blood hematocrit values of broiler chickens treated with boiled papaya leaves in drinking water are presented in Table 2.

Table 2. Haematocrit value (%) of blood of broiler chickens given boiled papaya leaves in drinking water.

	Treatment			
Repetition	P1	P2	P3	P4
1	23.45	24.60	26.76	28.78
2	27.60	27.67	27.45	27.23
3	24.87	23.56	24.67	30.56
4	24.21	27.54	28.80	27.89
5	26.81	25.90	25.50	26.56
Average	$25.38^{a} \pm 1.76$	$25.85^{ab} \pm 1.80$	$26.64^{ab} \pm 1.62$	$28.20^{b} \pm 1.55$

Note: Different superscripts on the same line indicate significant differences (P<0.05).

The results of the analysis of variance showed that giving boiled papaya leaves had a significant effect (P<0.05) on the blood haematocrit value of broiler chickens. Duncan's test results showed that the haematocrit value of broiler chickens in treatment P4 was significantly higher than the haematocrit value in treatment P1 (25.38%) but was not significantly different from treatments P3 (26.64%) and P2 (25.85%). This is due to the flavonoid, andrographolide and terpenoid content contained in papaya leaves, which causes erythrocyte levels to increase. Apart from that, Vitamin C and Iron also affect the haematocrit value. [8] Papaya leaves contain substances needed for the formation of haematocrit, including iron, manganese, cobalt, vitamins, amino acids and hormones which affect the number of erythrocytes, because haematocrit is a part of erythrocytes which functions as a proportion for measuring erythrocytes.

The average haematocrit value obtained in this study was 25.38%–28.20%, which is still within the normal range. [9] stated that the normal haematocrit value for chickens is between 22–35% with an average of 30%. The results of this study are almost the same as those reported by Edi *et al.* (2020)] that the haematocrit value of broiler chickens treated with dragon fruit peel waste through drinking water was 26.94 ± 0.78–27.66 ± 2.90%. The haematocrit value in this study was also higher than the research reported Suci *et al.* (2012) which stated that the haematocrit value with the addition of teak leaf extract phytobiotics in laying hens was 22.67 ± 3.21–27.00 ± 1.73%. This means that the compounds in papaya leaves can increase chicken blood haemoglobin.

3.3 *Differential leukocyte*

3.3.1 *Lymphocyte*

The results of research on the blood lymphocyte values of broiler chickens treated with boiled papaya leaves in drinking water are presented in Table 3. The results of the analysis of variance showed that giving boiled papaya leaves had a significant effect (P<0.05) on the blood lymphocyte values of broiler chickens. Duncan's test results showed that the lymphocyte value of broiler chickens in treatment P4 was significantly higher than the lymphocyte value in treatment P1 (48.47%) but was not significantly different from treatment P3 (50.18%) and P2 (49.50%). This is thought to be the presence of saponin compounds which are able to stimulate the proliferation process resulting in an increase in the number of lymphocytes. Saponin functions as an immunostimulant, namely stimulating leukocyte activity to increase body immunity (Harahap *et al.* 2014).

Table 3. Lymphocyte values (%) in the blood of broiler chickens given boiled papaya leaves in drinking water.

	Treatment			
Repetition	P1	P2	P3	P4
1	46.28	47.75	49.75	51.00
2	50.50	48.50	49.25	52.65
3	47.30	47.25	50.30	51.20
4	48.50	50.52	51.60	49.25
5	49.75	51.25	50.00	51.45
Average	$48.47^{a} \pm 1.73$	$49.05^{ab} \pm 1.75$	$50.18^{b} \pm 0.88$	$51.11^{b} \pm 1.22$

Note: Different superscripts on the same line indicate significant differences (P<0.05).

The average lymphocyte value obtained in this study was 48.47%–51.11%, which is still in the normal range. The percentage of lymphocytes in poultry blood ranges from 42–66%

(Fakhruddin *et al.* 2023). The results of the research carried out were higher, reported by Cahyaningsih *et al.* (2007) that the lymphocyte value in free-range chickens treated with Sambiloto extract was 20.59–24.59%. This indicates that water boiled in papaya leaves is slightly more effective in increasing lymphocyte values than water boiled in bitter leaves.

3.3.2 *Monocyte*

The results of research on the blood monocyte values of broiler chickens treated with boiled papaya leaves in drinking water are presented in Table 4.

Table 4. Monocyte value (%) of blood of broiler chickens given boiled papaya leaves in drinking water.

	Treatment			
Repetition	P1	P2	P3	P4
1	6.75	8.25	7.50	8.75
2	7.25	7.00	8.25	7.25
3	7.25	7.25	8.75	7.25
4	6.25	7.75	7.75	8.75
5	6.50	7.75	7.25	9.25
Average	$6.8^{a} \pm 0.45$	$7.6^{a} \pm 0.49$	$7.9^{ab} \pm 0.60$	$8.25^{b} \pm 0.9$

Note: Different superscripts on the same line indicate significant differences (P<0.05).

The results of the analysis of variance showed that giving boiled papaya leaves had a significant effect (P<0.05) on the blood monocyte values of broiler chickens. The Duncan test results showed that the P4 treatment was significantly higher than the monocyte value in the P1 treatment (6.8%) but was not significantly different from the P3 (7.9%) and P2 (7.6%) treatments. This is due to the content of tannin compounds in papaya leaves which have high anti-bacterial, anti-protozoal, anti-viral, anti-parasitic and anti-coccidia activity which can cause monocyte values to increase. Monocytes, in carrying out the function of the immune system, act as macrophages, namely swallowing and destroying cells, microorganisms and foreign objects that are pathogenic (Eroschenko *et al.* 2008).

The average monocyte value obtained in this study was 6.8%–8.25%, this value is still within the normal range. The number of monocytes in the blood of broiler chickens ranges from 3–9% of total leukocytes (Guyton & Hall 1997). The monocyte value from this study was higher than research conducted (Hen–drawan *et al.* 2019). The monocyte value of broiler chickens treated with seligi leaves was 2.6–1.8%. The results of this research were also higher than research conducted (Lokapirnasari & Yulianto 2014) which stated that the monocyte value of chickens treated with spirulina was 1.28 ± 0.00–0.00 ± 0.49%. This indicates that papaya leaf water is more effective in increasing blood monocytes which play a role in the immune system compared to seligi leaves and spirulina.

4 CONCLUSION

Based on the results of this study, it can be concluded that administering boiled papaya leaves through drinking water has a significant effect (P<0.05) on haemoglobin, haematocrit, lymphocyte and monocyte values.

5 SUGGESTIONS

Further research needs to be carried out to determine the effect of adding boiled papaya leaves to drinking water at a higher level or dose on the blood profile of broiler chickens.

REFERENCES

Arjuna D., T. Saili dan A.M. Tasse. 2019. Pengaruh pemberian air rebusan daun belimbing wuluh (*Averrhoa bilimbi* L) terhadap jumlah leukosit ayam broiler yang mengalami cekaman panas. *J. Anim. Agric. Sci.* 1 (1): 28–33).

Badaruddin R., H. Hafid, L.O. Nafiu, Syamsuddin, A. Indi dan F.A. Auza. 2022. Hemoglobin level and total differential blood leucocytes of broiler chicken given different probiotics. *Int J. Sci. Eng. Technol.* 9 (2): 224–230.

Cahyaningsih U., H. Malichatin dan Y.E. Hedianto. 2007. Diferensial leukosit pada ayam setelah diinfeksi Eimeria tenella dan pemberian serbuk kunyit (Curcuma domestica) dosis bertingkat. *Prosiding Seminar Nasional Teknologi Peternakan dan Veteriner di Bogor*, 21–22 Agustus. Pusat Penelitian dan Pengembangan Peternakan, Badan Penelitian dan Pengembangan Pertanian, Departemen Pertanian. Hlm. 593–599.

dr. Brahm U. *Buku Kedokteran EGC.* Jakarta.

Edi D.N., M.H. Natsir dan L.H. Djunaidi. 2020. Profil darah ayam petelur yang diberi pakan dengan penambahan fitobiotik ekstrak daun jati (*Tectona grandis* Linn. f). *Jurnal Peternakan.* 17 (2) : 96–102.

Eroschenko VP. 2008. *Fiore's Atlas Of Histology With Functional Correlations.* Edisi Kesebelas. Lippincott Williams & Wilkins. Philadelpia.

Fakhruddin D.A., S. Siswanto, D. Septinova dan P.E. Santosa. 2023. Gambaran total leukosit dan diferensial leukosit ayam kampung (*Gallus gallus domesticus*) dengan pemberian ekstrak sambilato (*Andrographis paniculata*). *Jurnal Riset dan Inovasi Peternakan.* 7 (1): 48–56.

Guyton, A. C. dan J. E. Hall. 1997. Sel Darah Merah, Anemia, dan Poloisitemia. Didalam Fisiologi Kedokteran. Terjemahan: dr. Irawati, dr. L. M. A. Ken Arita Tengadi dan dr. Alex Santoso. *Penerbit Buku Kedokteran*, E. G. C. Jakarta.

Harahap R.A. 2014. *Profil Darah Ayam Broiler Periode Finisher Yang Diberi Pakan Plus Formula Herbal.* Institut Pertanian Bogor. Bogor.

Hendrawan W.I.W.D., I.M. Merdana dan IW. Sudira. 2019. Pemberian infusa daun dadap terhadap profil leukosit ayam broiler fase grower-finisher yang mengalami stres transportasi. *Jurnal Indonesia Medicus Veterinus.* 8 (4): 464–473.

Hoffbrand A.V., dan J.E. Petit. 2005. *Kapita Selekta Hematologi. Edisi 4.* Penerbit Buku Kedokteran EGC. Jakarta.

Jain N.C. 1993. *Essential of Veterinary Hematology*. Philadelphia: Lea & Febiger.

Jannah PN., Sugiharto dan Isroli. 2017. Jumlah leukosit dan diferensiasi leukosit ayam broiler yang diberi minum air rebusan kunyit. *J. Ternak Tropika.* 8 (1): 15–19.

Lokapirnasari W.P. dan A.B. Yulianto. 2014. Gambaran sel eosinofil, monosit dan basofil setelah pemberian spirulina pada ayam yang diinfeksi virus flu burung. *Jurnal Veteriner.* 15 (4): 499–505.

Malik L.O.A.F., D. Zulkarnain dan R. Libriani. 2022. Profil hematologi ayam broiler yang diberi pakan mengandung enzim fitase dengan level berbeda. *Jurnal Ilmiah Peternakan Halu Oleo.* 4 (1): 27–32.

Melia D., Siswanto, P.E. Santoso dan S. Suharyati. 2021. Pengaruh pemberian jinten hitam (Nigella sativa) sebagai imunomodulator dalam air minum terhadap profil darah (Hemoglobin dan hematokrit) broiler betina. *Jurnal Riset Dan Inovasi Peternakan.* 5 (3):168–173.

Patimah T. dan H. Burhanuddin. 2020. Pengaruh penambahan ekstrak *Centella asiatica* L terhadap jumlah leukosit dan diferensiasi leukosit ayam petelur. *JNTTIP.* 2 (4): 234–241.

Rasbawati, Almahdali dan Munir. 2022. Pengaruh pemberian ekstrak daun pepaya (*Carica papaya* L) dalam air minum terhadap berat dan presentase karkas broiler. *Jurnal Ilmiah Peternakan* 4 (1): 1–6.

Rosmalawati, N. 2008. *Pengaruh Penggunaan Tepung Daun Sembung (Blumea balsamifera) dalam Ransum terhadap Profil Darah Ayam Broiler Periode Finisher.* Skripsi. Program Studi Ilmu Nutrisi dan Makanan Ternak Fakultas Peternakan Institut Pertanian Bogor, Bogor.

Sadaman. 2013. Status kesehatan ayam pedaging yang diberi limbah kulit buah naga (*Hylocereus undatus*) dalam air minum sebagai antioksidan. *Jurnal Penelitian Sosial Keagamaan.* 16 (1): 14–19.

Satyaningtijas, A.S., S.D. Widhyari dan R.D. Natalia. 2010. Jumlah eritrosit, nilai hematokrit, dan kadar hemoglobin ayam pedaging umur 6 minggu dengan pakan tambahan. *J. Kedokteran Hewan.* 4 (2): 69–73.

Setyawan D.I., Bidura dan A.A. Putra. 2014. Pengaruh pemberian ekstrak daun kelor dan bawang putih melalui air minum terhadap karkas broiler umur 2-6 minggu. *Jurnal Ternak Tropika.* 2 (2): 252–261.

Sherwood L. 2011. *Human Physilogy: From Cells to Systems.* 6th Ed. Diterjemahkan oleh

Suci D.M., Asella, L.W. Utami dan W. Hermana. 2018. Pengaruh pemberian ransum mengandung tepung daun mengkudu (morinda citrifolia linn) terhadap performa dan profil darah itik lokal periode grower. *Buletin Makanan Ternak.* 16 (1): 11–23.

Swenson, M.J. (1984). *Duke's Physiology of Domestic Animals.* 10th Ed. Ithaca and London: Publishing Associattes a Divisin of Cornell University.

Tamzil M.H., R.R. Noor, P.S. Hardjosworo, W. Manalu, C. Sumantri. 2014. Hematological response of chickens with different heat shock protein 70 genotypes to acute heat stress. *Int J Poult Sci* 13: 14–20.

Tiya Dwi N.A., R. Badaruddin, M. Akramullah, A. Bain dan N. Sandiah. 2021. Hemoglobin level and total leukocyte differential in laying hens fed with betel leaf juice (Piper betle linn). *Int J Sci Eng Technol.* 8(2): 81–86

Technological Innovations in Tropical Livestock Development for Environmental Sustainability and Food Security – P. Dhian Isnaeni et al. (eds)

Effect of duration of fumigation using potassium permanganate (KMnO4) and formalin on hatchability, viability of quail egg *Coturnix coturnix japonica*

M.A. Pagala*, H. Has & Risman
Department of Animal Science, Faculty of Animal Science, Universitas Halu Oleo, Kendari, Southeast Sulawesi, Indonesia

ABSTRACT: This study aims to analyze the effect of duration of fumigation using potassium permanganate (KMnO4) and formalin on hatchability and viability of quail egg embryos (*Coturnix coturnix japonica*). This study used 200 fertile quail eggs. This study used a completely randomized design (CRD) with 4 treatments and 5 replications. The treatments consisted of: P1 (Control without fumigation treatment), P2 (fumigation duration 5 minutes), P3 (fumigation duration 10 minutes) and P4 (fumigation duration 15 minutes). The variables observed were embryo viability, hatchability and embryo mortality. The results showed that the treatment of different fumigation durations on quail eggs had a significant effect ($P<0.05$) on hatchability and viability of quail egg embryos. It can be concluded that the best treatment was the P2 treatment with a fumigation duration of 10 minutes.

Keywords: Fumigation, Quail, Hatchability, Viability

1 INTRODUCTION

Quail farming is one of the egg-producing livestock which is quite popular and developed by the community. This is because it is supported by fairly good quail production, the production cycle is short and maintenance is quite easy. Sufficient egg productivity and high public preference for quail eggs provide great opportunities and profits for quail business actors.

Even though quail egg production is quite high, the process of handling egg hatching has quite complex problems. One of the problems is the risk of microorganism contamination of quail eggs so that it can disrupt the hatching process. Microorganism contamination usually comes from the cloaca, air, the infrastructure used to store the eggs and from the incubator used during hatching. Before eggs emerge from the cloaca, they are generally contaminated with microorganisms originating from the urinary tract and excretory tract (Hasanah *et al.* 2019). Prevention of contamination by microorganisms can be done by having eggs to be hatched cleaned or disinfected first before being placed in the hatching machine. Fumigation is one method that can be used to disinfect eggs. Fumigation aims to kill microorganisms found on the egg shell. Fumigation is an important procedure to ensure that the embryos in hatching eggs are protected from contamination by microorganisms which can cause embryo death. (Hariani *et al.* 2017).

The fumigation action needs special attention so that the results of the fumigation spread evenly over the surface of the egg shell. Apart from that, the duration of the fumigation must

*Corresponding Author: amrullah.pagala@uho.ac.id

DOI: 10.1201/9781003468943-9

also be appropriate because if it is too fast then the gas will not evenly hit the shell which causes the microorganisms to remain alive, but if it is too long then the substances contained in gas will also harm the egg embryo. Therefore, it is necessary to know the correct length of fumigation to produce optimal quail DOQ production.

2 MATERIALS AND METHOD

The research was carried out from February to March 2023 at the Animal Science Unit Laboratory, Faculty of Science, Halu Oleo University, Kendari City.

The materials used in this research were hatching machines, egg trays, egg binoculars, stationery, cameras, digital scales, measuring cups, petri dishes and 3 fumigation boxes measuring 25 cm × 25 cm × 25 cm. The materials used are 200 fertile quail eggs, Potassium Permanganate (KMnO4) and 37% Formalin, fertile quail eggs obtained from quail livestock on the Asfar Puyuh farm in Lombe Village, Gu District, Central Buton Regency which are 9 months old, with a ratio of mating males and females was 1:5, eggs are collected for 2 days and stored at room temperature for 6 days.

Activities carried out at the preparation stage include providing tools and materials that will be used during the research. Then before hatching, the hatching machine is first disinfected, after that a temperature stability test is carried out.

The fumigation treatment process for eggs was adapted from Hasana *et al.* 2017) with the following stages:

(1) Weigh 0.22 ml of formalin
(2) Weigh KMnO4 with a weight of 0.11 grams
(3) Put the hatching eggs into the fumigation box
(4) Put KMnO4 into the fumigation box
(5) Mix the formalin solution into the KMnO4 and close the box tightly
(6) Wait until the time has been adjusted to the treatment, after that the eggs are removed simultaneously and placed in the hatching machine

Hatching eggs that have been fumigated according to the treatment are then put into a hatching machine that has been temperature stabilized for two days with a hatching machine temperature of 380 0C. Every day the hatching eggs are rotated and water is added so that the temperature of the eggs is even and the humidity is maintained.

The data collection process was carried out in 3 stages, namely when the eggs were scanned at the age of 7 days to see the fertility of the eggs, then at the age of 14 days the observations were carried out to determine the viability of the embryos and when the eggs hatched to determine the hatchability of the eggs.

The research design used was a Completely Randomized Design (CRD) which consisted of 4 (four) treatments and 5 (five) replications and each experimental unit consisted of 10 (ten) eggs so that the total number of eggs used was 200 eggs. The treatments used were:

P0: Not fumigated
P1: Fumigation time 5 minutes
P2: Fumigation time 10 minutes
P3: Fumigation time 15 minutes

The variables observed in this study were hatchability, embryo viability. Hatchability is the percentage of eggs that hatch from the number of fertile embryos which is calculated using the following formula:

$$\text{Hatchability (\%)} = \frac{\text{Number of hatched eggs}}{\text{Number of fertile eggs}} \times 100\%$$

Embryonic viability is the percentage of fertile eggs from 7 days of hatching to 14 days of hatching, which is calculated using the following formula:

$$\text{Embryo viability (\%)} = \frac{\text{Number of fertile eggs that survive 14 daysi}}{\text{Number of fertile eggs hatched}} \times 100\%$$

The hatchability and embryo viability data obtained will be tabulated and then analyzed using variance to determine whether there is an effect of treatment. If the treatment has an effect, further tests will be carried out using the Duncan Multiple Range Test (DMRT).

3 RESULTS AND DISCUSSION

3.1 *Embryo vitality*

Embryo viability is the ability of the embryo to survive 14 days after the egg is in the hatching machine (Indrawati *et al.* 2015). Embryo viability for each treatment can be seen in Table 1.

Table 1. Percentage of viability of fumigated egg embryos with different time durations.

	Embryo Viability (%)			
repetition	P0	P1	P2	P3
1	83	67	78	50
2	71	83	75	50
3	86	83	89	50
4	71	83	78	50
5	83	83	75	57
Average	78.8 ± 7.22^a	79.8 ± 7.15^a	79 ± 5.78^a	51.4 ± 3.13^b

Note: Different superscripts on the same line indicate significant differences ($P<0.05$).

Based on the results of the analysis of variance, it shows that different fumigation duration treatments for quail eggs have a significant effect ($P<0.05$) on the viability of quail egg embryos. The average viability of embryos in this study was 51.4% – 79.8%. The results of this study were lower when compared to Middin's research which conducted research on fertility and hatchability of quail given herbal concoctions through drinking water at different doses which obtained an average Embryo viability is 94.5% (Middin *et al.* 2020). Further test results showed that treatment P0 was very significantly different from treatment P3 but treatment P0 did not show significantly different results from treatments P1 and P2. This shows that fumigation treatment with a duration of 15 minutes can reduce embryo viability, whereas treatments of 5 and 10 minutes do not reduce embryo viability. The high embryo mortality rate in the P3 treatment with a duration of 15 minutes is thought to be because fumigation that is too long will cause formalin to enter the egg's air sac, causing the air in the air sac to become polluted (mixed with formalin). In the early phase the embryo will continue to develop because the embryo does not need much oxygen, but after entering the final phase there are many embryos that die, this is because in the final phase the embryo needs a lot of oxygen which is obtained from the egg's air sac. Inappropriate fumigation can affect the growth of the embryo, so proper egg fumigation is necessary. The cause of embryos dying prematurely is due to poor egg storage, too long and too high a fumigation dose (Nuryati *et al.* 2002).

Treatments Pl and P2 did not reduce the viability of the embryo. This is thought to be because formalin has not yet entered the air sac but only killed the microorganisms found on the egg shell. Fumigation aims to kill or reduce contamination of microorganisms attached or attached to the surface of the egg (Hariani *et al.* 2017).

3.2 *Hatchability*

Egg hatchability is the number of eggs that hatch compared to the number of fertile eggs and is expressed in percent (Ningtyas *et al.* 2018). The hatchability of each treatment can be seen in Table 2.

Table 2. Percentage of hatchability of fumigated eggs with different time durations.

	Hatchability (%)			
Repetition	P0	P1	P2	P3
1	67	67	67	38
2	71	67	75	25
3	71	83	78	38
4	71	67	78	38
5	67	67	75	43
Average	69.4 ± 2.19^{a}	70.2 ± 7.15^{a}	74.6 ± 4.50^{a}	36.4 ± 6.73^{b}

Note: Different superscripts on the same line indicate significant differences (P<0.05).

Based on the results of the analysis of variance, it shows that different fumigation duration treatments for quail eggs have a very significant effect (P<0.05) on the hatchability of quail eggs. The average hatchability of eggs in this study was 36.4%–74.6%, this value is lower when compared to Kusuma's research which conducted research on the effect of fumigation using betel leaf water on hatchability of eggs and mortality of quail egg embryos which obtained an average hatchability namely 80.55%–96.91% (Kusuma *et al.* 2022). The low hatchability of eggs in this study is thought to be caused by substances contained in formalin entering the air sacs. Formalin has carcinogenic properties which can kill embryos and endanger health (Ramadhan *et al.* 2019). Formalin concentrations of 0.1–5.0 ppm can cause irritation of the nose and throat (BPOM 2008). Disinfection using chemicals at low concentrations cannot kill pathogenic bacteria in eggs, whereas at high concentrations it can kill the embryos in the eggs (Alkhakim *et al.* 2018).

Further test results showed that treatment P0 was very significantly different from treatment P2 but treatment P0 did not show significantly different results from treatments Pl and P2. This shows that fumigation treatment with a duration of 15 minutes can reduce egg hatchability, whereas treatments of 5 and 10 minutes do not reduce egg hatchability. The low average hatchability in the P3 treatment is thought to be due to long-term fumigation having an impact on reducing egg hatchability, this is because formalin will enter the air sacs of the eggs, causing the air in the egg sacs to become polluted. Formalin will react quickly with the mucus lining of the digestive tract and respiratory tract (Wardani and Mulasari 2016). Formaldehyde is a compound in the form of a gas that dissolves easily in water with a pungent odour, is more reactive and dangerous if inhaled because it can cause irritation to the respiratory tract, if it comes into contact with the skin, it will burn and if exposed in large quantities can cause death (Fadli *et al.* 2016).

Treatments Pl and P2 did not reduce egg hatchability, this is thought to be because formalin has not entered the air sac but only killed microorganisms found on the surface of the egg shell. Fumigation aims to kill or reduce contamination of microorganisms attached or attached to the surface of the egg (Hariani *et al.* 2017).

The egg air sac functions to provide air for the egg embryo, air is needed by the embryo so that the embryo remains alive and develops. Embryos need oxygen and emit carbon dioxide during their development process (Hasanah *et al.* 2019). The egg hatching process requires oxygen for survival and to affect the embryo (Junita *et al.* 2016).

4 CONCLUSION

Based on the research results, it can be concluded that the length of fumigation has a very significant effect on the hatchability and viability of quail egg embryos, the best length of fumigation is 10 minutes. Treatment with a fumigation duration of 15 minutes can reduce the hatchability and viability of quail egg embryos.

REFERENCES

[BPOM] Badan Pengawas Obat dan Makanan. 2008. *Formalin (Larutan Formaldehida)*. Jakarta (ID): BPOM

Alkhakim FH, MN Huda, GD Fitri, D Ambarwati, dan H Tistiana. 2016. Pengaruh ekstrak daun kersen terhadap daya tetas dan mortalitas telur itik hibrida. *Jurnal Ilmu-Ilmu Peternakan*. 26 (2): 8–13.

Fadli RA, MN Ibrahim, dan MS Sadimantara. 2016. Analisis kandungan zat pengawet formalin pada terasi yang diperdagangkandi pasar tradisional kota kendari.

Hariani F, Pagala MA, dan R Aka. 2017. Karakteristik telur tetas parenst stock ayam broiler yang difumigasi dan tanpa fumigasi. *Jurnal Ilmu dan Teknologi Peternakan Tropis*. 4(1):6–12.

Hasanah N, ND Wahyono, dan A Marzuki. 2019. Teknik manajemen penetasan telur tetas ayam kampung unggul kub di kelompok gumukmas jember. *Jurnal Uniska*. Kediri: 13–22.

Indrawati E, S Rahadi, T Saili, dan LO Nafiu. 2015. Fertilitas, daya hidup embrio, daya tetas dan bobot tetas telur ayam ras hasil inseminasi buatan dengan ayam tolaki. *Jurnal Ilmu dan Teknologi Peternakan Tropis*. 2 (2):10–18.

Junita H, A Hamdan, dan Sukendi. 2016. Pengaruh Suhu dan Oksigen Terhadap Penetasan Telur dan Kelulushidupan Awal Larva Ikan Pawas (Osteochilus hasselti C.V.). *Fakultas Perikanan dan Kelautan Universitas Riau*.

Kusuma R, PJPN Jefri, SG Hidayati, Zulkarnain, dan Erwin. 2022. Pengaruh fumigasi menggunakan air daun sirih terhadap daya tetas telur dan mortalitas embrio telur puyuh. *Jurnal Embrio* (14):48–62.

Middin RR, LO Nafiu, dan R Badaruddin. 2020. Fertilitas dan daya tetas burung puyuh (*coturnix-coturnix japonica*) yang diberi ramuan herbal melalui air minum dengan dosis berbeda. *Jurnal ilmiah peternakan halu oleo*. 2(1):114–118.

Ningtyas MS, Ismoyowati, dan IH Sulistyawan. 2013. Pengaruh temperatur terhadap daya tetas dan hasil tetas telur itik (*Anas plathyrinchos*). *Jurnal Ilmiah Peternakan*. 1(1):347–352.

Nuryati TS, M Khamim, dan PS Hardjosworo. 2002. Sukses Menetaskan Telur.

Ramadhan FK, Rukmiasih, dan R Afnan. 2019. Penggunaan ekstrak pelepah pisang ambon sebagai sanitizer kerabang terhadap daya tetas telur itik lokal. *Jurnal Ilmu Produksi dan Teknologi Hasil Peternakan*. 07(3): 88–95.

Wardani RI, SA Mulasari. 2016. Identifikasi formalin pada ikan asin yang dijual di kawasan pantai teluk penyu kabupaten cilacap. *Jurnal Kesehatan Masyarakat*. 10(1):43–48.

Technological Innovations in Tropical Livestock Development for Environmental Sustainability and Food Security – P. Dhian Isnaeni et al. (eds)
© 2025 The Author(s), ISBN 978-1-032-74373-8
Open Access: www.taylorfrancis.com, CC BY-NC-ND 4.0 license

Quality characteristics of eggs-derived superior native chicken in Kendari city

T. Saili*, L.O. Nafiu, A. Bain, N.S. Asminaya, R. Badaruddin & Y. Lestari
Department of Animal Science, Faculty of Animal Science, Universitas Halu Oleo, Kendari, Southeast Sulawesi, Indonesia

ABSTRACT: Each type of chicken exhibits eggs with distinct physical characteristics. Nevertheless, these disparities in both quantity and quality necessitate thorough examination. The objective of this study is to assess the quality attributes of superior Kampung chicken eggs in Kendari City. The research was conducted in September 2023 at the Poultry Farming Unit Laboratory, Faculty of Animal Science, Universitas Halu Oleo. The primary material utilized in this study comprised eggs from seven chicken strains: Kampung chickens, Arab chickens, KUB chickens, ULU chickens, Sensi chickens, Elba chickens, and Bangkok chickens, with 50 eggs from each strain. The assessed variables included egg weight, egg length, egg width, shell thickness, and egg index. The data were subjected to variance analysis to scrutinize the impact of strain on quantitative traits. Differences between treatments were assessed using Duncan's Multiple Range Test (DMRT) with IBM SPSS Statistics 25 software. The results of the variance analysis revealed a significant effect ($P<0.05$) of chicken strain on egg weight, egg length, egg width, and shell thickness, while no significant effect ($P>0.05$) was observed on the egg index. KUB chicken eggs exhibited the highest average weight (54.02 ± 4.70g), whereas Kampung chicken eggs displayed the smallest (42.92 ± 4.02g). Additionally, the study disclosed a significant impact ($P<0.05$) of chicken strain on the albumen index, yolk index, and Haug Unit. ULU chicken eggs recorded the highest yolk color score (11.10), whereas Elba chicken eggs exhibited the lowest (8.65). In conclusion, this research indicates that the quality of superior Kampung chicken eggs in Kendari City falls within the good category.

Keywords: Kampung chicken, egg characteristics, index, yolk, albumen

1 INTRODUCTION

Animal protein from livestock sources holds significance as it is more easily digested and absorbed by the human body. This is attributed to the amino acid content in livestock-derived animal protein, which closely aligns with the amino acid requirements of humans. Poultry is the primary choice for livestock farming in communities due to its relatively short maintenance period (Lidyawati *et al.* 2019). In Indonesia, local chickens consist of various breeds/strains, including native chickens, Bangkok chickens, Balitbangtan Superior Kampung Chickens (KUB), Elba chickens, Arab chickens, ULU chickens, and Sensi chickens (Madu *et al.* 2020).

Local chickens are the preferred choice as a protein source among communities. They are utilized as food due to their relatively easy maintenance, minimal land requirements, easily accessible and affordable feed, and ability to adapt quickly to the surrounding environment.

*Corresponding Author: takdir69@uho.ac.id

 DOI: 10.1201/9781003468943-10

Additionally, local chickens exhibit resilience to adverse environmental conditions and possess immunity against various diseases (Putri *et al.* 2020). Mahmud *et al.* (2017) have documented that poultry, including local chickens, are livestock raised for the production of both meat and eggs.

Eggs, as a food product derived from chickens, hold high value as a source of animal protein. Eggs are known for their delicious taste, easy digestibility, and high nutritional content, making them suitable for consumption by individuals of all age groups (Soeparno *et al.* 2011). Saliem *et al.* (2001) state that the consumption of eggs tends to be higher compared to other livestock products because eggs are easily obtained at a relatively low cost, making them affordable for individuals with lower purchasing power. However, it's worth noting that eggs remain a livestock product susceptible to damage.

Damage to chicken eggs can occur through various factors, including physical, chemical, and biological aspects, leading to alterations during the storage process. Therefore, when selecting Kampung chicken eggs, it is crucial to pay attention to their quality. The overall quality of a Kampung chicken egg is influenced by both the quality of its internal components (egg content) and the quality of its external shell (eggshell) (Sudaryani, 2000). Hence, understanding the characteristics and quality of eggs, along with the influencing factors, is of utmost importance from both the consumers' and producers' perspectives to sustain their business endeavors.

2 RESERARCH METHODS

This research was conducted at the Laboratory of Poultry Farming Unit and the Laboratory of Animal Product Technology, Department of Animal Science, Faculty of Animal Science, Halu Oleo University, Kendari. The research duration spanned one month. Instruments employed in the study included a digital scale, calipers, micrometer, and Yolk Color Fun. The research material encompassed chicken eggs from seven different superior native chicken strains, each consisting of 30 eggs, resulting in a total of 210 eggs being examined.

2.1 *Egg preparation*

There are 7 types of eggs used, including eggs from Kampung chickens, Sensi chickens, Elba chickens, KUB chickens, Arab chickens, Ulu chickens, and Bangkok chickens, each with a quantity of 30 eggs. These eggs were obtained from Alisa Farm in the Konda District and Fatan Farm in the Baruga District, Kendari City.

2.2 *Data collection and analysis*

The physical quality testing of eggs was conducted using 30 eggs each from Arab chickens, Kampung chickens, Ulu chickens, Sensi chickens, Elba chickens, KUB chickens, and Bangkok chickens. All the data were then compiled into a table for further descriptive analysis.

2.3 *Observation variable*

The variables for the physical quality of the egg exterior include egg weight, egg index, and shell thickness. In contrast, the quality variables for the interior involve the yolk index, albumen index, yolk color, and Haugh Unit (HU). Yolk color is measured using the yolk color fun. The calculation of the Haugh Unit value (HU) follows the formula proposed by Yuwanta (2004):

$$HU = 100 \log(H + 7,57 - 1,7.W0,37)$$

Information:

HU: Haugh Value of Egg Units
H: Height of egg white in thick part (mm)
G: Gravitational constant 32,20
W: Egg weight (g).

This research is planned to use a Completely Randomized Design (CRD) consisting of 7 treatments and 30 replications. The treatments in this study include S1 = Kampung Chicken, S2 = Ulu Chicken, S3 = Sensi Chicken (Selected Sentul), S4 = Elba Chicken, S5 = Superior Kampung Chicken from Balitbang (KUB), S6 = Arab Chicken, and S7 = Bangkok Chicken. The mathematical model is based on Steel and Torrie (1991):

$$Y\_ij = \mu + \pi\_i + \epsilon\_ij$$

Information:

Yij = Observation value of treatment to-i and to-j replication
μ = Middle value
ƛi = Influence of treatment to-i
ϵ_ij = Errors arising from treatment i and repeat to-j
i = Treatment to – i (1, 2, 3, 4, 5,6)
j = Repeat to –j (1, 2, 3, 4, 5)

The obtained data will be analyzed using an analysis of variance according to the research design. If the treatments yield a significant effect, further analysis will be conducted using Duncan's Multiple Range Test (DMRT). Data processing will be carried out using SPSS Version 26 software.

3 RESULT AND DISCUSSION

3.1 *Exterior characteristic of egg*

The external characteristics of chicken eggs evaluated include egg weight, egg length, egg index, and shell thickness. Data on the external characteristics of eggs obtained are presented in Table 1.

3.2 *Egg weight*

The analysis of variance results indicates that the chicken type significantly influences ($P<0.05$) egg weight. Furthermore, based on the DMRT test, it was found that the egg weight of KUB chickens is significantly higher ($P<0.05$) compared to the egg weight of

Table 1. Exterior characteristics of eggs based on superior chicken types in Kendari city.

Types of Chickens	Egg Weight (g)	Egg Index (%)	Shell Thickness (mm)
Kampung	42.92 ± 4.02^{e}	77.62 ± 11.07	0.52 ± 0.09^{a}
Ulu	48.20 ± 6.00^{bc}	76.64 ± 3.19	0.40 ± 0.05^{b}
Sensi	48.60 ± 4.19^{b}	78.52 ± 2.76	0.52 ± 0.07^{a}
Elba	46.94 ± 3.30^{cd}	77.26 ± 2.96	0.55 ± 0.10^{a}
Kub	54.02 ± 4.70^{a}	78.25 ± 2.49	0.41 ± 0.04^{b}
Arab	43.24 ± 2.85^{e}	77.02 ± 4.46	0.52 ± 0.17^{a}
Bangkok	46.32 ± 2.96^{d}	76.23 ± 5.41	0.36 ± 0.05^{b}

Note: different superscripts on the same column indicate significant difference between type of chicken.

native chickens, Ulu, Sensi, Elba, Arab, and Bangkok chickens. The order of the average egg weights from highest to lowest is as follows: KUB (54.02g ± 4.70), Sensi chicken eggs (48.60g ± 4.19), Ulu chicken eggs (48.20g ± 6.00), Elba chicken eggs (46.94g ± 3.30), Bangkok chicken eggs (46.32g ± 2.96), Arab chicken eggs (43.24g ± 2.85), and native chicken eggs (42.92g ± 4.02).

The findings of this study reveal egg weight values higher than those reported by Marlya *et al.* (2021), who documented native chicken egg weight at 39.82g and Arab chicken egg weight at 40.36g. The egg weight of Bangkok chickens in this study is nearly comparable to the research findings of Badaruddin *et al.* (2017), who recorded Bangkok chicken egg weight at 46.57g. According to Hartono *et al.* (2014), egg weight can be influenced by genetic factors and feed quality.

3.3 *Egg index*

The analysis of variance results indicates that the different chicken breeds do not have a significant effect (P>0.05) on the egg index. The mean egg indices for each chicken breed, in sequence, are as follows: native chicken (77.62 ± 11.07%), Ulu chicken (76.64 ± 3.19%), Sensi chicken (78.52 ± 2.76%), Elba chicken (77.26 ± 2.96%), KUB chicken (78.25 ± 2.49%), Arab chicken (77.02 ± 4.46%), and Bangkok chicken (76.23 ± 5.41%). The obtained results in this study range from 76.23% to 78.25%. The egg indices fall into the good category, aligning with Nasution's (2009) perspective that a good egg index falls within the range of 70%–79%.

According to Saddat and Adrizal (2009), an egg index between 70% and 79% is considered good. Additionally, eggs with an index of around 75% are round and have the potential to hatch at around 70–75%, while eggs with an elongated shape have a hatching potential of only about 30–35% (Sodak, 2011). In this context, the research results indicate that all seven types of eggs can be categorized as having normal conditions.

3.4 *Shell thickness*

The analysis of variance results indicates that the chicken breed significantly influences (P<0.05) the thickness of the eggshell. Based on the Duncan's Multiple Range Test (DMRT), it is observed that the eggshell thickness of Elba chicken is significantly higher (P<0.05) than that of Bangkok chicken (0.36 ± 0.05 mm), Ulu chicken (0.40 ± 0.05 mm), and KUB chicken (0.41 ± 0.04 mm). The mean eggshell thickness for each chicken breed, in sequence, is as follows: native chicken (0.52 ± 0.09 mm), Ulu chicken (0.40 ± 0.05 mm), Sensi chicken (0.52 ± 0.07 mm), Elba chicken (0.55 ± 0.10 mm), KUB chicken (0.41 ± 0.04 mm), Arab chicken (0.52 ± 0.17 mm), and Bangkok chicken (0.36 ± 0.05 mm). The mean eggshell thickness of native chicken, Sensi chicken, Elba chicken, and Arab chicken is nearly the same, suggesting that this similarity may be due to both types of chickens being raised under the same conditions—intensive farming with identical feed.

The eggshell thickness of Elba chicken (0.55 ± 0.10 mm) is significantly higher, with a difference of 0.19 mm compared to Bangkok chicken (0.36 ± 0.05 mm), a difference of 0.15 mm compared to Ulu chicken (0.40 ± 0.05 mm), and a difference of 0.14 mm compared to KUB chicken (0.41 ± 0.04 mm). This difference is suspected to be due to variations in the farming system. Elba chicken, native chicken, Sensi chicken, and Arab chicken in this study were intensively raised in battery cages with adequate nutritional feed, ensuring the calcium requirements for eggshell formation were met. According to the standards presented by Soeparno *et al.* (2011), eggshells are considered good when they reach a minimum of 0.33 mm. Therefore, the eggshell thickness of superior native chickens in Kendari, as indicated by this research, falls within the good category, ranging from 0.36 ± 0.05 mm to 0.55 ± 0.10 mm.

3.5 *Egg quality*

The quality of chicken eggs evaluated in this study includes the albumen index (egg white), yolk index (egg yolk), Haugh Unit, and yolk color. Data on the quality of chicken eggs obtained in this study are presented in Table 2.

Table 2. Egg quality based on chicken type.

Types of Chickens	Albumen Index	Yolk Index	Haugh Units	Yolk color
Kampung	0.07 ± 0.02^{c}	0.28 ± 0.12^{d}	74.03 ± 7.54^{c}	11.05 ± 1.43^{a}
Ulu	0.08 ± 0.02^{bc}	0.32 ± 0.08^{cd}	74.04 ± 11.94^{bc}	11.10 ± 0.72^{a}
Sensi	0.09 ± 0.02^{ab}	0.46 ± 0.05^{a}	79.06 ± 5.67^{ab}	9.15 ± 1.18^{bc}
Elba	0.10 ± 0.02^{a}	0.39 ± 0.06^{b}	82.62 ± 7.14^{a}	8.65 ± 1.50^{c}
Kub	0.10 ± 0.03^{a}	0.37 ± 0.10^{bc}	82.03 ± 7.18^{a}	10.70 ± 1.03^{a}
Arab	0.08 ± 0.02^{bc}	0.44 ± 0.04^{a}	72.77 ± 9.09^{d}	10.80 ± 1.58^{a}
Bangkok	0.08 ± 0.01^{c}	0.39 ± 0.02^{b}	78.19 ± 6.11^{abc}	9.80 ± 1.20^{b}

Note: different superscripts on the same column indicate significant difference between type of chicken.

3.6 *Albumen index*

The analysis of variance results reveals that the different strains of chickens significantly influence ($P<0.05$) the egg albumen index. Further, Duncan's Multiple Range Test (DRMT) indicates that the albumen index of Elba chicken significantly differs ($P<0.05$) from that of kampung chicken, Ulu chicken, Arab chicken, and Bangkok chicken. However, there is no significant difference ($P>0.05$) in the albumen index between Sensi chicken and KUB chicken.

The mean albumen indices for various chicken breeds, in sequential order, are as follows: kampung chicken (0.07 ± 0.02), Ulu chicken (0.08 ± 0.02), Sensi chicken (0.09 ± 0.02), Elba chicken (0.10 ± 0.02), KUB chicken (0.10 ± 0.03), Arab chicken (0.08 ± 0.02), and Bangkok chicken (0.08 ± 0.01). According to Yuwanta (2010), the fresh albumen index should ideally range from 0.050 to 0.174. Additionally, as the egg ages, the albumen diameter widens, leading to a decrease in the albumen index. Factors such as genetics, albumen height and diameter, and the duration of egg storage can influence the albumen index (Hartono *et al.* 2014). In this study, the albumen index ranges from 0.07 to 0.10. Purmaningsih (2010) reported that a good egg albumen index typically falls within the range of 0.05–0.17. Therefore, the findings of this research indicate that the egg albumen index is categorized as of good quality.

3.7 *Yolk index*

The results of the analysis of variance indicate that the superior kampung chicken breed significantly influences ($P<0.05$) the egg yolk index. Furthermore, based on Duncan's Multiple Range Test (DMRT), it is evident that the yolk index of Sensi chicken significantly differs ($P<0.05$) from that of Kampung, Ulu, Elba, KUB, and Bangkok chickens. However, there is no significant difference ($P>0.05$) in the yolk index between Arab chickens and the breeds above.

The average yolk index for various chicken breeds in sequence is as follows: Kampung chicken (0.28 ± 0.12), Ulu chicken (0.32 ± 0.08), Sensi chicken (0.46 ± 0.05), Elba chicken (0.39 ± 0.06), Arab chicken (0.37 ± 0.10), KUB chicken (0.44 ± 0.04), and Bangkok chicken (0.39 ± 0.02). Purwati *et al.* (2015) stated that fresh eggs should have a yolk index ranging from 0.33 to 0.50, with an average yolk index value of approximately 0.42. According to the SNI 01-3926-2008 standard (BSN, 2008), the fresh yolk index should range from 0.33 to 0.52

3.8 *Haugh unit*

The results of the analysis of variance indicate that superior native chicken breeds significantly influence ($P<0.05$) the Haugh Unit. According to Duncan's Multiple Range Test (DMRT), it is found that the Haugh Unit of KUB and Elba chickens is significantly higher ($P<0.05$) compared to the Haugh Unit of Kampung, Ulu, and Arab chickens.

Tugiyanti & Iriyanti (2012) state that Haugh Unit values can be used as a basis for assessing egg quality. Sodak (2011) emphasizes that several factors, including albumen viscosity, genetic factors, storage duration, temperature, and the age of the chicken, influence the Haugh Unit. An egg consists of three main parts: the eggshell, albumen (egg white), and yolk.

According to Purwati *et al.* (2015), eggs of good quality should have a Haugh Unit value of at least 75. The higher the Haugh Unit value, the better the quality of the egg. Thus, the results of this study indicate that the higher Haugh Unit in KUB and Elba chickens signify that the eggs from these breeds have better quality compared to eggs from Kampung, Ulu, and Arab chickens.

3.9 *Yolk color*

The analysis of variance results indicates that superior native chicken breeds significantly influence ($P<0.05$) the color of the egg yolk. Furthermore, based on Duncan's Multiple Range Test (DMRT), it is revealed that the yolk color of Ulu chickens is significantly higher ($P<0.05$) compared to the yolk color of Sensi, Elba, and Bangkok chickens. However, there is no significant difference ($P>0.05$) in the yolk color of Kampung, KUB, and Arab chickens.

The yolk color is measured using a yolk color fan consisting of 15 color series, with the lowest score being 1 (pale yellow) and the highest score being 15 (orange). The yolk color scores for Ulu and Kampung chickens are 11.10 ± 0.72 and 11.05 ± 1.43, respectively, which are higher than the yolk color scores for Bangkok (9.80 ± 1.20) and Elba (8.65 ± 1.50) chickens.

According to Hartono *et al.* (2014), yolk color is influenced by genetic factors and feed composition. Natural pigments affecting yolk color include xanthophylls found in green feed (Nur, 2015). Yolk pigments are influenced by the types of pigments in the diet, such as corn, which can deepen yolk color. Yolk pigment content belongs to the group of carotenoids, including xanthophylls, lutein, zeaxanthin, and small amounts of beta-carotene and cryptoxanthin (Winarno, 2002). The high yolk color score is attributed to the beta-carotene content. With an increase in beta-carotene content in the diet, yolk color intensity also increases, and a higher beta-carotene content in the diet can reduce cholesterol in eggs (Nuraini *et al.* 2008).

4 CONCLUSION

Based on the research findings, several conclusions can be drawn: (1) The average egg weight of KUB chickens is higher compared to eggs from Sensi, Ulu, Elba, Bangkok, Arab, and traditional Kampung chickens. Additionally, the egg index obtained in this study falls within the range of 76.23% to 78.25%, categorized as good. (2) The eggshell thickness of Elba chickens is superior compared to the other six superior Kampung chicken breeds. This indicates that the chicken breed significantly influences eggshell thickness. (3) Superior Kampung chicken breeds have a significant impact ($P<0.05$) on the variables of albumen index, yolk index, Haugh Unit, and yolk color. These results indicate that the different chicken breeds can affect the characteristics of egg quality, such as albumen index, yolk index, egg freshness (Haugh Unit), and yolk color. Thus, the overall research findings affirm that selecting superior Kampung chicken breeds has a significant impact on the physical characteristics and quality of eggs, opening opportunities for improved egg production with higher quality.

REFERENCES

Adrizal, A., & Nasution, S. (2009). Pengaruh pemberian level protein-energi ransum yang berbeda terhadap kualitas telur ayam buras. *Seminar Nasional Teknologi Peternakan dan Veteriner*, 613–618.

ATIK, P. (2010). *Pengaruh Penambahan Tepung Keong Mas (Pomacea Canaliculata Lamarck) Dalam Ransum Terhadap Kualitas Telur Itik*, [Thesis]. Universitas Sebelas Maret.

Hartona, T. A., Puger, A. W., & Nuriyasa, L. M. (2014). *Kualitas Telur Lima Jenis Ayam Kampung Yang Memiliki Warna Bulu Berbeda. Jurnal Peternakan Tropika*, 2(2), 153–162.

Haryono, H. (2000). Langkah-Langkah teknis uji kualitas telur konsumsi ayam ras. *Temu Teknis Fungsional Non Peneliti*, 175–184.

Lidyawati, A., Khopsoh, B., & Haryuni, N. (2019). Efek penambahan level vitamin e dan selenium dalam pakan terhadap performa ayam petelur yang diinseminasi buatan. *Jurnal Ilmiah Peternakan Terpadu*, 6(2), 106–110.

Madu, W. O. A., Napirah, A., & Saili, T. (2021). Pertumbuhan beberapa strain ayam lokal yang diberi pakan dengan level protein berbeda. *Jurnal Ilmiah Peternakan Halu Oleo*, 2(4), 441–445.

Mahmud, A. T. B. A., Afnan, R., Ekastuti, D. R., & Arief, I. I. (2017). Profil Darah, performans dan kualitas daging ayam persilangan kampung broiler pada kepadatan kandang berbeda (blood profile, performans and meat quality of crossed kampung broiler chicken In different stocking density). *Jurnal Veteriner*, 18(2), 247–256.

Nur, A. (2015). *Kualitas Telur Ayam Ras Yang Dipelihara Pada Sistem Free-Range Dengan Waktu Pemberian Naungan Alami Yang Berbeda* [Skripsi]. Universitas Hasanuddin.

Nuraini, N., Sabrina, S., & Latif, S. A. (2008). Performa ayam dan kualitas telur yang menggunakan ransum mengandung onggok fermentasi dengan neurospora crassa. *Media Peternakan*, 31(3), 195–202.

Purwati, D., Djaelani, M. A., & Yuniwarti, E. Y. W. (2015). Indeks Kuning Telur (IKT), Haugh Unit (HU) dan Bobot Telur pada Berbagai Itik Lokal di Jawa Tengah. *Jurnal Akademika Biologi*, 4(2), 1–9.

Putri, A. B. S. R. N., Gushairiyanto, G., & Depison, D. (2020). Bobot badan dan karakteristik morfometrik beberapa galur ayam lokal. *Jurnal Ilmu dan Teknologi Peternakan Tropis*, 7(3), Article 3.

Saliem, H. P., E. M. Lakolo, T. B., Purwantini, Ariani M., & Marisa, Y. (2001). Analisis ketahanan pangan tingkat rumah tangga dan regional. Laporan hasil penelitian. *Pusat Penelitian dan Pengembangan Sosial Ekonomi Pertanian.* Bogor.

Sudaryani, T. (2000). Kualitas Telur. *Penebar Swadaya*, Jakarta.

Sodak, J. F. (2011). Karakteristik Fisik dan Kimia Telur Ayam Arab Pada dua Peternakan di Kabupaten Tulungagung, Jawa Timur. [Skripsi]. *Institut Pertanian Bogor.*

Soeparno, R., Rihastuti A., Indratiningsih & Triatmojo, S. (2011). Dasar Teknologi Hasil Ternak. *Fakultas Peternakan Universitas Gadjah Mada University Press P.O. Box 14*, Bulaksumur, Yogyakarta.

Steel, R. G. D. & Torrie, J. H. (1991). Prinsip dan Prosedur Statistika: suatu pendekatan biometrik. *Gramedia Pustaka Utama*, Jakarta.

Yuwanta, T. (2004). Dasar Ternak Unggas (5th Ed.). *Yogyakarta.* Kanisius.

Technological Innovations in Tropical Livestock Development for Environmental Sustainability and Food Security – P. Dhian Isnaeni et al. (eds)

Natural increase of kacang goats (*Capra aegagrus hircus*) in Bombana Regency

R. Aka, A.S. Aku*, R.M. Anton & N.A. Lestari
Department of Animal Husbandry, Faculty of Animal Husbandry, Halu Oleo University, Indonesia

ABSTRACT: This study was conducted to analyze the natural increase of kacang goats in Bombana Regency, Southeast Sulawesi Province. The research location was determined using stratified sampling method and three districts were selected based on the category of goat's population, namely low population category (district Rumbia), medium population category (district Lantari Jaya), and high category (district Mata Oleo). The research sample was select-ed using the purposive sampling method, the criteria used farmers who have kacang goat does who have given birth more than once and have at least two years of farming experience. The data obtained during the research, namely birth rate, mortality rate and natural increase of the kacang goats' population for one year were tabulated, analyzed and explained descriptively quantitatively. The results showed that the birth rate for one year was 522 heads (67.61%) while the mortality rate was 145 heads (16.09%). The natural increase value of the kacang goats' population in Regency Bombana in 2015 was 51.52%.

Keywords: Kacang goats, Natural Increase, Bombana Regency

1 INTRODUCTION

Southeast Sulawesi Province has several livestock development policies, one of which is the Ruminant Livestock Development Program. One of the districts in Southeast Sulawesi Province designated as a development area for ruminant livestock (cattle, buffaloes and goats) is Bombana Regency. The population of cattle, buffaloes and goats in Regency Bombana in 2022 was 54,496, 794 and 4,821 respectively (BPS-Statistics of Bombana Regency 2023).

In general, the goat rearing system practiced by the community in Bombana Regency is still traditional, namely extensive and semi-intensive. In the extensive rearing system, kacang goats are reared by grazing without considering the availability of cages and feed, as the animals are released in areas with natural food sources such as agricultural areas and plantations (Amin *et al.* 2021). The extensive husbandry system can make goats susceptible to disease and easily stolen by others (Satriawan *et al.* 2023). Semi-intensive goat rearing is done by grazing on grassland (pasture) in the morning until the afternoon. During the grazing period, the farmers will tie the goats to certain tree trunks and also to those that are not tied by letting the goats graze on the pasture. In the afternoon, the farmer herds the goats into the cage (Amin *et al.* 2021). In addition, the maintenance system raises many problems for farmers, including those directly related to livestock productivity, namely the growth rate (body weight gain) and the number of goat kids born each year. An aspect that has a great influence on livestock productivity in terms of the number of goat kids born each year is the

*Corresponding Author: achmad.s.aku@uho.ac.id

DOI: 10.1201/9781003468943-11

population structure, birth rate, mortality rate, re-productive activity of the mother and natural increase.

Natural increase is the difference between the birth rate and the death rate of livestock within a given period (one year). Natural increase can indicate an increase or decrease in the livestock population within a year. The natural increase of the population can be influenced by several factors, including the number of does, litter size, mortality rate and birth rate of goat kids. Based on this description, it is necessary to conduct a study on the natural increase of the kacang goats' population in Bombana Regency so that the dynamics of the goat population in a given period of time (one year) can be known.

2 MATERIALS AND METHODS

2.1 *Population and sample*

The population of this study is all goats kept by farmers in Bombana Regency with selected districts as the sample. In Each district will take three villages will be sampled, taking into account the largest goats population.

The sample respondents are farmers in three districts: district Rumbia representing the lowest population, district Lantari Jaya representing the middle population, and district Mata Oleo representing the highest population. The number of respondents in each village was 10 farmers and if there were less than 10 farmers then all farmers were used as respondents with predetermined criteria.

2.2 *Location determination and sampling technique*

The research sampling technique in determining the district research location was carried out using the stratified sampling method according to Suprapto (2010), the number of livestock in 22 districts was stratified into low population, medium population and high population categories. Within each category, one district was randomly selected.

Population strata are determined by taking the range of the highest goat population (PT) minus the lowest population (PR) = (K population) and then dividing by three to give the strata interval (1/3 K). The range of strata is determined as follows: (1) low population = PR to PR + 1/3 K; (2) medium population = PR + 1/3 K + 1 to PR + 2/3 K; (3) high population = PR + 2/3 K + 1 to PR + K (Sani 2008).

Sites at district level were identified using purposive sampling following Suprapto (2010) by selecting the village with the largest goat population in a district. In each district, 3 villages were selected for the survey. A sample of three villages was selected in Rumbia district representing the lowest population of Lantowonua, Doule and Lameroro villages, Lantari Jaya district representing the medium population of village Lantari, Pasare Apua and Anugrah villages and Mata Oleo district representing the highest population of village Liano, Pomontoro and Tambako Island villages.

2.3 *Data collection technique*

The type of data collected in this study is divided into two, namely primary data and secondary data. Primary data is obtained through direct interviews using questionnaires and direct observations in the field, while secondary data is data obtained from offices and agencies related to the research.

2.4 *Data analysis*

Data obtained in the form of both primary and secondary data were tabulated and then analyzed. Natural increase (NI) was calculated using the formula (Hardjosubroto 1999):

(1) The proportion goat births to the total sample population in a given period was calculated using the formula:
B = C/N × 100%.
Description:
B: Percentage of goat births in the total sample population.
C: number of goat births in a period (tails)
N: total population sample (tails)
(2) The percentage of goat mortality in the total population sample was calculated using the formula:
D = (TM)/(N + TM) × 100%.
Description:
D: percentage of deaths in the total sample population.
TM: number of animals that died in one year (head)
N: total sample population (head)
(3) The natural increase value is calculated using the formula
NI = B − D
Description:
NI: Natural increase value
B: Percentage of goat births in the total population sample in one year (%)
D: Percentage of cattle mortality in the total population sample within one year within one year.

3 RESULTS AND DISCUSSION

3.1 *Birth rate*

The birth rate of pea goats is the number of animals born to each mother that gave birth in the last period or per year.

Table 1. Birth rate of kacang goats in Bombana Regency.

Parameters	District			Number
	Rumbia	Lantari Jaya	Mata Oleo	
Total sample population (tails)	199	237	336	772
Total parent population (tails)	58	57	82	197
Percentage of breeding stock in total population (%)	29.15	24.05	24.40	25.51
Number of breeding females giving birth (tails)	38	45	70	153
Number of goat kids at birth (tails/year)	129	164	229	522
Percentage of births (%)				
Single	0	0	2.11	0.70
Twin two	51.92	58.82	54.74	55.16
Twin three	48.08	41.18	43.16	44.14
Percentage of mothers having given birth in the parent population (%)	65.51	78.94	85.36	77.66
Percentage of mothers having given birth in the population (%)	19.09	18.98	20.83	19.81
Percentage of goat births in total population (%)	64.82	69.19	68.15	67.61

The results showed that the total population of local goats in Regency Bombana was 197 mothers and the number of mothers who gave birth during the year (January-December) was 153 tails (19.81% of the total population and 77.66% of the total population of mothers) with the number of kids born as high as 522 tails (67.61% of the total population). The number of mothers, the number of mothers who gave birth and the birth rate is higher when compared to the results of the research by Wulandari *et al.* (2020) the number of mothers of local goats in three sub-districts of East Kolaka Regency was 94 heads, the number of mothers who gave birth was 67 tails at 71% and the number of cemetery mothers was 67 tails at 71.27% and the number of goat kids born was 131 tails (52.4% of the total population); and lower than the findings of Zalima *et al.* (2021), the number of local goat herds in West Muna Regency was 107 tails, the number of lambing mothers was 92 tails at 85.98% and the number of goat kids born was 346 tails (76.72% of the total population). According to Harmoko *et al.* (2022), the percentage of goat kids born was 28.67%.

The high birth rate in this study was influenced by several factors: the percentage of productive mothers who gave birth was quite high at 77.66% of the total number of mothers, and in general, kacang goat mothers in Bombana Regency are prolific, giving birth to twins (55.16%) and triplets (44.14%) as shown in Table 1. In addition, the kidding interval of goats in Bombana Regency is 8–9 months, so that some kacang goats can give birth twice a year, especially goats that give birth at the beginning of the year (January-March). The results of this study are similar to those reported by Wulandari *et al.* (2020) that the lambing interval of kacang goats in East Kolaka is 8.19 months, the kiding interval of local goats in Siompu district is 8.2 months, and in Lapandewa district is 8.19 months (Basman *et al.* 2015), the kidding interval of kacang goats in Siompu District, South Buton is 8.2 months and can be said to be still within the normal range (Nurjani *et al.* 2020); the kidding interval of saburai goats in Tanggamus Regency is or 10.35 ± 1.66 months (Ananta *et al.* 2020) and 8.30 ± 0.03 months (Adhianto *et al.* 2016).

3.2 *Mortality rate*

The mortality rate of kacang goats is the number of goats that die compared to the total population at the beginning of the year and the number of births during the year for each respondent farmer.

Table 2. Mortality rate of kacang goats in Bombana Regency.

Parameters	District			Number
	Rumbia	Lantari Jaya	Mata Oleo	
Total sample population (tails)	199	237	336	772
Mortality of goats (tails/year)	39	53	53	145
Percentage of goat mortality in total population (%)	16.38	18.27	13.62	16.09

The results showed that the mortality rate of kacang goats in Bombana Regency was 16.09%, which was higher than that reported by Harmoko *et al.* (2022). The mortality rate of goats in Lakor Subdistrict, Southwest Maluku Regency was 6.54%, while the mortality rate of Kacang goats in North Konawe Regency was 13.96% (Wati *et al.* 2014). However, it is lower than the findings of Wulandari *et al.* (2020), the mortality rate of goats in East Kolaka Regency was 17.67%, and the findings of Zalima *et al.* (2021), the mortality rate of goats in West Muna Regency was 16. 72%; Afriani *et al.* (2019) the average mortality rate of kacang goats in Kubu Jaya is 10%; Sulastri *et al.* (2020) the average mortality rate of kacang goats in North Kolaka District is 13.48%.

The mortality rate of kacang goats in Bombana Regency was caused by the death of goat kids born with triplets during the preweaning period, which was 58.96%. The results of this study are higher than those reported by Widianingsih and Yani (2000) that the mortality of goat kids, especially during the preweaning period, can reach 10-50%, and the results of research reported by Tampubolon and Nasution (2023) that the preweaning mortality of kacang goats in Bargottopong village, Padangsidimpuan City, which are semi-intensively reared, was 14.29%. The high preweaning mortality rate in Bombana Regency is due to competition for colostrum and milk from the mother and lack of attention from the farmer when the mother gives birth. Kacang goats that cannot compete die because they do not re-ceive colostrum as an antibody and mother's milk at the preweaning age. In addition to goat kid deaths, deaths also occurred in post-weaning, young and adult goats (41.04% of the total goat population that died). Skin diseases (scabies) and accidents caused by extensively reared goats were the most common causes. The mortality rate is due to animal diseases such as scabies, which is difficult to control, lack of attention by farmers in handling births, lack of knowledge about feed management and maintenance of goats.

3.3 *Natural increase of the population*

The natural increase of a population is calculated from the difference between deaths and births within a given period (one year).

The results showed that the natural increase of the peanut goat population in Bombana Regency is quite high (51.52%), which is higher than the natural increase of 22.13% reported by Harmoko *et al.* (2022). The high natural increase in the population of kacang goats in Bombana Regency is due to the high birth rate (67.61%) and low mortality rate (16.09%). However, this natural increase is smaller than the natural increase of Peranakan Etawah goat population in Kaligesing and Sendowo breeding centres by Susilo (2001), which averaged 53.80%; Aprilinda *et al.* (2016) natural increase value in Karang Endah village, Terbanggi Besar district, Central Lampung Regency, namely PE goats 38.30%, Rambon 29.33% and Kacang 27.35% (including high category). The results of natural increase of Kacang goats in Bombana Regency can be categorised in the high range (51.52%). The value of natural in-crease is generally divided into three groups, where the range of natural increase value 0.00-15.00% is low, the range of natural increase value 15.01–30.00% is medium, while the range of natural increase value 30.01–45.90% is high (Putra *et al.* 2017).

The results showed that the natural increase of the peanut goat population in Bombana Regency is quite high (51.52%), which is higher than the natural increase of 22.13% reported by Harmoko *et al.* (2022). The high natural increase in the population of kacang goats in Bombana Regency is due to the high birth rate (67.61%) and low mortality rate (16.09%). However, this natural increase is smaller than the natural increase of Peranakan Etawah goat population in Kaligesing and Sendowo breeding centres by Susilo (2001), which averaged 53.80%; Aprilinda *et al.* (2016) natural increase value in Karang Endah village, Terbanggi Besar district, Central Lampung Regency, namely PE goats 38.30%, Rambon 29.33% and Kacang 27.35% (including high category). The results of natural increase of Kacang goats in Bombana Regency can be categorised in the high range (51.52%). The value of natural in-crease is generally divided into three groups, where the range of natural increase value 0.00-15.00% is low, the range of natural increase value 15.01-30.00% is medium, while the range of natural increase value 30.01-45.90% is high (Putra *et al.* 2017).

Table 3. Natural increase of kacang goats in Bombana Regency

Parameters	District			Number
	Rumbia	Lantari Jaya	Mata Oleo	
Percentage of goat births in total population (%)	64.82	69.19	68.15	67.61
Percentage of goat mortality in total population (%)	16.38	18.27	13.62	16.09
Natural increase (%)	48.44	50.92	54.53	51.52

4 CONCLUSION

It can be concluded that the natural increase of kacang goats in Bombana Regency is 51.52%.

PREFERENCES, SYMBOLS AND UNITS

Afriani, D., A. Tohardi and Zakiatulyaqin. 2019. Productivity of pea goats (*Capra aegagrus*) in Rasau Jaya Iii village, Rasau Jaya district, Kubu Raya regency. *Journal of Agricultural Science Equator*. 8(2). 1–7. http://dx.doi.org/10.26418/jspe.v8i2.32064.

Amin, L., Aka, R and Sani, L.O.A. 2021. Characterization of qualitative traits of local goats in Siompu district. *JIPHO*, 3(2). 209–216. http://dx.doi.org/10.56625/jipho.v3i2.18034.

Aprilinda, S., Sulastri, and Suharyati, S. 2016. Reproductive status and production estimation of goat breeds in Karang Endah village, Tebanggi Besar district, Central Lampung Regency. *Journal of Integrated Animal Science*, 4(1), 51–58. http://dx.doi.org/10.23960/jipt.v4i1.p%25p.

Adhianto. K., Hamdani, M. D.I., Sulastri, and Listiana, I. 2016. Production performance of male Saburai goats in two seedling source areas in Tanggamus Regency. *Animal Husbandry Science*, 14 (92), 22–29. https://doi.org/10.20961/sainspet.v14i2.4342.

Basman, Saili, T. and Ba'a, L.O. 2015. Kid crop and mortality of bean goat kids in mainland and island areas of Buton Regency. *JITRO*, 2(2), 39–53. http://dx.doi.org/10.33772/jitro.v2i2.3800.

BPS-Statistics of Bombana Regency. 2023. Bombana Regency in Figures. Rumbia.

Fikri, A.M., Adhianto, K., Husni, A. and Qisthon, A. 2020. Performance of Saburai goats reared by farmers in Gisting village, *Tanggamus Regency. Journal of Animal Husbandry Research and Innovation*, 4(2), 98–103. https://doi.org/10.23960//JRIP.2020.4.2.98.

Harmoko, H. Jesajas, J. Makatita, J. M. Lainsamputty and R. L. Dolewikou. 2022. Population dynamics of Lakor goats in Lakor district, *Southwest Maluku Regency. Journal of Tropical Animal and Veterinary Science*, 12(1), 107–113. https://doi.org/10.46549/jipvet.v12i1.287.

Nurjani, Ba'a, L.O. and Sani, L.O.A. 2020. Observation of reproductive potential of female goats traditionally reared in Siompu district, South Buton Regency. *JIPHO*, 2(1), 74–81. http://dx.doi.org/10.56625/jipho.v2i1.11193.

Putra, D.E., Sarbaini and T. Afriani. 2017. Estimation of buffalo breeding potential in Ulakan Tapakis district, Padang Pariaman regency, West Sumatra province, Indonesia. *Veterinary Journal*, 18(4), 624–633. https://doi.org/10.19087/jveteriner.2017.18.4.624.

Sani, L.A. 2008. Labour Effort of transmigrant and local families in beef cattle raising in south konawe district. Thesis. *Faculty of Animal Husbandry*, Gadjah Mada University. Yogyakarta.

Satriawan, L.O., Sandiah, N., Aka, R. 2023. Goats rearing system in Binongko district, Wakatobi Regency. *JIPHO*, 5(4), 284–289. http://dx.doi.org/10.56625/jipho.v5i4.41853.

Suprapto, J. 2010. Statistical theory and applications. *Erlangga*. Jakarta.

Susilo, P., 2001. Estimation of Peranakan Ettawa goat production in Kaligening and Sendowo breeding centres. Doctoral thesis. Faculty of Animal Husbandry, Gadjah Mada University. Yogyakarta.

Tampubolon, Y.K., and Nasution, Z. 2023. Productivity of peanut, blingon and Peranakan etawa goats under semi-intensive management. *Journal of Animal Science*, 07(02), 59–65. http://dx.doi.org/10.31604/jac.v7i1.8590.

Wati, L., Aka, R., and Saili, T. 2014. Kacang goats (*Capra hircus*) kid crop in North Konawe Regency. *JITRO*, 1(1), 9–15. http://dx.doi.org/10.33772/jitro.v1i1.356.

Widaningsih and Yani, N. 2000. Tips for reducing mortality of goats and sheep in the preweaning period. *Livestock Research Centre. Bogor*.

Wulandari, S., Aka, R., and Nafiu, L.O. 2020. Litter size and mortality of local goats in East Kolaka Regency. *JIPHO*, 2(4), 427–431. http://dx.doi.org/10.56625/jipho.v2i4.16934.

Zalima, W.O.Z., Aka, R. and Rahman.2021. Kid crop Kacang goats in West Muna Regency, Southeast Sulawesi. *IJAAS*, 3(3), 24–27. http://dx.doi.org/10.33772/ijaas.v3i3.

Technological Innovations in Tropical Livestock Development for Environmental Sustainability and Food Security – P. Dhian Isnaeni et al. (eds)
© 2025 The Author(s), ISBN 978-1-032-74373-8
Open Access: www.taylorfrancis.com, CC BY-NC-ND 4.0 license

Quality of frozen semen sexing Brahman cross bovine using *Ophiocephalus striatus* albumin extract

Nurcholis* & S.M. Salamony
Department of Animal Husbandry, Faculty of Animal Agriculture, Musamus University, Indonesia

A. Baharun
Department of Animal Science, Faculty of Animal Agriculture, Djuanda University, Indonesia

ABSTRACT: Sperm sexing as several problems, such as decreased sperm motility, damage to cell membranes, and the high price of Bovine Serum Albumin (BSA). A study is needed to reduce the risk of sperm damage and sperm capacity using cheap albumin. This study aimed to determine sperm quality, the proportion of X and Y sperm using the albumin column method with *Ophiocephalus striatus* fish albumin extract (OSAE). Semen was collected using an artificial vagina from three Brahman cross bovine. *Ophiocephalus striatus* fish albumin extract, albumin columns were made in different concentrations according to P0 BSA (5% top :10% bottom), P1 OSAE (2% top: 4% bottom), P2 OSAE (3% top: 5% bottom), dan P3 OSAE (4% top: 6% bottom), P4 (7% top: 9% bottom). The parameters observed included sperm motility, sperm viability, sperm abnormalities, X and Y sperm proportions. Analysis was carried out using one-way analysis of variance (ANOVA). The results showed that the proportion of X and Y sperm using BSA 5%: 10% (67% : 73.5%) was higher ($P<0.05$) compared to OSAE 2%: 4% (39.20% : 75.50%), OSAE 3%: 5% (50.87%: 73.20%), OSAE 4%:6% (61.25%: 68.60%) and OSAE 7%:9% (64.64%: 66.78%). Post-thawing sperm motility and viability of P1 were highest (67.60%) than other treatments. Sperm viability (74.61%) and sperm abnormalities in P4 were highest (8.7%) than those of other treatments. In conclusion, the use of OSAE 4%:6% effective for separating the highest proportion of X and Y sperm, and OSAE 2%:4% produce the highest sperm motility and sperm viability after freezing.

Keywords: Separation, Sperm, Ophiocephalus striatus, Albumin

1 INTRODUCTION

The application of artificial insemination (AI) technology has been proven to be able to increase business efficiency in accordance with the goals and desires of breeders. The implementation of AI in Merauke has had an impact on improving livestock quality (Nurcholis *et al.* 2019). in Merauke, small breeders such as Ongole Crossbreed (OC) and Brahmancross (BC) because this type of livestock is able to adapt to extreme environments. OC cattle are resistant to the climate in Merauke (Nurcholis *et al.* 2021). Generally, breeders prefer male cattle, because of their fast growth. This is in accordance with keeping male livestock, namely beef livestock. Selection of the gender of the female desired as a superior parent.

Sex selection in livestock can be done using the sperm separation method. Sex selection requires sperm separation technology to produce calves of the desired sex (Khamlor *et al.* 2014) The process of sperm sexing in several types of cattle has been carried out, such as OC

*Corresponding Author: nurcholis@unmus.ac.id

DOI: 10.1201/9781003468943-12

cattle (Mardi *et al.* 2020) and Limousin cattle (Kusumawati *et al.* 2018). The methods for sperm sexing are column albumin gradient (Maulana *et al.* 2019; Wolf *et al.* 2008) swim up (Meitei *et al.* 2021), Percoll gradient (Arias *et al.* 2017; Machado *et al.* 2009), immunological selection of X- and Y (Quelhas *et al.* 2021).

Each of the separation methods has advantages and disadvantages in the field. Therefore, it is necessary to find out the method for separating sperm quickly and cheaply. Separating sperm using a bovine serum albumin (BSA) column has advantages over manual separation methods. Bovine serum albumin is weak in that it is expensive but easy to apply in the field. Based on the existing problems, an alternative is needed to overcome these problems, including utilizing the potential of fish albumin (Maulana *et al.* 2019). Gastor fish (local name in Merauke), scientific name *Ophiocephalus striatus*, has an advantage because of its high albumin content. (Tungadi 2020) states that Gastor fish albumin is 30.20% per 100 mg. The albumin content in *Ophiocephalus striatus* fish is thought to be high and can be used for sperm differentiation processes such as the use of albumin in eggs and human serum albumin (HSA). The role of fish albumin in the splitting process is to filter X and Y sperm in the column. Therefore, this study aimed to examine sperm quality, and the proportion of X and Y sperm separated using OSAE.

2 MATERIALS AND METHODS

2.1 *Animal and ethical approval*

Three BC bulls for four years were reared intensively by breeders and in individual cages. Cattle semen was collected twice weekly using an artificial vagina (AV) with a water temperature of 50-55°C. This research was carried out at the Merauke Agricultural Quarantine and Musamus University. Processing of cattle semen refers to the Indonesian national standard SNI: 4869-1:2021 (BSN, 2021) for frozen cattle semen. The sperm separation flow is illustrated in Figure 1. Ethical feasibility of animals The Faculty of Veterinary Medicine, Gadjah Mada University (UGM) approved this research through decision No.23/EC-FKH-2022.

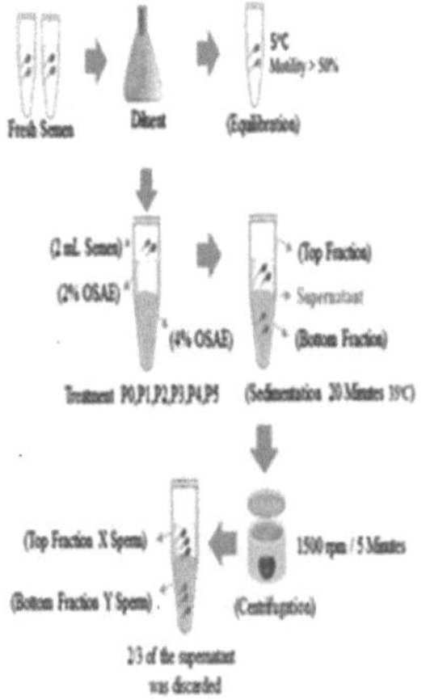

Figure 1. Sperm separation flow is illustrated.

2.2 *Semen evaluation*

Semen evaluation is the only effective method for detecting bull fertility (Tanga *et al.* 2021). The semen assessment processes were macroscopic, including volume, consistency, colour and pH (6.4-8 scale using paper indicators). All microscopic evaluations used a binocular microscope (Olympus CX43, Japan) integrated with a monitor. This evaluation included sperm mass movement, sperm motility, sperm viability, sperm concentration, sperm morphology, and sperm membrane integrity.

Observation of sperm motility (%) using a microscope with a magnification of 200x and 400x (IAEA 2005). Mix 5 drops of 0.9% NaCl with 1 drop of fresh semen. Motility value determination using 0-100% (Nurcholis *et al.* 2021).

Observation of sperm viability (%) and sperm abnormalities (%) were observed before making preparations for Eosin Negrosin (EN) (IAEA 2005). They were dripping 4-5 EN to 1 drop of fresh semen, homogenizing, and preparing a smear. Validity was evaluated with 200x magnification, and live sperm did not absorb colour, while dead sperm did absorb the colour. The minimum count was 200 sperm cells. Evaluate abnormalities in sperm by dividing normal and abnormal sperm multiplied by 100% (Nurcholis *et al.* 2021). The post-sexing evaluation process also used this method.

Observation of sperm concentration x (106) was carried out by looking at 5 boxes on a Neubauer slide chamber (0.100 mm and 0.0025 mm, German brand). The observation method is done by looking at one box in the middle, 2 boxes at the top left and right, and two at the bottom left and right. Observation under a microscope with a magnification of 100 x or 200 x. The concentration is calculated by looking at the sperm heads in the box which are counted as 1, while the sperm heads which are on the boundary are counted as ½. The sperm counting formula is the number of boxes 5 x 5 fields of view x 5 dilution factors (1:200) x 10,000 (Nurcholis *et al.* 2021).

Sperm membrane integrity (%) can be observed by hypoosmotic swelling (HOS) (Ramu and Jeyendran 2013). 50 μL semen was added to 1000 μL HOS solution (1.351 g fructose and 0.735 g sodium citrate in 100 mL distilled water with an osmolarity of 150 m). The mixture was homogenized and then incubated at 37oC for 30 minutes in a water bath. The evaluation was conducted randomly in 10 fields of view to observe a minimum of 250 sperm. Calculations were performed using a phase-contrast binocular microscope with a magnification of 400 times. The intact sperm plasma membrane is marked with a coiled or inflated tail, while damaged sperm is marked with a straight tail. The percentage of sperm membrane integrity was calculated by comparing the number of reacting sperm (positive HOS) divided by the number of counted sperm x 100%.

2.3 *Preparing OSAE*

Ophiocephalus striatus (OS) fish albumin was obtained from a modified extraction process according to (Romadhoni *et al.* 2016). A total of 250 grams of OS fish meat was cleaned with distilled water. The fish meat was steamed with distilled water in a ratio of 1:1 on a hotplate at 60 degrees Celcius for 10 minutes, and the resulting extract was filtered. Separation of crude protein and lipid extracts was carried out by mixing n-Hexane solution with a ratio of 1:1 for 35 minutes at room temperature. This extract was put into a tube until two layers were formed. The bottom layer was taken and centrifuged at 9,000 rpm for 20 minutes. The centrifugation results were allowed to stand until the supernatant appeared at the bottom, taken and filtered to become OSAE. Store at -20°C before use.

2.4 *Treatment sexing sperm using OSAE*

Sperm sexing treatment with control proportions P0 BSA (5% top:10% bottom), P1 OSAE (2% top: 4% bottom), P2 OSAE (3% top: 5% bottom), dan P3 OSAE (4% top: 6% bottom), P4 (7% top: 9% bottom). Semen was diluted (1:1 ratio), then 1 ml was taken to be added to the gradient and incubated for 20 minutes at 35°C temperature. Then, washing was done by taking 1 ml of semen in the top and bottom layers, and each sample was put in 3 ml of diluent. Centrifugation was carried out at 1500 rpm for 5 minutes. 2 ml of supernatant was discarded, and 2 ml of pellet was left, mixing diluent. The lower layer fraction is indicated as Y-chromosome sperm, and the upper layer fraction as X-chromosome sperm (Kaiin *et al.* 2017). The parameters measured were the proportion of X and Y sperm from both top and bottom fractions, sperm motility, sperm viability, and sperm abnormalities. The semen that has been separated is then frozen. The clotting process is carried out using procedures according to Nurcholis *et al.* 2021. Semen dilution is carried out using Andromed® CSS One-step (Un Paso) REF: 13503/1200.

2.5 *Data analysis*

All data on the quality of fresh and frozen semen and the proportion of sperm with X and Y chromosomes were presented in the form of mean and standard error (SE) and analyzed using one-way ANOVA, to identify between treatments using Duncan ($P<0.05$) with the help of software SPPS ver 22.

3 RESULTS AND DISCUSSION

3.1 *Fresh semen quality of Brahman cross bovine*

The quality of fresh semen of Brahman cross bovine in general was presented in Table 1. The average fresh semen volume of three Brahman cross bulls was 4.7, with pH between 6.5, thick and moderate consistency. Microscopic observations showed sperm mass movement (+ ++), sperm motility between 82.5% sperm viability between 87.6%, sperm concentration 1027x(106)/mL, normal sperm was 96.5%, and abnormal sperm was between 3.5%. In general, fresh semen from Brahman-cross cattle was of decent quality for further processing. In general, the fresh semen using one-way ANOVA, to identify between treatments using Duncan ($P<0.05$) with the help of software SPPS ver 22.

The Semen volume of Brahman-cross cattle was an average of 4.7 ml. The semen volume of Brahman-cross (BC) local was 4.93 ml (Islam *et al.* 2018). It was due to due to differences in the type of livestock, feed, environment, and genetics. According to (Bhave *et al.* 2020), genetics and the environment affect the production and quality of cattle semen. The pH value of fresh semen was within normal limits, i.e. 6.5. The pH of fresh semen for cattle generally is 6.4 – 6.6 (Prastiya *et al.* 2023). Semen pH is usually correlated with sperm motility (Dhumal *et al.* 2021). The motility and viability of fresh semen sperm are 70% and

Table 1. Fresh semen quality of BC bovine.

Characteristics	Average (SE)
Macroscopic	
Volume(ml)	4.7 ± 0.69
pH	6.5 ± 0.18
Colour	Cream
Consistency	Moderate
Microscopy	
Movement of Sperm	+++
Total Sperm Motility (%)	82.5 ± 1.65
Sperm Viability (%)	87.6 ± 1.05
Sperm concentration $\times$ (10^6)	1027 ± 80.93
Morphology	
Normal sperm (%)	96.5 ± 0.80
Abnormal sperm (%)	3.5 ± 1.19

80%, respectively (Nurcholis *et al.* 2021). The quality of fresh semen in this study complies with Indonesian national standards (SNI 4869-1:2021).

3.2 *Proportion of X and Y sperm*

Sperm sexing is an attempt to change the natural proportion of Y and X spermatozoa (50%:50%) into the desired proportion using the sexing method. The results of research on the proportion of X and Y sperm in BC bovine are shown in Table 2. The use of BSA (5%:10%) has a proportion of 67%:73.50%, which indicates that there is more separation of the Y chromosome at the bottom. The use of OSAE (2%: 4%) produces a higher proportion of Y chromosome sperm than X, ie (39.20 %: 75.50%). This finding shows that a large proportion of Y-chromosome sperm is found in the bottom fraction. This is caused by the movement of Y sperm that being faster and more energetic to penetrate the albumin column separator.

Table 2. Proportion of X and Y sperm.

	Proportion of Sperm (%)		
Fractionof Treatment	X		Y
No Sexed	52.60		47.40
		X Fraction (Top)	
BSA 5%	67.00±0.25		33.00±0.20
OSAE 2%	39.20±0.14		60.80±1.15
OSAE 3%	50.87±0.10		49.13±0.90
OSAE 4%	61.25±0.08		38.75±0.05
OSAE 7%	64.64±1.00		35.36±0.90
		Y Fraction (Bottom)	
BSA 10%	26.50±0.15		73.50±0.12
OSAE 4%	24.50±0.25		75.50±0.25
OSAE 5%	26.80±0.10		73.20±0.10
OSAE 6%	31.40±0.15		68.60±0.10
OSAE 9%	33.22±0.05		66.78±1.12

BSA: Bovine Serum Albumin; OSAE: *Ophiocephalus striatus* Albumin Extract

According to (Prasad *et al.* 2010), Y sperm move faster and X sperm move more slowly because they have a lot of chromatins in their heads so their heads are larger. This sperm separation result is lower than Maulana *et al.* (2019), the proportion of X and Y sperm in SO bulls using Channalbumin 2%:4% (42.33%:79.13%). This difference is thought to occur due to differences in the albumin used and the process.

3.3 *Brahman cross bull sperm quality post-thawing*

The quality of post-thawing sperm from sexing semen shows that there are differences between X and Y sperm ($P<0.05$). In Table 3, X sperm with BSA treatment (control) had the highest motility reaching 69.50%, followed by P1 and P2. The use of OSAE 4%-7% in sperm separation has an impact on X sperm motility ranging from 54%. Sperm viability in this study was normal. The abnormality of post-thawing sperm is quite high, damage in general is due to the centrifugation and washing processes during sperm separation. However, the quality of sperm X post-thawing is within normal limits based on SNI4869-1:2021.

Table 3. Sperm quality post-thawing (X Sperm).

Characteristics Sperm X	P0	P1	P2	P3	P4
Sperm Motility (%)	69.50±0.15[a]	67.60±0.10[b]	66.45±0.50[b]	54.75±1.19[c]	54.55±1.15[c]
Sperm Viability (%)	78.50±0.25[a]	74.61±1.10[b]	73.70±0.10[b]	60.12±1.30[c]	61.15±1.10[c]
Sperm Abnormality (%)	5.00±0.25[a]	4.60±0.20[a]	4.80±0.25[a]	7.90±0.25[b]	8.07±1.15[b]

BSA: Bovine Serum Albumin; OSAE: *Ophiocephalus striatus* Albumin Extract

Table 4. Sperm quality post-thawing (Y Sperm).

Characteristics Sperm Y	P0	P1	P2	P3	P4
Sperm Motility (%)	68.70±0.10[a]	66.40±0.10[b]	6.25±0.50[b]	55.75±1.10[c]	5.55±1.20[c]
Sperm Viability (%)	78.70±0.20[a]	75.00±1.00[b]	4.70±0.10[b]	62.25±1.15[c]	2.10±1.00[c]
Sperm Abnormality (%)	4.50±0.20[a]	4.50±0.75[a]	4.95±0.35[a]	6.00±0.20[b]	7.35±1.50[b]

BSA: Bovine Serum Albumin; OSAE: *Ophiocephalus striatus* Albumin Extract, Difference a,b,c in the same row (P<0.05)

The research results in Table 4 show that Y sperm motility in Brahman-cross bulls diluted using Andromed® has the highest value, namely 68.70%, followed by P1 and P2. The use of OSAE in sperm separation affects the motility level of Y sperm. This can happen because the sperm has expended a lot of energy to penetrate the albumin layer so that the motility is lower when compared to X sperm.

The results of this study were higher than the findings of (Teken *et al.* 2020), the average motility of post-thawing cow sperm resulting from sexing using Andromed® diluent (62.50%). Maulana *et al.* 2019 stated that the motility of X sperm using channalbumin was 2% and 4% on average (65%–64%), and Y sperm was 59%. This difference can be influenced by fresh cement, and the diluent used.

In addition, sperm motility and sperm viability are influenced by plasma fluid and mitochondrial function which produces ATP for movement. Semen plasma released after semen collection can increase the number of live sperm after separation and sorting (Steinhauser *et al.* 2016). The sperm sexing process can cause damage to the sperm cell membrane, this occurs due to lipid peroxidation. It was due to the antioxidants in sperm cells are not balanced with Reactive Oxygen Species (ROS). Oxidative stress causes damage to sperm DNA and sperm membranes. The impact is decreased sperm motility (Ribas-Maynou & Benet 2019).

High post-thawing sperm abnormalities because of the semen sexing process. Centrifugation and washing can be the main trigger for increased abnormalities caused by laboratory errors. Post-thawing sperm abnormalities in this study were quite high, reaching 8.07%. X sperm and 7.3 Y sperm. This means that there is an increase in abnormalities of 3–5%. This condition is not included in the primary abnormality category. However, the normal limit for sperm abnormalities is 10%. According to (Utami *et al.* 2014) the tolerance limit for sperm abnormalities is 12–23%.

4 CONCLUSION

The use of OSAE 4%:6% can be used to replace BSA because it has X and Y sperm sorting levels. Using BSA with Andromed® diluent produces the best motility. However, the use of OSAE 2%:4% with the addition of Andromed® diluent produces the best post-thawing sperm quality followed by 4%:6% with an average of 66–67%. Therefore, it is recommended to continue until the AI process.

AUTHORS' CONTRIBUTIONS

Nurcholis played a role in research formulation, data collection, data processing and methods. Abdullah Baharun played a role in analyzing the data and discussion results. Syetiel M Salamony played a role in collecting field data and discussions. The authors declare no conflict of interest.

ACKNOWLEDGEMENTS

Acknowledgements to Kemendikbudristek-Indonesia for the PFR scheme for providing research funding no. Contract 136/E5/PG.02.00.PL/2023.

REFERENCES

Arias, M. E., Andara, K., Briones, E., & Felmer, R. (2017). Bovine sperm separation by swim-up and density gradients (Percoll and BoviPure): Effect on sperm quality, function and gene expression. *Reproductive Biology*, *17*(2), 126–132. https://doi.org/10.1016/j.repbio.2017.03.002

Bhave, K. G., Thilak Pon Jawahar, K., Kumarasamy, P., Sivakumar, T., Joseph, C., Shirsath, T., Deshmukh, P., & Venkataramanan, R. (2020). Genetic and non-genetic factors affecting semen production and quality characteristics of Gir cattle breed under semi-arid climate. *Veterinary World*, *13*(8), 1714–1718. https://doi.org/10.14202/vetworld.2020.1714-1718

Dhumal, S. S., Naik, P., Dakshinamurthy, S., & Sullia, K. (2021). Semen ph and its correlation with motility and count-a study in subfertile men. *Jornal Brasileiro de Reproducao Assistida*, *25*(2), 172–175. https://doi.org/10.5935/1518-0557.20200080

Islam, M., Apu, A., Hoque, S., Ali, M., & Karmaker, S. (2018). Comparative study on the libido, semen quality and fertility of Brahman cross, Holstein Friesian cross and Red Chittagong breeding bulls. *Bangladesh Journal of Animal Science*, *47*(2), 61–67. https://doi.org/10.3329/bjas.v47i2.40236

Kaiin, E., Gunawan, M., Octaviana, S., & Nuswantara, S. (2017). *Verifikasi molekuler metode sexing sperma sapi dengan kolom BSA (Bovine Serum Albumin)*. *3*, 241–245. https://doi.org/10.13057/psnmbi/m030214

Khamlor, T., Pongpiachan, P., Sangsritavong, S., & Chokesajjawatee, N. (2014). Determination of sperm sex ratio in bovine semen using multiplex real-time polymerase chain reaction. *Asian-Australasian Journal of Animal Sciences*, *27*(10), 1411–1416. https://doi.org/10.5713/ajas.2014.14223

Kusumawati, E. D., Rahadi, S., Isnaini, N., Wahjuningsih, S., Abdullah, A. G., Agustina, R., & Susilawati, T. (2018). Effect of different extender on the quality of sexing sperm before freezing in limousin cattle. *IOP Conference Series: Materials Science and Engineering*, *434*(1). https://doi.org/10.1088/1757-899X/434/1/012102

Machado, G. M., Carvalho, J. O., Filho, E. S., Caixeta, E. S., Franco, M. M., Rumpf, R., & Dode, M. A. N. (2009). Effect of Percoll volume, duration and force of centrifugation, on in vitro production and sex ratio of bovine embryos. *Theriogenology*, *71*(8), 1289–1297. https://doi.org/10.1016/j.theriogenology.2009.01.002

Mardi, I., Yekti, A. P. A., Kuswati, K., Luthfi, M., & Susilawati, T. (2020). Kualitas semen beku sexing sapi peranakan ongole menggunakan volume semen awal yang berbeda. *Jurnal Ilmu dan Teknologi Peternakan Tropis*, *7*(3), 238. https://doi.org/10.33772/jitro.v7i3.12203

Maulana, T., Said, S., Arifiantini, R. I., & Setiadi, M. A. (2019). Sex sorting sperm of sumba ongole bulls by using snakehead fish (Channa striata) albumin extract. *Journal of the Indonesian Tropical Animal Agriculture*, *44*(1), 106–113. https://doi.org/10.14710/jitaa.41.1.106-113

Meitei, H. Y., Uppangala, S., Sharan, K., Chandraguthi, S. G., Radhakrishnan, A., Kalthur, G., Schlatt, S., & Adiga, S. K. (2021). A simple, centrifugation-free, sperm-sorting device eliminates the risks of centrifugation in the swim-up method while maintaining functional competence and DNA integrity of selected spermatozoa. *Reproductive Sciences*, *28*(1), 134–143. https://doi.org/10.1007/s43032-020-00269-5

Nurcholis., F. A., Arifiantini, R. I., & Salamony, S. M. (2021). Supplementation of pandanus conoideus oil in cryopreservation diluents for maintaining the semen quality of ongole grade bull. *Tropical Animal Science Journal*, *44*(2), 146–151. https://doi.org/10.5398/TASJ.2021.44.2.146

Nurcholis., Salamony, S. M., Muchlis, D., & Prahesti, K. I. (2019). System application of artificial insemination technology to the welfare level of cattle breeders in Merauke. *IOP Conference Series: Earth and Environmental Science*, *343*(1). https://doi.org/10.1088/1755-1315/343/1/012169

Prasad, S. C., Rangasamy, S., & Satheshkumar, S. (2010). Sex preselection in domestic animals - current status and future prospects. *Veterinary World*, *3*(7), 346–348. https://doi.org/10.5455/vetworld.2010.346-348

Prastiya, R. A., Suprayogi, T. W., Debora, A. E., Wijayanti, A., Amalia, A., Sulistyowati, D., & Nugroho, A. P. (2023). Green tea extract addition into a tris-based egg yolk extender improves bali bull sperm quality. *Animal Bioscience*, *36*(2), 209–217. https://doi.org/10.5713/ab.22.0184

Quelhas, J., Santiago, J., Matos, B., Rocha, A., Lopes, G., & Fardilha, M. (2021). Bovine semen sexing: Sperm membrane proteomics as candidates for immunological selection of X- and Y-chromosome-bearing sperm. *Veterinary Medicine and Science*, *7*(5), 1633–1641. https://doi.org/10.1002/vms3.540

Ribas-Maynou, J., & Benet, J. (2019). Single and double strand sperm DNA damage: Different reproductive effects on male fertility. *Genes*, *10*(2). https://doi.org/10.3390/genes10020105

Romadhoni, A. R., Afrianto, E., Pratama, R. I., & Grandiosa, R. (2016). Extraction of snakehead fish [*Ophiocephalus striatus* (Bloch, 1793)] into fish protein concentrate as albumin source using various solvent. *Aquatic Procedia*, *7*, 4–11. https://doi.org/10.1016/j.aqpro.2016.07.001

Steinhauser, C. B., Graham, J. K., Lenz, R. W., & Seidel, G. E. (2016). Removing seminal plasma improves bovine sperm sex-sorting. *Andrology*, *4*(6), 1131–1137. https://doi.org/10.1111/andr.12245

Tanga, B. M., Qamar, A. Y., Raza, S., Bang, S., Fang, X., Yoon, K., & Cho, J. (2021). Semen evaluation: Methodological advancements in sperm quality-specific fertility assessment - A review. *Animal Bioscience*, *34*(8), 1253–1270. https://doi.org/10.5713/ab.21.0072

Teken, G. E., Yusuf, M., Said, S., & Toleng, A. L. (2020). The quality of sexed sperm separated using bovine serum albumin column and extended using tris aminomethane at different temperatures. *IOP Conference Series: Earth and Environmental Science*, *492*(1). https://doi.org/10.1088/1755-1315/492/1/012067

Tungadi, R. (2020). Potensi ikan gabus (*Ophiocephalus striatus*) dalam mempercepat penyembuhan luka. *Jambura Fish Processing Journal*, *1*(1), 46–55. https://doi.org/10.37905/jfpj.v1i1.4505

Utami, T., Tophianong, C., & Tarsisius. (2014). Pengaruh suhu thawing pada kualitas spermatozoa sapi pejantan the effect of thawing temperature on sperm quality of friesian holstein. *Jurnal Sain Veteriner*, *32* (1), 32–39.

Wolf, C., Brass, K., Rubin, M. I., Pozzobon, S., Mozzaquatro, F., & De La Corte, F. (2008). Effect of sperm selection by "Swim-Up" technique on the sex ratio of in vitro produced ovine embryos. *The Iraqi Journal of Veterinary Medicine*, *37*(2), 175–179. https://doi.org/10.30539/iraqijvm.v37i2.279

Technological Innovations in Tropical Livestock Development for Environmental Sustainability and Food Security – P. Dhian Isnaeni et al. (eds)

Portrait of body weight of swamp buffalo based on weighing and using a rondo measuring tape in South Konawe district

L.O. Nafiu*, T. Saili, M. Abadi, R. Badaruddin & F.A. Auza
Department of Animal Science, Faculty of Animal Science, Halu Oleo University, Indonesia

ABSTRACT: This research aimed to analyze the body weight of swamp buffalo based on weighing and using a rondo measuring tape in different sub-districts, sexes and ages in South Konawe Regency. The parameters observed included: body weight at the age of 1–12 years which is weighed directly and using a rondo measuring tape. The study showed that the body weight of swamp buffalo in South Konawe Regency is significantly affected by age ($P<0.05$). The average body weight of swamp buffalo in South Konawe Regency based on weighing 467.38 ± 146.57 kg. It was lower than the body weight of a rondo measuring tape which is 532.47 ± 200 and weighed 60 kg with an average difference of 65.09 kg and an average deviation of 13.93%. Female swamp buffalo tend to have a higher body weight than that of male buffalo. Based on the result, it can be concluded that the rondo measuring tape is less accurate for estimating the body weight of swamp buffalo in the South Konawe District.

Keywords: Swamp buffalo, body weight, weighing, rondo measuring tape

1 INTRODUCTION

Domestic meat production capabilities are currently unable to meet people's meat needs. Imports of frozen meat and feeder cattle from abroad in 2022 will amount to 265,065 tons or 37.67% of total needs (Livestock and Animal Health Statistics 2022). Beef imports have increased from year to year (Nafiu *et al.* 2017 and 2020a). One of the government's steps to fulfil meat needs is to increase domestic meat production from buffalo. Buffalo livestock plays an important role in increasing national meat production, considering that its performance is not much different from beef cattle and its existence has been integrated with the social, economic and cultural life of the community (Nafiu *et al.* 2015).

Swamp buffalo have several advantages, including being able to adapt to a fairly bad environment by using low-quality feed and having a good response to improvements in feed (dan 2018; Nafiu *et al.* 2017), and can be used as a source of labour and food diversity (Dude *et al.* 2011 and Sembiring *et al.* 2013). However, the buffalo farming business also has several weaknesses, such as a lack of public and government attention to increasing buffalo production and low reproductive performance (Nafiu *et al.* 2013; Nafiu *et al.* 2020b and Nafiu *et al.* 2020c).

National buffalo population trends have fluctuated. In 2020 the population of buffalo in Indonesia was 1,154,226, to 1,143,189 in 2021, then to 1,170,209 in 2022 (Livestock Statistics and Animal Health, 2022). In recent years, the development of the buffalo population in Southeast Sulawesi Province has been quite encouraging. In 2019 the buffalo population was only 2,162, increasing to 2,668 in 2022 (BPS Southeast Sulawesi 2023) with an average increase rate of 7.80% per year.

*Corresponding Author: ldnafiu@gmail.com

DOI: 10.1201/9781003468943-13

South Konawe Regency is one of the swamp buffalo development areas in Southeast Sulawesi Province. The development of the buffalo population in this area in the last four years has been quite rapid. In 2019 the population was 191 heads, growing to 351 heads in 2022 (BPS Southeast Sulawesi 2020 and 2023) with an average increase rate of 27.95% per year. Most of the buffalo population in South Konawe Regency is concentrated in Mowila and Angata Districts with a total of 291 head in 2022 or covering 82.91% (BPS South Konawe 2023). Mowila and Angata sub-districts can be used as buffalo development centres in South Konawe Regency.

Morphometric characteristics, especially body weight, are important basic information in the buffalo farming business because they have high economic value and greatly determine selling value. However, determining the weight of buffalo in rural areas is difficult because adequate weighing equipment is not available. Recently, the body weight of ruminant livestock, including buffalo, has been estimated using a rondo measuring tape. The use of a rondo measuring tape in estimating body weight needs to be evaluated for accuracy. This study aimed to evaluate the body weight of swamp buffalo based on weighing and using a rondo measuring tape in the South Konawe Regency.

2 RESEARCH METHODOLOGY

This research was carried out in South Konawe Regency, covering two sub-districts, namely: Mowila District and Angata District. The research location was determined purposively because the sub-district has the highest buffalo population in the South Konawe Regency. Field observations were carried out for 3 months, August – October 2023.

The material used was 150 swamp buffalo aged 1–12 years, consisting of 37 male buffalo and 113 female buffalo. Other materials used are a list of questions and writing tools. The equipment used includes: (1) digital scales with a capacity of 1500 kg for weighing the buffalo's body weight, (2) clamp cage measuring 1 m X 2 m for weighing and measuring body dimensions, and (3) random measuring tape for measuring chest circumference.

2.1 *Observed variables*

The observed variables and their measurement methods are as follows:

(1) Body weight was measured by placing the buffalo on a digital scale (kg).
(2) Chest circumference was measured by circling a measuring tape just behind the scapula, using a rondo measuring tape (cm).

The age of the buffalo is determined based on information from the farmer/livestock worker and based on the condition of the buffalo's teeth and horns.

2.2 *Data*

Body weight data is grouped based on sub-district area, sex and age of the buffalo. The data obtained was analyzed to the mean, standard deviation and coefficient of diversity based on Walpole (1982), using the following equation:

$$\bar{X} = \frac{\sum_{i=1}^{n} Xi}{n} \qquad s = \sqrt{\frac{\sum_{n-1}^{n} (X_i - \bar{X})^2}{n-1}}$$

$$VC = \frac{s}{\bar{X}} \times 100\%$$

Where:
$\bar{X}$ = Means   s = Standard Deviation
$\bar{X}_i$ = the sample size of variable x   n = number of samples
VC = Variation Coefficient

To analyze the sources of variation in factors such as sub-district area, sex and age of buffalo, use analysis of variance "General Linear Model (GLM)", with a mathematical equation model as follows:

$$Y_{ijk} = u + A_i + B_j + AB_{ij} + \epsilon_{ijk} Y_{ijk} = u + A_i + B_j + AB_{ij} + \epsilon_{ijk}$$

Y_{ijk} = Observation value of Factor A at level-i, Factor B at level-j and replication at k
u = Mean
A_i = Effect of Factor A at level i
B_j = Effect of Factor B at level j
AB_{ij} = interaction of factor A and factor B
ϵ_{ijk} = The effect of the error on Factor A at level-i, Factor B at level-j and the k replication.

The buffalo's body weight needs to be corrected to obtain uniform data for each age class. Buffalo less than 1-year-old is corrected to 1 year old, less than 2 years old is corrected to 2 years old, less than 3 years old is corrected to 3 years old and buffalo less than 4 years old is corrected to 4 years old.

$$BW_{year} = \left(\frac{BWG}{month} \times \frac{Age_{month} * Age_{year}}{AC_{year}}\right) + BiW$$

$$BWG/month = \left(\frac{BW - BiW}{month}\right)$$

Where:
BWG = body weight gain   AC = Age Class   BiW = Birth weight.

To calculate the magnitude of the deviation from estimating body weight using a rondo measuring tape against weight, use the following equation:

$$Deviation_{(\%)} = \left(\frac{MW - WW}{WW}\right) \times 100\%$$

Where:
MW = Measuring weight   WW = Weighing weight.

3 RESULTS AND DISCUSSION

3.1 *The influence of district area and age on body weight of swamp buffalo*

A portrait of buffalo body weight based on weighing results and using a rondo measuring tape according to sub-district area, sex and age of buffalo in South Konawe Regency in Table 1.

The average body weight of buffalo based on weighing is 468.43 ± 151.37 kg, and a rondo measuring tape was 539.19 ± 205.99, or 65.09 kg. The prediction resulted in a lower number than that of direct weighing using a digital scale, with a 13.93% deviation. The deviation from body weight estimation based on the rondo measuring tape obtained in this study was lower than the finding of Naibaho *et al.* (2016) which obtained an estimation bias of 23.50%. However, estimating body weight using the Schoorl and Smith formula obtained smaller deviations which were 9.45% and 4.60% respectively (Naibaho *et al.* 2016).

The body weight of swamp buffalo obtained in this study was higher than that of swamp buffalo in Bombana Regency, namely 452.50 ± 121.00 on Kabaena Island and

377.30 ± 100.06 kg in South Poleang District (Nafiu *et al.* 2015). Chantalakhana and Skunmum (2002) reported that the body weight of adult swamp buffalo in Thailand ranges from 350 to 650 kg. Likewise, Shackleton and Harestad (2003) reported that the body weight of swamp buffalo in China is 250 kg, and in Myanmar around 300 kg.

Table 1. The average and standard deviation of swamp buffalo body weight based on weighing (weighing weight) and based on rondo measuring tape (measuring weight) (kg) according to district and age in South Konawe Regency.

			Weighing Weight		Measuring Weight		
Sub District	Age (year)	Replication (n)	Mean ± Sd	VC (%)	Mean ± Sd	VC (%)	Deviation (%)
Angata	1	14	248.07 ± 50.76	20.46	226.43 ± 67.55	29.83	8.72
	2	7	344.00 ± 72.64	21.12	345.14 ± 53.34	15.45	0.33
	3	8	410.38 ± 57.83	14.09	500.88 ± 99.27	19.82	22.05
	4	4	547.00 ± 36.68	6.71	652.75 ± 45.50	6.97	19.33
	5	5	580.80 ± 56.33	9.70	719.00 ± 55.01	7.65	23.79
	6	31	582.77 ± 69.42	11.91	690.48 ± 71.69	10.38	18.48
	Total	69	468.43 ± 151.37	32.31	539.19 ± 205.99	38.20	15.11
Mowila	1	13	220.38 ± 44.18	20.05	218.62 ± 58.83	26.91	0.80
	2	10	355.40 ± 71.46	20.11	325.40 ± 63.90	19.64	8.44
	3	7	458.29 ± 61.21	13.36	456.43 ± 116.85	25.60	0.41
	4	3	565.67 ± 99.14	17.53	646.00 ± 128.42	19.88	14.20
	5	5	539.00 ± 41.94	7.78	673.67 ± 118.76	17.63	24.99
	6	43	552.70 ± 75.18	13.60	652.26 ± 90.06	13.81	18.01
	Total	81	466.48 ± 143.29	30.72	526.74 ± 196.99	37.40	12.92
Total	1	27	234.74 ± 48.87^{a}	20.82	222.67 ± 62.41	28.03	5.14
	2	17	350.71 ± 69.89^{b}	19.93	333.53 ± 58.85	17.65	4.90
	3	15	432.73 ± 62.37^{c}	14.41	480.13 ± 106.33	22.15	10.95
	4	7	555.00 ± 63.63^{d}	11.46	649.86 ± 80.90	12.45	17.09
	5	10	559.90 ± 51.74^{d}	9.24	694.27 ± 93.93	13.53	24.00
	6	74	565.30 ± 73.86^{d}	13.07	668.49 ± 84.39	12.62	18.25
	Total	150	467.38 ± 146.57	31.36	532.47 ± 200.60	37.67	13.93
Average Body Weight Deviation Based on Rondo Measuring Tape: 13.93%							
Effect of Sub-district			ns		ns		
Effect of Age			**		**		
Interaction of Sub-district and Age			ns		ns		

Note: ns = not significant (P>0,05); ** = Significant (P<0,05). VC = Variation Coefficient (%) Sd = Deviation standard.

Based on the results, the sub-district area has no significant effect (P>0.05) on the body weight of swamp buffalo in the South Konawe Regency. However, the age of the buffalo has a significant effect (P<0.05) on body weight. As the age increases, the buffalo's body weight becomes higher, but after 6 years or more the buffalo's body weight relatively increases and decreases.

The average body weight of adult swamp buffalo obtained in this study ranged from 432.73 to 565.30 kg. This is higher than Gerli *et al.* (2014) who reported that the average body weight of female swamp buffalo at the Siborongborong Pig and Buffalo BPTU, North Tapanuli Regency, North Sumatra aged 2–3.5 years was 223.65 ± 16.28 and aged 3.5–7.0 years was 398.00 ± 38.46 kg, male swamp buffalo aged 2–3.5 is 305.17 ± 16.44 kg and aged 3.5–7.0 yo is 462.17 ± 43.67 kg. Meanwhile, Sumantri *et al.* (2021) reported that the body weight of Kalimantan swamp buffalo for males with an average age of 3.4 years was

392.7 ± 104 kg. The body weight of a 2-year-old Sumbawa swamp buffalo is 268.0 kg, a 3-year-old is 306.4 kg, a 4-year-old is 319.1 kg and a 5-year-old is 359.5 kg (Anggraeni and Triwulanningsih 2007).

3.2 *Influence of sex and age on body weight of swamp buffalo*

The average and standard deviation of swamp buffalo body weight based on body weight results and rondo measuring tape (kg) according to sex and age in South Konawe Regency in Table 2.

Table 2. Average and Standard Deviation of Swamp Buffalo Body Weight Based on Weighing and Using a Rondo Measuring Tape (kg) According to Sex and Age in South Konawe Regency.

			Weighing Weight		Measuring Weight	
Sex	Age (year)	Replication (n)	Mean ± Sd	VC (%)	Mean ± Sd	VC (%)
Male	1	14	226.71 ± 46.90	20.69	215.93 ± 61.25	28.37
	2	6	334.83 ± 68.80	20.55	302.00 ± 58.60	19.40
	3	7	396.86 ± 47.49	11.97	463.00 ± 115.00	24.84
	4	2	553.50 ± 41.72	7.54	644.00 ± 19.80	3.07
	5	3	576.67 ± 97.77	16.95	663.00 ± 160.10	24.15
	6	5	568.20 ± 46.79	8.23	608.60 ± 128.00	21.03
	Total	37	368.62 ± 147.87	40.11	389.08 ± 194.51	49.99
Female	1	13	243.38 ± 51.33	21.09	229.92 ± 65.30	28.40
	2	11	359.36 ± 72.22	20.10	350.73 ± 53.88	15.36
	3	8	464.13 ± 58.60	12.63	495.13 ± 103.57	20.92
	4	5	555.60 ± 75.08	13.51	652.20 ± 98.47	15.10
	5	8	575.63 ± 54.19	9.41	706.00 ± 68.59	9.72
	6	68	562.57 ± 74.55	13.25	672.90 ± 79.93	11.88
	Total	113	99.72 ± 131.43	26.30	579.42 ± 179.88	31.04
Total	1	27	234.74 ± 48.87	20.82	222.67 ± 62.41	28.03
	2	17	350.71 ± 69.89	19.93	333.53 ± 58.85	17.65
	3	15	432.73 ± 62.37	14.41	480.13 ± 106.33	22.15
	4	7	555.0 ± 63.63	11.46	649.86 ± 80.90	12.45
	5	11	575.91 ± 62.99	10.94	694.27 ± 93.93	13.53
	6	73	562.96 ± 72.77	12.93	668.49 ± 84.39	12.62
	Total	150	467.38 ± 146.57	31.36	532.47 ± 200.60	37.67
Average Body Weight Deviation Based on Rondo Measuring Tape: 13.93%						
Effect of Sex			ns		ns	
Effect of Age			**		**	
Interaction of Sex and Age			ns		ns	

Based on Table 2, age has a significant effect (P<0.05) on weight weighing and measuring weight of swamp buffalo. However, sex and its interaction with age have no significant effect (P>0.05) on the body weight of swamp buffalo in South Konawe Regency.

The results of this study also found that male swamp buffalo had a lower body weight compared to female swamp buffalo, although statistically, it was not significantly different (P>0.05). This may be caused by the following factors: (1) adult male buffalo with good performance have been sold, (2) generally male buffalo are only kept and remain in the population until the age of 3 years, and (3) male buffalo with low body weight performance low is maintained longer in the population. Nafiu *et al.* (2015) reported that breeders in Bombana Regency generally sell male swamp buffalo that have good performance, for example, high body weight, because buyers are interested in them and are willing to pay high prices. The higher the body weight and better the body condition of the male buffalo, the higher the selling value. As a result, male livestock with high performance will be sold quickly, while those with less performance will still be kept and produce offspring (Nafiu *et al.* 2015).

The average body weight of male buffalo for all age classes (1-12 years) was 368.62 ± 147.87 kg, while female buffalo was 499.72 ± 131.43 kg. This is higher than Galib *et al.* (2017) who reported the results of their research on swamp buffalo in Babakan District, Cirebon Regency, that the average body weight of male buffalo was 376.30 ± 3.90 and female 409.30 ± 5.10 kg. Meanwhile, the body weight of a female Surti buffalo aged 1 year is 130.96 ± 2.59 and male is 130.05 ± 2.84 (Pandya *et al.* 2015). Dahlan *et al.* (2019) reported that the average body weight of adult male buffalo (aged 3 years or more) on Kabaena Island, Bombana Regency was 503.8 ± 70.5 kg, while that of females was 527.0 ± 43.2 kg. Pipiana (2010) reported that the body weight of buffalo on Moa Island at the same age was 295.09 kg. The opposite situation was reported by Sumantri *et al.* (2022) that adult male Kalimantan swamp buffalo (kalang buffalo) have an average body weight of 380.2 ± 110 kg, which is higher for female buffalo, namely 312.4 ± 116 kg.

The results of this study are relatively not much different from the body weight of swamp buffalo in Sragen Regency, Central Java aged 3 years, namely 445.2 ± 11.9 in males and 516.7 ± 7.7 in females (Nastiti *et al.* 2023). Likewise with the research results of Mufiidah *et al.* (2013) who reported the average body weight of swamp buffalo in Tempursari Regency was 406.82 ± 9.97 kg and male buffalo in Serang was 300.3 ± 39.90 kg (Komariah *et al.* 2018).

Variations in body weight of swamp buffalo from various regions may be caused by the following factors: (1) differences in agro-climatic and agroecosystem conditions, (2) the buffalo rearing system applied, (3) availability of feed both in quantity and quality, (4) variations in age, (5) sex ratio, and (6) breeding and reproductive management applied. Besides that, male buffalo usually sell quickly. Nafiu *et al.* (2015) reported that the high number of male buffalo sales in Bombana Regency affected reducing the average weight of male cattle. Negative selection occurs in male buffalo so that their genetic quality decreases. Robbani *et al.* (2010) reported the same situation in swamp buffalo in Bogor Regency and concluded that in general female buffalo in Cibungbulang, Pamijahan, Nanggung and Sukajaya subdistricts had body weights that tended to be higher than male buffalo.

4 CONCLUSION

Based on the results it can be concluded that: (1) the average body weight of swamp buffalo in South Konawe Regency is significantly ($P<0.05$) influenced by age, but not significantly ($P>0.05$) influenced by sub-district area and sex, (2) the average body weight of swamp buffalo in South Konawe Regency based on weighing results (weighing weight) is 467.38 ± 146.57 kg, lower than the body weight using a rondo measuring tape (measuring weight) which is 532.47 ± 200, 60 kg with an average difference of 65.09 kg and an average deviation of 13.93%. Female swamp buffalo tend to have a higher body weight than male buffalo, although statistically, it is not significantly different ($P>0.05$). The Rondo measuring tape is less accurate for estimating the body weight of swamp buffalo in South Konawe Regency.

ACKNOWLEDGEMENTS

The author expresses his deepest thanks and appreciation to all parties involved in the research, especially the Head of LPPM UHO who funded the research and the students involved in the research.

REFERENCES

Anggraeni, A. & Triwulanningsih, E., 2007. Keragaan bobot badan dan morfometrik tubuh kerbau Sumbawa terpilih untuk penggemukan. *Seminar dan Lokakarya Nasional Usahaternak Kerbau*; 124–131.

BPS South Konawe Regency, 2023. South Konawe Regency in Figures for 2022. *BPS South Konawe Regency*, Andolo.

BPS Southeast Sulawesi, 2023. Southeast Sulawesi in Figures for 2022. *BPS Southeast Sulawesi, Kendari*, Kendari

BPS Southeast Sulawesi, 2020. Southeast Sulawesi in Figures for 2019. *BPS Southeast Sulawesi*, Kendari

Chantalakana, C, and P. Skunmun. 2002. *Sustainable smallholder animal systems in the tropics*. 1 Edition, Kasetsart University Press. Bangkok.

Dahlan, R., Nafiu dan, L. O., Aku, A. S., 2019. Korelasi antara ukuran-ukuran tubuh dan bobot badan ternak kerbau di Pulau Kabaena Kabupaten Bombana. *Ind. J. Anim. Agric. Sci.*, 1(1): 21–27. 9154-25590-1-PB.pdf

Direktortat Jenderal Peternakan dan Kesehatan Hewan, 2023. *Statistik Peternakan Republik Indonesia Tahun 2022. Direktortat Jenderal Peternakan dan Kesehatan Hewan*, Kementerian Pertanian Republik Indonesia, Jakarta.

Dude, C. Sumantri, H. Martojo, dan A. Anang. 2011. Keragaan sifat kualitatif dan kuantitatif kerbau lokal di Propinsi Banten. *Jurnal Ilmu Ternak*, 11 (2): 61–67.

Galib, I., C. Sumantri dan A. Gunawan. 2017. Aplikasi ukuran linier tubuh sebagai penduga bobot badan pada kerbau rawa. *Jurnal Ilmu Produksi dan Teknologi Hasil Peternakan* Vol. 05(1): 41–45. January 2017. ISSN 2303-2227. 19626-Article Text-60280-1-10-20180124.pdf

Gerli, Hamdan dan A. H. Daula. 2014. Karakteristik morfologi ukuran tubuh kerbau murrah dan kerbau rawa di BPTU Siborongborong. *J. Peternakan Integratif* Vol. 1 (3): 276–287. 3973-11481-1-PB (1).pdf

Komariah, Burhanuddin, and N. Permatasari. 2018. Potential and development analysis of swamp buffalo in Serang District. *Jurnal Ilmu Produksi dan Teknologi Hasil Peternakan* 06(3):90–97.

Mufiidah, N., M. N. Ihsan, and H. Nugroho. 2013. The productivity of female swamp buffaloes (Bubalus bubalis carabanesis) in terms of reproductive performance and body measurements at Tempursari Subdistrict Lumajang Regency. *Jurnal Ternak Tropika* 14 (1):21–28. Produktivitas-Induk-Kerbau-Rawa-Bubalus-Bubalis-Carabanesis-Ditinjau-Dari-Aspek-Kinerja-Reproduksi-Dan-Ukuran-Tubuh-Di-Kecamatan-Tempursari-Kabupaten-Lumajang.pdf

Nafiu, L.O., dan T. Saili, 2013. Portrait of reproductive management implementation on buffalo breeding in Bombana District. *Proceeding: Buffalo International Conference 2013-"Buffalo and Human Welfare"*. Makassar 4-5 November 2013: pp 122–131. http://karyailmiah.uho.ac.id/karya-ilmiah.php?read=8625

Nafiu, L.O., T. Saili and A. Bain. 2015. Morphometric portrait of swamp buffalo in Bombana. *Journal: Proceeding: International Seminar: Improving Tropical Animal Production for Food Security*. pp 94–107. Kendari 3-5 November 2015. ISBN 978-602-8161-91-6. http://ojs.uho.ac.id/index.php/P-ISITAPFFS/article/view/1132/780

Nafiu, L.O., T. Saili, A. Madiki, R. ahman, Suparman dan R.Badaruddin. 2017. Growth performance of young bull buffalo in feed improvement program. *Proceedings: International Conference: Preparing Human Resources for Global Enterpreneurship*. Kendari 21 Oktober 2017: pp 48–56. ISBN: 978-602-51921-0-4. http://karyailmiah.uho.ac.id/karya-ilmiah.php?cari=la+Ode+nafiu

Nafiu, L.O., T. Saili, A. Bain, Muhidin, M. Rusdin and R. Badaruddin. 2018. Response of selected heifer buffalo to feed improvement in Bombana Regency, Indonesia. *Pakistan Journal of Nutrition* -Volume 17, Issue 12, Bulan November 2018 pp 683–688. ISSN 1680-5194. https://scialert.net/abstract/?doi=pjn.2018.683.688

Nafiu, L.O., M. Abadi, L.O.A. Sani, I. Salam. 2020. Smallholder farm-based buffalo breeding in Bombana Regency was reviewed from a financial feasibility aspect. *International Journal of Scientific & Engineering Research*. Volume 11, Issue 1, Bulan Januari, Tahun 2020, pp 1228–1232. ISSN 2229-5518. https://www.ijser.org/research-paper-publishing-january-2020.aspx

Nafiu, L.O., T. Saili, A. Bain, F. Nasiu, M. Abadi and R. Badaruddin. 2020. Selection of cow buffalo and its effect on reproductive characteristics of swamp buffalo. *Journal: IOP Conference Series: Earth and Environment Science International Conference: Improving Tropical Animal Production for Food Security*. ITAPS IOP Conf. Series: Earth and Environmental Science Volume 465, Nomor 1 (2020) 012043:1-7. Online ISSN 1755-1315. Print ISSN 1755-1037. https://iopscience.iop.org/article/10.1088/1755-1315/465/1/012043/pdf

Nafiu, L.O., Muzuni, M. A. Pagala, W. Kurniawan, dan S. Rahadi. 2020. Identification of growth genes diversity of swamp buffalo using RFLP in Kabaena Island, Bombana District, Southeast Sulawesi,

Indonesia. *Biodiversitas* 21 No 5 pp 1901–1907. ISSN: 1412-033X. E-ISSN: 2085-4722. https://smujo.id/biodiv/article/view/5087

Naibaho, T., Hasnudi dan Hamdan. 2016. Pengembangan model pita ukur dan rumus pendugaan bobot badan berdasarkan lingkar dada pada ternak kerbau. *Jurnal Peternakan Integratif* vol. 4 (2): 173–183. April 2016. file:///C:/Users/lenovo/Downloads/2793-Article%20Text-8718-1-10-20191103%20(1).pdf

Nastiti, N. A., J. Riyanto, R. Dewanti, M. Cahyadi, A. K. Wati, W. Pawestri, and Y. Yant. 2023. Reproduction and Production Performance of Swamp Buffalo (Bubalus bubalis) at the Small-Scale Holder Farmer in Sragen Regency, Central Java, Indonesia. *Jurnal sain Peternaan Indonesia*, vol. 18(3):140–147. (PDF) Reproduction and Production Performance of Swamp Buffalo (Bubalus bubalis) at the Small-Scale Holder Farmer in Sragen Regency, Central Java, Indonesia (researchgate.net)

Pandya, G.M., C.G. Joshi, D.N. Rank, V.B. Kharadi, B.P. Bramkshtri, P.H. Vataliya, P.M. Desai and J.V. Solanki. 2015. Genetic analysis of body weight traits of surti buffalo. *Buffalo Bulletin* (June 2015) vol. 34 (2): 189–195. Body_Weight_Buffalo_Bulletein_Surti_Buffalo.pdf

Pipiana. J., Endang Baliarti., dan I Gede Suparta Budisatria. 2010. Kinerja kerbau betina di Pulau Moa, Maluku. *Buletin Peternakan* vol. 34(1):47–54, ISSN 0126-4400. Pipiana.pdf

Robbani, A. R., Jakaria, dan C. Sumantri. 2010. Karakteristik fenotipik kerbau rawa di Kabupaten Bogor (Phenotypic Characteristic of Swamp Buffalo in Bogor District). *Seminar dan Lokakarya Nasional Kerbau* 2010: 49–56. Karakteristik fenotipik Kerbau rawa di kabupaten bogor (ipb.ac.id)

Sembiring, F., Hamdan dan E. Mirwandhono. 2013. Analisis morfometrik kerbau lumpur (*Bubalus bubalis*) Kabupaten Karo Sumatera Utara *(morphometric analysis of swamp buffalo (Bubalus bubalis*) *Karo District North Sumatra. J. Peternakan Integratif* vol. 1 (2); 134–145. 2222–7092-1-PB.pdf

Shackleton D., Harestad A. 2003. *Bovids, Buffaloes and Bison. Di dalam: M. Hutchins, editor. Grzimek's Animal Encyclopedia. Ed ke-2*. Farmington Hills: Gale groups.

Sumantri, I., Habibah, A. Dwijatmiko, R.G. P. Hidayanto. 2021. Model estimasi bobot badan dan produksi karkas kerbau Kalimantan Selatan yang dipelihara dengan sistem kalang. *Prosiding Seminar Nasional Lingkungan Lahan Basah* Vol. 6(2): p-ISSN 2623-1611, e-ISSN 2623-1980. April 2021. 634-954-1-PB (1).pdf

Sumantri, I., T.S.M. Widi, N. Widyas, Habibah and H. Albana. 2022. *Morphometrics and carcass production of Kalimantan swamp buffalo under extensive production system (Klang)*, Livestock Research for Rural Development 34 (3): 2022. LRRD3432022.pdf

Walpole, R. 1982. Pengantar Statistika. Terjemahan: B. Sumantri. P.T. Gramedia, Jakarta. Download Buku Pengantar Statistika Walpole Pdf – Berbagai Buku

Technological Innovations in Tropical Livestock Development for Environmental Sustainability and Food Security – P. Dhian Isnaeni et al. (eds)
© 2025 The Author(s), ISBN 978-1-032-74373-8
Open Access: www.taylorfrancis.com, CC BY-NC-ND 4.0 license

Identification of growth hormone releasing hormone in Gayo Buffalo (*Bubalus bubalis*) using PCR-RFLP

A. Sofia
Department of Animal Science, Faculty of Agriculture, Syiah Kuala University, Indonesia

E.M. Sari* & M.A.N. Abdullah
Department of Animal Science, Faculty of Agriculture, Syiah Kuala University, Darussalam, Aceh Cattle and Local Livestock Research Center, Indonesia

Gholib & S. Wahyuni
Faculty of Veterinary, Syiah Kuala University, Indonesia

ABSTRACT: The objectives of this research were to the identification of GHRH gen in Gayo buffalo using the PCRRFLP method. GHRH is a hypothalamic hormone which stimulates growth hormone secretion in the pituitary gland. Growth Hormone Releasing Hormone is a hormone that stimulates the synthesis and secretion of Growth Hormone which influences growth. Therefore, the GHRH gene is a genetic characteristic that can be used as a basis for selecting livestock. The objective of this study was to identify polymorphisms Growth Hormone-releasing hormone (GHRH) gene of the Gayo buffalo. A total of 15 blood samples from Aceh Tengah were used to determine polymorphism using the PCR-RFLP method and were detected using endonuclease HaeIII. The isolated DNA using a pair of primers 5'-GTA AGG ATG GCT CTG CCA GGT3 'and GHRH reverse 5'-TGC ATG ATG CTG TCC CTC TGG A-3' produced fragments as long as 451 bp. In this study, there were GHRH/HaeIII genotypes AA genotypes 100%, AB genotype 0% and BB genotype 0%. It could verify that the Gayo buffalo is monomorphic.

1 INTRODUCTION

Ruminants like buffaloes can be employed for labour, milk production, and meat production. In addition, buffalo have a significant percentage of carcasses (Kristanto *et al.* 2006). One of the regencies in Aceh Province is Central Aceh Regency, which had 13,372 Gayo buffalo in population in 2018 (Dinas Peternakan dan Kesehatan Hewan Peternakan 2018).

According to the Republic of Indonesia's Minister of Agriculture's Decree No. 302/Kpts/SR.120/5/2017, issued May 4, 2017, Gayo buffalo is an animal genetic resource from Aceh. The physiological traits of Gayo buffalo include their resistance to harsh conditions, including food and water, their placid and submissive nature, their tolerance for parasitic diseases (fleas, ticks, and worms), their ability to travel great distances in search of food and their their water, and their ability to live in groups under the leadership of Ulu Tawar (a term from the Gayo language). In terms of consumption, the Gayo Highlanders favour buffalo meat over beef. They believe that buffalo meat tastes better than beef (Sari 2020).

Buffalo's population growth, productivity, and output are still below ideal levels at the moment. Buffalo's genetic quality improvement is still far behind that of other cattle, though. As

*Corresponding Author: ekameutiasari@usk.ac.id

DOI: 10.1201/9781003468943-14

an alternative to the selection, improvement based on genetic markers can be applied. The MAS (Marker Assisted Selection) strategy, which bases selection on DNA traits that govern economic variables, is one of the selection strategies that is presently under development.

Hormone Growth Released Growth hormone, which affects growth, is synthesized and secreted by hormones, which are hormones. Thus, a genetic trait that can serve as a foundation for cattle selection is the GHRH gene.

2 MATERIALS AND METHODS

2.1 *DNA isolation*

Samples (15) of fresh blood were isolated with Genomic DNA Genomic DNA was extracted from fresh meats using Pure Link TM Genomic DNA Mini Kits and protocol. DNA extracts were electrophorized on 1% agarose gel stained with SYBRTM Safe (Invitrogen) staining solution. DNA bands were visualized and documented by Gel Imager.

2.2 *Polymerase chain reaction*

The GHRH Gene fragment is PCR amplified using forward primer (5′→3′) GTA AGG ATG CCA GCT CTG GGT[3] and reverse primer (5′→3′) TGC CTG CTC TCC TGG A-3'. A 25 µl PCR reaction containing 1 µl of each primer (final concentration of 50 pmol), 12.5 µl of GoTaq Green PCR master mix (Promega Corporation, Madison, WI), and 120 ng of DNA template was prepared and run using a Bio-Rad thermal-cycler. The PCR conditions used were initial denaturation (1 cycle) at 95 °C for 5 minutes, followed by 40 cycles of three-step PCR reactions consisting of denaturation at 95° for 45 seconds, annealing at 60 °C for 45 seconds and extension at 72 °C for 45 seconds, and ended with a final extension at 72 °C for 5 minutes.

2.3 *Restriction fragment length polymorphism*

The PCR products were digested with HaeIII enzyme for 48 hours at 37 °C. The reaction was prepared by mixing 15 µl of the PCR product with 2.5 ml of 10x digestion buffer, 16.5 µl of nuclease-free water, and 1 IU of Btg I enzyme (Invitrogen). The products were electrophorized in 2,5% agarose gel at 85 Volt for 60 minutes, stained with ethidium bromide, and viewed using a digital gel imager.

2.4 *Data analysis*

The diversity of individual genotypes can be determined from the DNA band found. Each sample is compared based on the same size (marker) and the allele frequency is calculated. Allele frequencies are calculated based on the formula Nei (1987).

$$X_i = \frac{2^{nii} + \sum n_{ii}}{2n}$$

Where: X_i = allele frequency of -i; n_{ii} = Number of individuals with genotype ii; n_{ij} = Number of individuals with genotype ij; n = Total individual sample

3 RESULTS AND DISCUSSION

3.1 *DNA isolation*

The study found that Figure 1 below shows the outcomes of DNA isolation from 15 Gayo buffalo blood samples that were electrophoresed using a 1% agarose visualization using a gel imager. Figure 1 illustrates how the DNA band derived from the separation of DNA from Gayo buffalo blood samples exhibits bright, transparent DNA fragments that are less thick or thin in the agarose well. According to Susanti (2017), higher-quality DNA is obtained if the results of DNA isolation indicate that the DNA is thicker and brighter; conversely, lower-quality DNA is obtained if the results of DNA isolation reveal that the DNA is thinner.

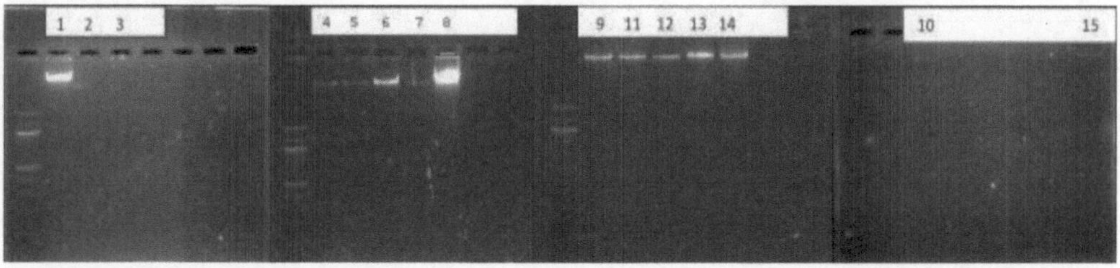

Figure 1. DNA isolation.

From all the separated samples, some had thin bands, and some had stains at the base of the bands where the DNA was found. Anam (2010), believes that the smear that forms on the agarose gel suggests that material other than DNA has been extracted, resulting in a smear beneath the DNA band.

3.2 *Amplification of GHRH gene*

A DNA molecule can be readily and quickly multiplied using the PCR process (Aslinda 2016). Using the Polymerase Chain Reaction (PCR) technique, Growth Hormone Releasing Hormone (GHRH) fragments in DNA Gayo buffalo blood samples were amplified. The PCR results were amplified using two primers. GHRH reverse 5'-TGC CTG CTC ATG ATG TCC TGG A - 3'FSH gene with a primer length of 451 bp and GHRH forward 5'-GTA AGG ATG CCA GCT CTG GGT3'.

Using primers that followed Moody *et al.* (1995) in cattle, the GHRH gene in Gayo buffalo was successfully amplified by PCR (Polymerase Chain Reaction). The effectively amplified native buffalo GHRH gene (Figure 2) had a bp size of 451 and matched the reference DNA sequence.

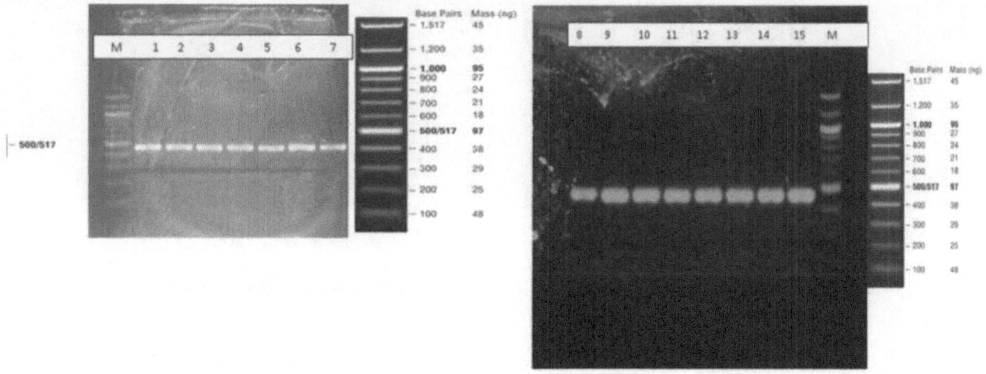

Figure 2. Amplification of GHRH gene.

The PCR reagent material, the circumstances under which the primer is attached to the genomic DNA (target gene), and the state of the PCR machine all play a significant role in the success of the GHRH gene amplification. Viljoen *et al.* (2005) state that the proper concentration and interaction of PCR components are essential for successful DNA amplification. Hemoglobin, an inhibitor that can prevent the Taq polymerase enzyme from working, has an impact on the outcome of DNA amplification as well. Primer attachment temperature, primer concentration, target DNA concentration, and Mg2+ concentration are frequently adjusted in PCR optimization.

3.3 *Detection of GHRH gen in gayo buffalo using PCR-RFLP*

Buffalo cattle have AA genotype if (band) DNA with length 312 pb. The BB genotype is indicated by the presence of four fragments namely 194, 94 pb and 45 pb. Genotype AB shows the livestock has different combinations of genes from its two parents.

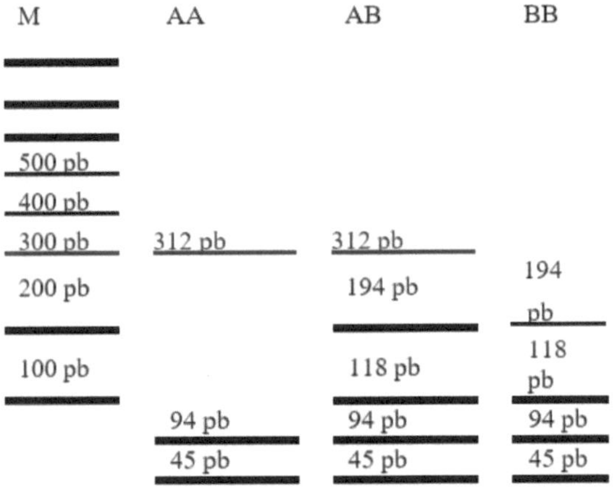

Figure 3. Zymogram of electrophoretic pattern showing the genotypes AA, BB, AB.

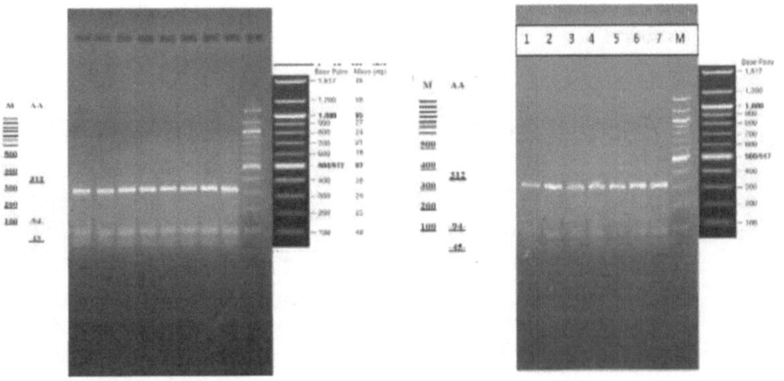

Figure 4. GHRH Gene Fragments using PCR-RFLP method with HaeIII enzymes.

Using the RFLP approach, the GHRH gene diversity in Gayo buffalo was found. HaeIII, a restriction enzyme that can identify four base-cutting sites, was employed in this study. When five pieces of length 312 PB are found in a DNA band measuring 312 long, buffalo cattle are considered to have the AA genotype. Buffalo cattle with the homozygous genotypes AA and BB indicate that both parents contribute equally (alleles), but animals with the heterozygous genotype AB indicate that the cattle genetic makeup differs from that of their parents.

3.4 *Diversity of GHRH gen in gayo buffalo using PCR-RFLP*

The results of this study show that the GHRH gene in Gayo Buffalo is monomorphic (various) across all groups from four regions of Aceh. If an allele has an allele frequency of 0.99 (99%) or less, it is considered monomorphic. When two or more alleles (often more than 1%) are present in a population, genetic diversity arises (Nei.M 1987)

According to Figure 4, two cutting patterns— two bands—are formed. The band that is below the amplification product (homozygous +/+) is referred to as monomorphic (+/+). There is only one allele, the + allele, based on this kind of genotype. The study identified the following genotypes: BB (0%), AB (0%) and AA (100%).

Table 1. Diversity of GHRH-HaeIII gen.

Sample Code	Genotype	Percentage (%)
1 – 15	AA	**100**
	AB	-
	BB	-

Table 2. Genotype frequency of an allele frequency value for GHRH-HaeIII gen.

Sample Code	Genotype	Percentage (%)	Allele Frequency	Genotype frequency
1 – 15	AA	**100**	**1**	**0**
	AB	-	**0**	**0**
	BB	-	**0**	**0**

In this investigation, the AA genotype had a genotype frequency value of 100% for Gayo buffalo, whereas the AB genotype was absent from 15 samples. The findings of this investigation deviate from those of multiple other research that claimed the GHRH gene's AA genotype was infrequently detected. According to research done in 2003 by Dybus *et al.* homozygous $GHRH^A/GHRH^A$ calves had lower birth weights ($p \leq 0.01$) than homozygous GHRHB/GHRHB and $GHRH^B/GHRH^B$ cattle. Moody *et al.* (1995) reported that the fat percentage of FH cattle is influenced by the GHRH allele. Their research demonstrated a correlation between the milk production features of FH cattle and the variety of GHRH/HaeIII. The analysis indicates that the allele frequency of the GHRHs gene in the Gayo Buffalo is monomorphic (uniform), or, to put it another way, that an allele is considered monomorphic if its frequency is equal to or lower than 0.01 (1%) of the total. Numerous processes, including selection, gene mutation, mixing of two populations with different gene frequencies, internal and external crossover, and genetic drift, influence differences in gene and allele frequencies that arise (Yuniarsih 2011).

The findings of this investigation support those of Ishak *et al* (2012), who work on the diversity of the FSH beta-subunit gene as determined by the PCR-RFLP technique. Using Pst1, a restriction enzyme. Whereas no variations (monomorphic) were observed in Bali cattle, only variations (polymorphic) were found in FH, Brahman, Limousine, and Simmental cattle. Genetically, there are a variety of reasons why this might occur, including insufficient sample size, non-occurrence of random mating, population selection, and genetic drift, that is alterations in a small population's gene pool brought about by chance. Due to the bottleneck effect, which results in the formation of new populations and columns with a small number of individuals, genetic drift can happen in many tiny populations (Warwick 1994).

4 CONCLUSION

Drawing from the findings of the conducted research, the subsequent deductions can be made: The GHRH gene was first cut in the Gayo Buffalo, a single genotype truncated homozygous (+/+) was discovered that the gene genotype distribution is monomorphic (uniform) at the start of the GHRH gene cut in Gayo Buffalo.

REFERENCES

Anam, K. 2010. Isolation of Genomic DNA. *Biotechnology*. Agricultural Institute Bogor.

Aslinda, W. dan A. Ahmad. 2016. Isolation and Caracterization Agarose from the Red Makroalga Euchema cottoni for Separating DNA Fragments. *Online Journal of Natural Science*, 5 (3): 307–317.

Kristianto, L. K. 2006. Development of Kalang Buffalo breeding to support agribusiness and agritourism in East Kalimantan. *Proceedings*.

Dybus, A., M. Kmieć, Z. Sobek, W. Pietrzyk & dan B. Wiśniewski. 2003. Associations between growth hormone-releasing hormone (GHRH) and pituitary transcription factor 1 (PIT1) genes and production traits of Limousine cattle. *Arch. Tierz., Dummerstorf* 46 (6): 527–534.

Dinas Kesehatan Hewan dan Peternakan, 2018

Ishak, A. B. L. 2012. Identification of Diversity in The FSH Gene Beta Sub-unit of Gene FSH receptor dan GH Gene of Male Bali Cattle as Marker of Sperm Quality [Disertation]. [Bogor (Indonesia)]: Bogor Agricultural

Nei, M. 1987. *Molecular Evolutionary Genetics*. Columbia University Press. New York.

Sari, E. M., dan M. A. N. Abdullah. 2020. Genetic resource local Gayo buffalo livestock Syiah Kuala University Press. Banda Aceh.

Susanti, D. 2017. *Diversity of Growth Hormone (GH|MspI) in Coastal and Simental Cattle Using PCR-RFLP*. Thesis. Faculty of Animal Husbandry Andalas University. Padang.

Yuniarsih, P., Jakaria, dan Muladno. 2011. Ekspolaration in The Growth Hormone Exon 3 Gene of Etawah (PE), *Saanen dan PESA Crossbread Goats Using PCR-SSCP*. IPB, Bogor.

Warwick, E. J., J. M. Astuti dan W. Hardjosubroto. 1994. Livestock Breeding. Edisi V. Gadjah Mada University Press, Yogyakarta. 45–97.

Technological Innovations in Tropical Livestock Development for Environmental Sustainability and Food Security – P. Dhian Isnaeni et al. (eds)
© 2025 The Author(s), ISBN 978-1-032-74373-8
Open Access: www.taylorfrancis.com, CC BY-NC-ND 4.0 license

Characteristics of qualitative and quantitative traits of village chickens in Gu district, Buton Tengah regency

A. Indi*, Barlinton, R. Badaruddin & LO. Munadi
Department of Animal Science, Faculty of Animal Science, Halu Oleo University, Indonesia

ABSTRACT: This study aimed to determine the qualitative and quantitative characteristics of free-range chickens in Gu District, Central Buton Regency. A total of 300 free-range chickens, comprising 134 roosters and 166 hens, were used for this study. The parameters observed included qualitative characteristics such as coat color, comb shape, and shank color, as well as quantitative characteristics like body weight, chest circumference, back length, wing length, femur length, tibia length, shank length, and beak length. The data were analyzed using descriptive statistical analysis by calculating the mean, standard deviation, and coefficient of variance. The study found that free-range chickens in Gu District, Central Buton Regency, had colorless feathers (53.67%), Columbian feather patterns (31.33%), plain feather patterns (50.67%), silver flickering (66.67%), pea comb shapes (58.00%), and white/yellow shanks (77.67%). Quantitative characteristics comprised a body weight of 1688.95 grams for roosters and 1418.69 grams for hens. The chest circumference was 28.27 cm in roosters and 29.29 cm in hens. The back length was 19.88 cm in roosters and 18.58 cm in hens. The wing length measured 21.61 cm in roosters and 20.88 cm in hens. The femur length was 10.32 cm in roosters and 9.22 cm in hens. The tibia length was 11.51 cm in roosters and 10.59 cm in hens. The shank length for rooster chickens was 9.76 cm, and for hens, it was 9.74 cm. The beak length measured 2.03 cm in rooster chickens and 1.84 cm in hens. The external characteristics of village chickens in the Gu District, Central Buton Regency, include variations in feather color and pattern, comb shape, and leg color. Quantitatively, there are differences in body weight and dimensions between roosters and hens, with roosters tending to have more considerable body weight and dimensions. The population of village chickens in the area exhibits genetic diversity that reflects variations in morphological aspects and body size of the chickens.

1 INTRODUCTION

One of the sources of genetic wealth in Indonesia's local livestock is the village chicken. Village chickens have advantages compared to commercial breeds; they can be raised with either limited or substantial capital, and their care is easy due to their excellent adaptability. Generally, village chickens excel in terms of disease resistance and heat resistance and have better meat and egg quality compared to commercial breeds. However, village chickens also have some weaknesses, such as difficulty obtaining good breeding stock and low productivity, exacerbated by seasonal disease factors such as Newcastle disease. Newcastle Disease (ND) is a highly contagious viral disease in chickens with a high mortality rate. Newcastle Disease (ND) is a highly infectious disease with a high mortality rate caused by the Paramyxovirus genus, Paramyxoviridae family. ND is commonly referred to as *pseudo-fowl pest, pseudovogel-pest, atypical gefugelpest, pseudo-poultry plague, avian pest, avian distemper, ranches disease, tetelo disease, Korean fowl plague*, and a*vian pneumoencephalitis*. This disease can affect poultry, and

*Corresponding Author: amiluddin.indi@uho.ac.id

DOI: 10.1201/9781003468943-15

chickens are highly susceptible to ND infection. In poultry, ND is acute, rapidly spreading, and frequently followed by neurological disorders (Susanti *et al.* 2021). It raises concerns about the declining population of village chickens, and there is a risk that those with specific traits may face extinction (Sujionohadi & Setiawan 2000).

Qualitative traits are characteristics controlled by one or two gene pairs where the differences between their phenotypes are distinct, non-additive, and exhibit continuous variation. Typically, the relationship among chickens is most commonly codominant or incompletely dominant (Noor 2008). External genetic characteristics can be neutral, beneficial, or detrimental, depending on the environment in which the livestock is raised. The environment has no bearing on some significant qualitative traits used to identify a chicken breed, such as feather color, comb color, shank color, and comb shape. Quantitative traits, on the other hand, are measurable characteristics based on the morphological size of the animal's body, serving as the foundation to determine the diversity of morphological body size inherited in subsequent generations. The environment, such as feed and farming practice, has a big impact on many genes that influence these traits. The most economically valuable traits in village chickens are quantitative (Noor 2008). Some quantitative characteristics with economic value in village chickens include body weight, thigh length (femur), calf length (tibia), shank length (tarsometatarsus), and claw circumference. These characteristics can be used as predictors of growth and body weight. These traits are essential in economically assessing village chickens' growth and productivity. Farmers can make more accurate selections of breeding stock with high growth and productivity potential by measuring and understanding quantitative traits. Focusing on qualitative traits can help maintain superior characteristics such as resistance to diseases and heat in the context of village chickens. However, it is important to note that the husbandry environment also plays a significant role in expressing quantitative traits. Therefore, a balanced selection of both traits can provide a holistic approach to breeding efforts to produce resilient, productive, and economically viable village chickens.

2 MATERIAL AND METHODS

The tools used in this research include a measuring tape, a digital scale, writing tools, and a camera. The materials used consist of 300 village chickens, with 134 roosters and 166 hens (chicken aged 6 months to 2 years). Data on qualitative traits were analyzed descriptively, and the observation variables included (1) feather color, (2) shank color, and (3) comb shape. The data that was obtained was analyzed using the descriptive method. To determine the percentage of qualitative traits, the Supranto (1990) equation (1) was applied.

$$p = \frac{\sum x_i}{n} \times 100\% \tag{1}$$

To determine the mean and standard deviation of quantitative traits, the Sudjana (1989 equation (2) was employed.

$$\bar{x} = \frac{\sum x_i}{n} \qquad s = \frac{\sqrt{(\sum (x_i - \bar{x}))}}{n - 1} \tag{2}$$

3 RESULTS AND DISCUSSION

3.1 *Feather phenotype*

3.1.1 *Fur color*

Based on Table 1, village chickens in Gu district, Central Buton Regency, had a frequency of colored feathers in roosters at 52.99% and hen at 40.96%. Meanwhile, for non-colored

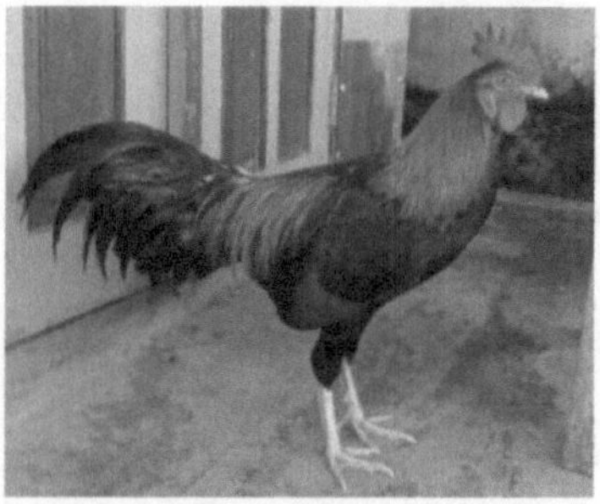

(a)

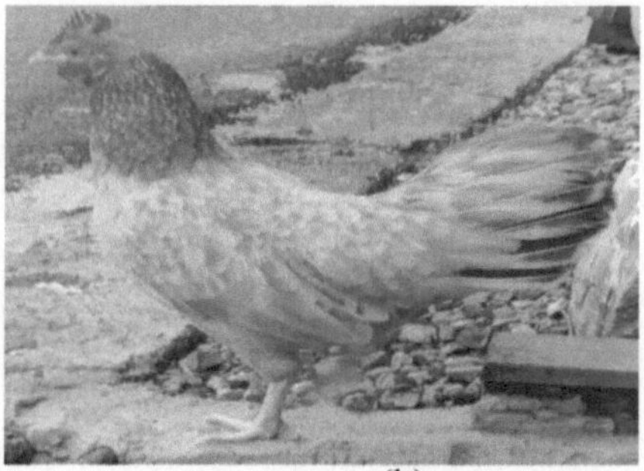

(b)

Figure 1. (a). Performance of male native chickens, (b). Performance of female native chickens.

feathers, the frequency was 47.01% in roosters and 59.64% in hen. There were more colored feathers on roosters and hen in Gu district, Central Buton Regency. Woli *et al.* (2020) found similar results in the Kusambi Subdistrict, West Muna Regency, where most of the feathers were colored (66.49% of roosters and 59.79% of hen). The results suggested a strong genetic link to the feather color pattern in village chickens in these areas.

3.1.2 *Feather pattern*

According to Table 1, the frequency of the Columbian feather pattern was predominant among rooster village chickens in Gu district, Central Buton Regency, at 47.76%, while at 29.10%, black at 13.43%, and wild at 9.70%. White feather patterns made up 31.33% of hen village chickens, while black feather patterns made up 25.90%, wild feather patterns made up 24.70%, and Columbian feather patterns made up 18.07%. The feather pattern in chickens was a major factor in determining the identification process alongside body shape and size, comb shape, and the color of leg scales.

Table 1. Feather phenotype of village chickens in Gu District, Central Buton regency.

	Frequency phenotype					
	Rooster = 134		Hen = 166		Average	
Phenotype	N	%	N	%	N	%
Fur color						
Colorless (II)	63	47.01	98	59.04	161	53.67
Colored (I)	71	52.99	68	40.96	139	46.33
Feather pattern						
Wild (E+-)	13	9.70	41	24.70	54	18.00
Columbian (Ee)	64	47.76	30	18.07	94	31.33
Black (E-)	18	13.43	43	25.90	61	20.33
White (I-cc)	39	29.10	52	31.33	91	30.33
Feather pattern						
Striated (B-)	77	57.46	71	42.77	148	49.33
Plain (Bb)	57	42.54	95	57.23	152	50.67
Feather flicker						
Silver (S-)	80	59.70	120	72.29	200	66.67
Gold (Ss)	54	40.30	46	27.71	100	33.33

Information: N = Sample

The importance of research on the feather color pattern of rooster village chickens in Gu Sub-district, Central Buton Regency, became evident with the dominance of the Columbian feather pattern at 47.76%. Understanding this variation provided insights into the genetic diversity that could be explored to enhance our knowledge of local village chickens. More research was needed to figure out the genetic factors that led to the dominance of the Columbian feather pattern, how they affected superior traits, and the ability of village chickens in the area to adapt. Furthermore, this research also revealed differences in the dominance of feather patterns between rooster and hen village chickens in the Gu district. Although the Columbian feather pattern remained the most dominant in rooster chickens, in hen, the white feather pattern occupied the dominant position with a percentage of 31.33%. Sexual dimorphism in the genetic expression related to feather color patterns caused this difference. Further research on the genetic factors supporting sexual dimorphism in this feather pattern could provide a deeper understanding of the genetic inheritance mechanism in village chickens.

3.1.3 *Plumage pattern*

According to Table 1, rooster village chickens in Gu district, Central Buton Regency, had a frequency of striped feather patterns at 57.46% and plain feather patterns at 42.54%. In comparison, hen village chickens had a frequency of plain feather patterns at 57.23% and striped at 42.77%.

3.1.4 *Feather kerlib*

According to Table 1, the majority of the feather gleam on rooster village chickens in Gu district, Central Buton Regency, was silver (59.70%) and gold (40.30%). In comparison, the majority of hen were silver (72.29%) and gold (27.71%). The results of this study differed from those of Nafiu *et al.* (2020), who reported that rooster village chickens had gold feather gleam at 88.50% and silver at 17.50%, whereas hen village chickens had silver feather gleam at 17.50% and gold at 88.50%. The feather gleam study of rooster village chickens in the Gu district, Central Buton Regency, was very different from the study by Nafiu *et al.* (2020) in the Lasusua Subdistrict. There were significant differences in the distribution of feather colors, with silver and gold being the most common. In the Gu district, silver feathers made up 59.70% of rooster village chickens, and gold feathers made up 40.30%. It was different from Nafiu *et al.'s* (2020) finding that gold feathers shone at 88.50%. It suggests that there were significant differences in genetic inheritance and color variation between village chicken populations in both regions. Similarly, striking differences were also observed in hen village chickens. In the Gu district, silver feather gleam dominated at 72.29%, while gold feather gleam was at 27.71%.

3.2 *Shape of the comb*

Table 2 revealed three types of comb shapes in village chickens in Gu district, Central Buton Regency: the single comb, pea comb, and rose comb. According to the research, the single

Table 2. The shape of the comb of native chickens in Gu District, Central Buton regency.

	Frequency phenotype					
	Rooster = 134		Hen = 166		Average	
Phenotype	N	%	N	%	N	%
Single (Rrpp)	75	55.97	49	29.52	124	41.33
Pea (nP_)	57	42.54	117	70.48	174	58.00
Rose (R_pp)	2	1.49			2	0.67

Information: N = Sample

comb made up 55.97% of the rooster village chickens' combs, with the pea comb coming in second at 42.54% and the rose comb coming in third at 1.49%. In contrast, the pea comb dominated hen village chickens at 70.48% and the single comb at 29.52%. The research results indicating three types of comb shapes in village chickens in Gu district, Central Buton Regency, namely the single comb, pea comb, and rose comb, provided an interesting overview of morphological variations in local village chickens. According to data analysis, the single comb made up 55.97% of the rooster village chickens' combs, with the pea comb coming in second at 42.54% and the rose comb coming in third at 1.49%.

3.3 *Shank color*

Table 3 shows that village chickens in Gu district, Central Buton Regency have two shank colors: yellow/white and black/gray. Yellow/white and black/gray were the dominant shank colors in rooster village chickens, at 82.84% and 17.16%, respectively. Similar to this, yellow/white accounted for 73.49% of the shank color in hen village chickens, and black/gray accounted for 26.51%. Amlia *et al.* (2019) explained that in Buton Regency, village chickens had white or yellow shanks dominating in roosters at 87% and in hen at 69%. Hassan *et al.* (2022) reported that the shank color in rooster chickens was yellow at 26%, black at 25%, gray at 25%, white at 24%, and green at 5%. White was the most prevalent color in hen (53%), followed by green (24%), yellow (19%), gray (2%), and black (2%).

Table 3. Shank color of native chickens in Gu District, Central Buton regency.

	Frequency phenotype					
	Rooster = 134		Hen = 166		Average	
Phenotype	N	%	N	%	N	%
White/Yellow (Id-)	111	82.84	122	7.49	233	77.67
Black/Grey (Idid)	23	17.16	44	26.51	67	22.33

Information: N = Sample

3.4 *Quantitative properties*

Measurement tools could identify quantitative traits, and many gene pairs, as well as environmental factors, influenced these traits.

3.4.1 *Body weight*

Based on Table 4, the body weight of village chickens in Gu district, Central Buton Regency, for roosters was 1688.95 ± 229.55 grams with coefficient of variation (CV) of 13.59%, and for hen, it was 1418.69 ± 247.11 grams with a CV of 17.42%. The diversity values of village chickens in this study for roosters were classified as moderate, while for hen they were classified as high. As stated by Rahmadhani *et al.* (2022), diversity values could be considered high if they were greater than or equal to 15%. The diversity of village chickens could be categorized into three levels: high (CV $\geq$ 15%), moderate (5% < CV < 15%), and low (CV $\leq$ 5%). The body weight of rooster village chickens obtained in this study was almost similar when compared to the quantitative traits of village chickens in the Mawasangka District exhibit coefficients of variation ranging from 8% to 21.4%. The average body weight for males is 1,378.67 gram ± 248.94 gram with a coefficient of variation (CV) of 18.06%, while for females, it is 1,095.53 gram ± 165.39 gram with a CV of 15.10% (Faldano *et al.*

Table 4. Quantitative characteristics of free-range chickens in Gu District, Central Buton Regency.

	Sex			
Variable	Rooster (N=134)	CV%	Hen (N=166)	CV%
BW (gram)	1,688.95 ± 229.55	13.59	1,418.69 ± 247.11	17.42
CC (cm)	28.27 ± 3.85	13.61	29.29 ± 2.03	6.94
BL (cm)	19.88 ± 1.59	8.01	18.50 ± 1.48	8.01
WL (cm)	21.61 ± 1.40	6.47	20.88 ± 1.35	6.49
FL (cm)	10.32 ± 1.08	10.46	9.22 ± 0.95	10.27
TL (cm)	11.51 ± 1.38	12.03	10.59 ± 1.28	12.13
ShL (cm)	9.76 ± 1.28	13.16	9.74 ± 1.38	14.21
BeL (cm)	2.03 ± 0.31	15.21	1.84 ± 0.25	13.58

Information: BW (body weight), CC (chest circumference), BL (back length), WL (wing length), FL (femur length), TL (tibial length), ShL (shank length), BeL (beak length), CV (coefficient of variation)

2023). The average body weight of rooster village chickens reached 1688.95 ± 229.55 grams with a coefficient of variation (CV) of 13.59%, while hen village chickens had an average body weight of 1418.69 ± 247.11 grams with a CV of 17.42%. The CV analysis indicated that the level of diversity in the body weight of hen village chickens was classified as high. In contrast, it was classified as moderate in rooster village chickens.

3.4.2 *Chest circumference*

Based on Table 4, the chest circumference of village chickens in Gu district, Central Buton Regency, for roosters was 28.27 ± 3.85 cm with a coefficient of variation (CV) of 13.61%, and for hen, it was 29.29 ± 2.03 cm with a CV of 6.94%. The chest measurements of the village chickens in this study were very dissimilar from those that Woli *et al.* (2020) reported for the village chickens in Kusambi Subdistrict, West Muna Regency. The roosters' measurements were 14.48 cm ± 1.929 cm with a CV of 13.32%, and the hen measurements were 26.75 cm ± 2.139 cm with a CV of 7.995%. The CV analysis indicated that the level of diversity in chest circumference in rooster village chickens was moderate, while in hen village chickens, it was low.

3.4.3 *Back length*

Based on Table 4, the back length of village chickens in Gu district, Central Buton Regency, for roosters was 19.88 ± 1.59 cm with a coefficient of variation (CV) of 8.01%, and for hen, it was 18.50 ± 1.48 cm with an 8.01% CV. Tamzil & Indarsih (2020) reported that the body length of rooster village chickens was 18.54 cm, and hen were 17.63 cm. However, the back length of village chickens obtained in this study was higher compared to Nafiu *et al.* (2020), who reported that the back length of village chickens in the Lasusua Subdistrict for roosters was 14.17 cm and hen were 12.23 cm. Researchers suspected that the high back length of village chickens in the study was due to the wider age range of the chickens (6 months to 2 years) compared to the literature, which only used chickens at seven months of age. Therefore, the village chickens in the study had more diversity in back length, resulting in a higher average back length.

3.4.4 *Wing length*

Table 4 shows that rooster village chickens in Gu district, Central Buton Regency, had a wing length of 21.61 ± 1.40 cm with a coefficient of variation (CV) of 6.47%, while hen village chickens had a wing length of 20.88 ± 1.35 cm with a 6.49% CV. It was consistent with Woli *et al.* (2020), who stated that observed genetic and environmental factors caused differences in livestock for various traits. The wing length of village chickens in Gu district, Central Buton Regency, as indicated in Table 4, showed significant differences between rooster and hen chickens. The average wing length of rooster village chickens was 21.61 ± 1.40 cm with a coefficient of variation (CV) of 6.47%, while hen village chickens had an average wing length of 20.88 ± 1.35 cm with a CV of 6.49%. The CV analysis classified the level of diversity in the wing length of village chickens in both genders as low.

3.4.5 *Femur length*

Table 4 shows that rooster village chickens in Gu district, Central Buton Regency, had a femur length of 10.32 ± 1.08 cm with a coefficient of variation (CV) of 10.46%, while hen village chickens had a femur length of 9.22 ± 0.95 cm with a 10.27% CV. Hidayat *et al.* (2017) reported that the femur length of village chickens for roosters was 11.75 cm, and for hen, it was 9.91 cm. The body weight of the chickens may have influenced this difference, resulting in a nearly equal femur length in each region. Table 4 shows significant differences in the femur length of village chickens between roosters and hen in Gu district, Central Buton Regency. The average femur length of rooster village chickens was 10.32 ± 1.08 cm with a coefficient of variation (CV) of 10.46%, while hen village chickens had an average femur length of 9.22 ± 0.95 cm with a CV of 10.27%. The CV analysis classified the level of diversity in femur length in both genders of village chickens as high.

3.4.6 *Tibial length*

Table 4 shows that rooster village chickens in Gu district, Central Buton Regency, had a tibia length of 11.51 ± 1.38 cm with a coefficient of variation (CV) of 12.03%, while hen had a tibia length of 10.59 ± 1.28 cm with a 12.13% CV. The results obtained were lower compared to Milas *et al.* (2020), who reported that the tibia length of rooster village chickens was 13.80 cm and hen were 12.60 cm. Thus, the tibia length in each livestock varied differently among individual animals. The average tibia length of rooster village chickens was 11.51 ± 1.38 cm with a coefficient of variation (CV) of 12.03%, while hen village chickens had an average tibia length of 10.59 ± 1.28 cm with a CV of 12.13%. CV analysis classified the level of diversity in tibia length as high in both genders of village chickens.

3.4.7 *Shank length*

Table 4 shows that rooster village chickens in Gu district, Central Buton Regency, had a shank length of 9.76 ± 1.28 cm with a coefficient of variation (CV) of 13.16%, while hen had a shank length of 9.74 ± 1.38 cm with a 14.21% CV. However, Amlia *et al.* (2016) reported that the shank length for rooster village chickens was 8.58 cm, and for hen, it was 7.06 cm, which was shorter than the actual shank length.

3.4.8 *Beak length*

Based on Table 4, it was found that the beak length of village chickens in Gu district, Central Buton Regency, for roosters, was 2.03 ± 0.31 cm with a coefficient of variation (CV) of 15.21%, and for hen, it was 1.84 ± 0.25 cm with a 13.58% CV. The average beak length of rooster village chickens was 2.03 ± 0.31 cm with a coefficient of variation (CV) of 15.21%, while hen village chickens had an average beak length of 1.84 ± 0.25 cm with a CV of 13.58%. CV analysis indicated that the level of diversity in beak length in both genders of village chickens was classified as high. This difference reflected the variation in the morphology of the beaks of local village chickens in the Gu district. The beak length is one of the morphological characteristics that can influence feeding behavior and the adaptation of chickens to their environment. There was also a lot of variation in the length of the beaks, which showed that breeding could be used to improve certain traits, like how well they ate or how well they handled certain environmental conditions.

4 CONCLUSION

These are the conclusions that can be drawn based on the results of this research: For village chickens in Gu district, Central Buton Regency, the most common qualitative traits were non-colored feathers (53.67%), Columbian feather pattern (31.33%), plain feather pattern (50.67%), silver feather glint (66.67%), pea comb shape (58.00%), and white/yellow shank color (77.67%). For village chickens, the most common quantitative trait was winging length, which varied moderately between roosters (6.47%) and hen (6.49%). Meanwhile, the qualitative traits of village chickens were predominantly characterized by non-colored feathers, Columbian feather pattern, plain feather pattern, silver feather glint, pea comb shape, and white/yellow shank color. The diversity in feather color and pattern, comb shape, and shank color provided a clear picture that could be used as identification characteristics in the breeding and conservation of local village chickens.

REFERENCES

Amlia, M. A. & Aka, P. R. 2016. Study of the qualitative and quantitative characteristics of free-range chickens in Lasalimu district, Buton Regency. *Jurnal Ilmu Dan Teknologi Peternakan Tropis 3*(1): 31–39.

Faldano, M. L. A., Badaruddin, R., & Sandiah, N. 2023. Qualitative and quantitative characteristics of village chickens in Mawasangka district. *Halu Oleo Animal Husbandry Scientific Journal*, *5*(4): 318–323.

Hassan, D., Laya, N. K., Ardiantoro, F. I. A., & Dako, S. 2020. Frequency analysis of qualitative characteristics of village chickens. *Animal Science*, *4*(2): 126–132.

Hidayat, Z. 2017. Study of characteristics and body sizes of merawang f2 chickens in petaling village, Bangka Belitung islands. *Bandar Lampung 19–20 Oktober* 2016.

Milas, E. S., Saerang, J. L., Lambey, L. J., & Takaendengan, B. J. 2020. Phenotypic characteristics of several quantitative traits of native chickens in Minahasa. *Zootec*, *40*(2): 603–614.

Nafiu, L, D., Abadi, M. & Wati, I. 2020. Charateristics of qualitantitative and qualitative properties of chicken village in the sub-district Lasusua, orth Kolaka district. *International Journal of Agricultures and Business*. *1*(2): 64–74.

Noor. 2008. External genetic characteristics and morphology of free-range chickens. *Jurnal Ilmu Ternak dan Lingkungan*. Universitas Patimura. Ambon.

Rahmadhani, P., R Badaruddin., & Aka, R. 2022. Phenotypic diversity and estimation of genetic distance of super native chickens using morphometric analysis. *Jurnal Ilmiah Peternakan Halu Oleo*. *4*(1): 13–18.

Sudjana, M. A. 1989. *Statistical Methods, Edisi Kelima*. Bandung: Tarsito

Sujionohadi, K. & Setiawan, A, L. 2000. *Laying village chickens*. Jakarta: Penebar Swadaya.

Supranto, J. 1990. Statistics Theory and Applications, *Edisi Kelima*. Jakarta: Erlangga.

Susanti, W. G., Wicaksono, A., & Basri, C. 2021. The Incidence of Newcastle Disease Amongst Backyard Chicken Farms in District of Barru. *Jurnal Ilmu Pertanian Indonesia*, *26*(3): 379–385.

Woli, L, O., Nafiu, L, O., & Syamsuddin. 2020. External genetic characteristics of free-range chickens in Kusambi District, West Muna Regency, Southeast Sulawesi Province. *Jurnal Ilmiah Peternakan Halu Oleo*, *2*(3): 228–237.

Technological Innovations in Tropical Livestock Development for Environmental Sustainability and Food Security – P. Dhian Isnaeni et al. (eds)

Gas production kinetics, dry matter and organic matter digestibility *in vitro* of liquid smoke mineral block

T.L. Aulyani*, Andy, Ismail & Arwan
Gowa Agriculture Development Polytechnic, Gowa Indonesia

R.A. Nurfitriani
Animal Production Study Program, Department of Animal Science, Politeknik Negeri Jember, Jember, East Java, Indonesia

A.B. Kimestri
Department of Animal Science, Faculty of Animal Science, Universitas Halu Oleo, Kendari, Southeast Sulawesi, Indonesia

ABSTRACT: This research aims to evaluate the supplementation of liquid smoke to mineral blocks on the kinetics and total gas production and Dry Matter Digestibility (DMD) and Organic Matter Digestibility (OMD) *in vitro*. Mineral blocks are feed additives that can be given to livestock with limited feed. The addition of liquid smoke to mineral blocks is expected to provide an antioxidant effect that improves the fermentation process and digestibility. One indicator of feed quality is the kinetics and total gas production produced during the fermentation process. Meanwhile, the higher the digestibility, the more feed that can be consumed. The experimental design was completely randomized with 3 treatments and 5 replications. The treatment was P1; control P2: Mineral Block Liquid Smoke 1% P3: Mineral block liquid smoke 2%. Data analysis used ANOVA and Duncan's advanced test. The parameters measured were gas production kinetics, DMD, and OMD. Based on research results, it is known that the addition of 1–2% liquid smoke mineral blocks can increase total gas production compared to without the addition of liquid smoke. The 1% addition of liquid smoke to the mineral block produces a total gas production value compared to other treatments. Meanwhile, the addition of 1% liquid smoke to mineral blocks significantly increases KCBO. Based on the research above, it was concluded that the supplementation level of liquid smoke added to mineral blocks was 1% and at the same time increased the quality of the basal diet.

Keywords: Liquid Smoke, *in vitro*, Mineral block

1 INTRODUCTION

In general, the main problem raised by the partners of the livestock group was the provision of feed. Cutting and carrying, cutting elephant grass or paddy straw, and giving it to cattle at home is the consequence of livestock custody requiring farmers to provide forage (Abustam *et al.* 2020). One of the contents of forage that is important for livestock is minerals. However, the minerals in the forage cannot fully meet the standard needs of livestock as a result of which some livestock experience mineral deficiencies. Mineral deficiencies cause livestock health problems such as bone brittleness and reproductive disorders. One

*Corresponding Author: tutikla49@gmail.com

DOI: 10.1201/9781003468943-16

alternative that could be a solution is making mineral blocks. Mineral blocks are a supplement that can increase livestock productivity, especially livestock that is fed low-quality feed (only forage). Mineral block supplementation using liquid smoke is one way to increase the nutritional value of mineral blocks. Liquid smoke is a product of the wood pyrolysis process, it's consisted of water, phenol, guaiacol, vanillin, catechol, syringol, carboxaldehyde furans, isoeugenol, pyrone, acetic acid, formic acid, and other carboxylic acids (Andy *et al.* 2020). Fenol contains liquid smoke known as an antibacterial agent that can control microbial growth and length of storage. liquid smoke is a complex mixture consisting of substances that can inhibit the growth of pathogenic bacteria such as E. coli, Staphylococcus aureus, and Candida albicans and functions as a natural antibiotic (Yamauchi *et al.* 2010).

Wood vinegar/pyroligneous acid/liquid smoke/bio-oil is a liquid product from the wood pyrolysis process. It consists of a complex mixture of water, phenol, guaiacol, vanillin, catechol, syringe, carboxaldehyde furans, isoeugenol, pyrone, acetic acid, formic acid, and other carboxylic acids [5]. Liquid smoke with a pH of 2.5–2.8 can function as an insecticide, fungicide, bactericide, and deodorant to treat foul odors from pets (Akakab 2006). The use of liquid smoke for livestock has not been widely used. Therefore, it is necessary to evaluate livestock performance first in a laboratory to minimize risks to livestock health. This evaluation can be carried out using *in vitro* methods. The *in vitro* method is a feed evaluation method using artificial stomachs of ruminant livestock on a laboratory scale. *In vitro*, testing needs to be carried out to find out the quality of the feed provided. Gas kinetics, Dry Matter Digestibility (DMD), and Organic Matter Digestibility (OMD) where measurement can describe whether a feed ingredient can be fermented properly. Apart from that, Dry Matter Digestibility (DMD) and Organic Matter Digestibility (OMD). This research aims to determine the function of adding liquid smoke to mineral blocks on gas kinetics and Dry Matter Digestibility (DMD) and OMD) *in vitro*.

2 MATERIALS AND METHODS

2.1 *Treatments*

Mineral Block Supplement was a modification of Urea Molasses Mineral Block (UMMB). This modification replaced molasses with coconut water and added liquid smoke (Abustam *et al.* 2018). This study used three treatments, to all three, liquid smoke was added at a concentration of 10% (with P0/control) 0%, (P1) 1%, and (P2) 2% in the formulation (w/w). The composition of the feed material in the mineral block is shown in Table 1.

Table 1. Composition of the feed material in mineral block (Abustam *et al.* 2018) with modification.

		Composition (g/kg) at levels of liquid smoke concentration of 10%		
No	Feed materials	(P0) 0%	(P1) 1%	(P2) 2%
1	Coconut water	30	29	28
2	Urea	5	5	5
3	Rice barn	30	30	30
4	Corn	10	10	10
5	Copra meal	10	10	10
6	Tapioca flour	10	10	10
7	Mineral mix	2	2	2
8	Salt	3	3	3
9	Liquid smoke	0	1	2

2.2 *In vitro incubation*

The samples were further incubated *in vitro* with buffered-rumen fluid in four replicates, represented by 5 incubation units per replicate, and conducted for 48 h at 39°C. Gas production was recorded after incubation of 2, 4, 6, 8, 10, 12, 24, dan 48 h. Gas production kinetics was conducted by Menke & Steinngas (1998) and calculated following the equation $p = a + b(1 - e^{-ct})$ (Wereszka & Michałowski 2012); with (a + b) = theoretical maximum of gas production; c = gas production rate. The dry matter and residual samples after 48 h incubation were used to estimate dry matter digestibility (DMD) and organic matter digestibility (OMD) of feed and Total Protozoa (Diaz *et al.* 1993).

2.3 *Parameter measured*

The experiment used a completely randomized design (CRD) with 5 replications, the treatments tested were P0: mineral block; P1: Mineral block + 1% liquid smoke; P2: mineral block + 2% liquid smoke. The parameters observed are: 1). Gas production kinetics 2). Total gas production 3). DMD and 4). DMO (AOAC 2005). Processing data by utilizing analysis of variance (ANOVA) and testing between averages used Duncan, With SPSS.27.

3 RESULTS AND DISCUSSION

3.1 *Gas production*

Data on gas production after 24 hours, 36 hours, and 48 hours of incubation can be seen in Table 2. Total Gas production 24-, 36- and 48-hour incubation ranged from 33.75 ml to 48.50 ml. The addition of liquid smoke in the mineral block increased gas production compared to controls but it was not significantly different (P>0.05). Not only total gas production, maximum gas production, and gas production rate were also not significantly different among treatments. This is thought to be because liquid smoke does not affect the bacterial ecosystem that digests feed in the rumen. This result was in agreement with the results reported by Saenab *et al.*, using biochar and smoke (liquid smoke) from cashew nut shells (Saenab 2018). Although the pH of liquid smoke was 3.75, respectively, they did not cause any negative effect on total gas production as the buffer solution added to the rumen liquor could maintain the pH of the rumen fermentation solution.

Table 2. Gas production after 24 hours, 36 hours, and 48 hours and total gas production.

Treatments	24 h (ml)	36 h (ml)	48 h (ml)	Total gas production (ml/300 mg DM)
P0	33.75 ± 0.50	41.63 ± 0.75	45.88 ± 1.11	9.42 ± 0.26
(P1) 1% LS	36.50 ± 0.41	44.38 ± 1.60	48.50 ± 2.45	10.09 ± 0.56
(P2) 2% LS	35.25 ± 1.55	42.25 ± 2.18	45.38 ± 2.50	9.35 ± 0.59

3.2 *Dry Matter Digestibility (DMD) and Organic Matter Digestibility (OMD)*

Dry matter digestibility, organic matter digestibility, and total protozoa are presented in Table 3. The analysis showed that the addition of Liquid Smoke showed no significant reduction in DMD values compared to control (p >0.05) smoke levels did not significantly reduce DMD compared to controls. Liquid smoke level 1–2% of mineral block ingredients also did not hurt rumen fermentation both in total gas production and gas production rate. This is supported by Saenab *et al.* who described that the addition of liquid smoke from cashew nut shells did not affect any digestibility and gas production (Saenab 2018).

Table 3. Dry matter digestibility, organic matter digestibility, and total protozoa.

Treatments	DMD (%)	OMD (%)	Total Protozoa ($\times 10^5$ /ml)
P0	34.41 ± 1.31	49.72 ± 0.49^{b}	1,51 ± 0.06^{c}
(P1) 1% LS	34.90 ± 2.05	50.11 ± 0.83^{c}	1,33 ± 0.08 ^{b}
(P2) 2% LS	32.90 ± 0.92	46.62 ± 0.55^{a}	1,17 ± 0.11^{a}

Note: DMD = dry matter digestibility, OMD = organic matter digestibility. Different superscripts in the same column show a significant difference at P<0.05. Statistical analysis of each product is tested separately for control.

The content of total phenol in liquid smoke in this experiment was 3.12%, not only did not hurt total gas production and gas production rate, it also did not affect DMD and OMD. Jayanegara reported that phenols at concentrations of more than 5% depressed livestock performance (Jayanegara 2009), so their use in rations needed to be low level. Furthermore, phenolic compounds can interact with proteins that are present in the cell wall or membrane and various enzymes of pathogenic microbes, hence, destroying microbes (Kondo *et al.* 2014).

Table 3 illustrates the effect of the liquid smoke mineral block on protozoa counts. Increasing the level of liquid smoke addition caused a decrease in protozoa count. This decrease in the number of protozoa causes a decrease in DMD and OMD (Newbold 2015). Protozoa have a role in the rumen fermentation process because they can degrade the main components of the feed. One of the ciliated protozoa that have an important role in the rumen is the Diploplastron affine which is common in livestock and can digest cellulose and carbohydrates from grain (Wereszka and Michałowski 2012) Furthermore, holotrich protozoa, although in small amounts, also have enzymes that are responsible for cellulose and hemicellulose degradation. Mosconi *et al.* the decline in protozoa populations also negatively impacts the digestion of fiber which is the main function of the rumen (Mosoni *et al.* 2011).

4 CONCLUSIONS

It is concluded that the addition of liquid smoke on the mineral block had the potency of feed additives in the rumen. Supplementation of the liquid smoke mineral block as a feed additive reduces protozoa without affecting total gas production and gas production rate. The best composi-tion for liquid smoke seen from KCBO and Protozoa is 1% LS.

ACKOWLEDGEMENTS

This study was supported by Politeknik Pembangunan Pertanian Gowa, Ministry of Agriculture, Republic of Indonesia. The authors are also grateful to all staff in the Nutrition Biochemistry Laboratory Universitas Gadjah Mada for their excellent technical assistance throughout the experimental period.

REFERENCES

Abustam, E., Said, M. I., & Yusuf, M. (2018). The effect of antioxidant activity of liquid smoke in feed supplement block on meat functional of muscle longissimus dorsi. *IOP Conference Series: Earth and Environmental Science*, *119*(1). https://doi.org/10.1088/1755-1315/119/1/012046

Abustam, E., Yusuf, M., Said, M. I., & Nahariah, N. (2020, April). The effect of liquid smoke on the properties of Bali beef performance in the feed block during fattening. In *IOP Conference Series: Earth and Environmental Science* (Vol. 492, No. 1, p. 012040). IOP Publishing.

Akakabe, Y., Tamura, Y., Iwamoto, S., Takabayashi, M., & Nyuugaku, T. (2006). Volatile organic compounds with characteristic odor in bamboo vinegar. *Bioscience, Biotechnology, and Biochemistry*, *70*(11), 2797–2799.

Andy, Abustam, E., Malaka, R., & Purwanti, S. (2020). A review of encapsulated liquid smoke. *IOP Conference Series: Earth and Environmental Science*, *492*(1). https://doi.org/10.1088/1755-1315/492/1/012061Anim.Sci. 27 1571–1576

Diaz, A., Avendano, M., & Escobar, A. (1993). Evaluation of Sapindus saponaria as a defaunating agent and its effects on different ruminal digestion parameters. *Livest. Res. Rural Dev*, *5*(2), 1–6.

Jayanegara, A., Makkar, H. P., & Becker, K. (2009). The use of prin ipal component analysis in identifying and integrating variables related to forage quality and methane production. *Journal of the Indonesian Tropical Animal Agriculture*, *34*(4), 241–247.

Kondo, M., Hirano, Y., Ikai, N., Kita, K., Jayanegara, A., & Yokota, H. O. (2014). Assessment of anti-nutritive activity of tannins in tea by-products based on in vitro rumen fermentation. *Asian-Australasian Journal of Animal Sciences*, *27*(11), 1571.

Menke, K.H. and H. Steinngas. 1998. Estimation of energetic feed value obtained from chemical analysis and in vitro gas production using rumen fluid. *Anim Res. Dev*, 28:7–55.

Mohan, D., Pittman Jr, C. U., & Steele, P. H. (2006). Pyrolysis of wood/biomass for bio-oil: a critical review. *Energy & fuels*, *20*(3), 848–889.

Mosoni, P., Martin, C., Forano, E., & Morgavi, D. P. (2011). Long-term defaunation increases the abundance of cellulolytic ruminococci and methanogens but does not affect the bacterial and methanogen diversity in the rumen of sheep. *Journal of Animal Science*, *89*(3), 783–791.

Newbold, C. J., de la Fuente, G., Belanche, A., Ramos-Morales, E., & McEwan, N. R. (2015). The role of ciliate protozoa in the rumen. In *Frontiers in Microbiology* (Vol. 6, Issue NOV). Frontiers Research Foundation. https://doi.org/10.3389/fmicb.2015.01313

Saenab, A., K.G, W., & Wina, E. (2018). Manipulation of rumen fermentation by bioindustrial products of cashew nut shell (Anacardiumoccidentale) to reduce methane and enhance other products. *Jurnal Ilmu Ternak Veteriner* 23(2) 61–70.

Tilley, J. M. A. (1963). A two-stage technique for the *in vitro* digestion of forage crops. *Grass and Forage Science*, *18*(2), 104–111.

Wereszka, K., & Michałowski, T. (2012). The ability of the rumen ciliate protozoan Diploplastron affine to digest and ferment starch. *Folia microbiologica*, 57, 375–377.

Yamauchi, K., Ruttanavut, J., & Takenoyama, S. (2010). Effects of dietary bamboo charcoal powder including vinegar liquid on chicken performance and histological alterations of the intestine. *In Journal of Animal and Feed Sciences* (Vol. 19).

Technological Innovations in Tropical Livestock Development for Environmental Sustainability and Food Security – P. Dhian Isnaeni et al. (eds)
© 2025 The Author(s), ISBN 978-1-032-74373-8
Open Access: www.taylorfrancis.com, CC BY-NC-ND 4.0 license

Utilization of Guanidino-acetic Acid (GAA) and Betaine on the weight and size of the digestive organs of native chickens grower phase

S. Purwanti*, M. Yusuf, J.A. Syamsu, N. Lahay, M. Nadir & A.A. Yamin
Department of Animal Nutrition, Faculty of Animal Science, Hasanuddin University, Indonesia

Z. Dwiyana
Department of Biology, Faculty of Mathematics and Natural Sciences, Hasanuddin University, Indonesia

R.G. Laras
Behn Meyer Chemicals, Indonesia

Sumiati
Department of Nutrition and Feed Technology, Faculty of Animal Science, Bogor Agricultural University, Bogor

J.A. Syamsu
Research and Development Center for Livestock Resources and Tropical Animals, Hasanuddin University, Indonesia

ABSTRACT: Native chickens are potential poultry livestock and genetically have high adaptability to the environment. The addition of Guanidino-acetic Acid (GAA) and Betaine can stimulate livestock growth and affect the health of the digestive tract. A healthy digestive tract is characterized by the development of weight and length of the digestive organs. Optimal development of digestive organs will maximize the function of the digestive system and nutrient absorption will increase. This research aims to determine the effect of a combination of GAA and Betaine on the weight and size of the digestive organs of native chickens. This research was conducted from April until June 2023. Maintenance and sampling are carried out in a mini closed house cage, Faculty of Animal Science, Hasanuddin University, Makassar. This research used 120 ULU native chickens. The experimental design used was a Completely Randomized Design (CRD) with 4 treatments and 5 replications. The treatment structure used is P0: Commercial ration (without the addition of GAA and Betaine), P1: Commercial ration + 0,06% GAA + 0,1% Betaine, P2: Commercial ration + 0,12% GAA + 0,1% Betaine, and P3: Commercial ration + 0,18% GAA + 0,1% Betaine. Data analysis using analysis of variance (ANOVA). The results of this research showed an insignificant effect ($P > 0.05$) on the weight and size of the digestive organs. The addition of a combination of Guanidino-acetic Acid (GAA) and betaine in feed has not yet affected the weight and size of the digestive organs of 10-week-old ULU native chickens.

Keywords: betaine, digestive organs, grower phase, guanidino-acetic acid, native chicken

1 INTRODUCTION

Native chickens are potential poultry breeds and genetically have a high ability to adapt to the environment (Sasmito 2022), however, native chickens have a slow growth rate so to

*Corresponding Author: sripurwanti@unhas.ac.id

 DOI: 10.1201/9781003468943-17

obtain high productivity, feed modification is required. Several ways can be done to increase the productivity of native chickens, one of which is by providing Guanidino-acetic Acid (GAA) and Betaine.

The use of GAA can be applied through livestock rations. GAA is a precursor to creatine which plays a role in energy metabolism. The use of GAA in poultry feed is more often used than creatine. Even though it has a different way of working than antibiotics, GAA has the potential to be an alternative to AGP for improving body weight and improving feed conversion ratio (FCR) (Hardiyanto *et al.* 2022).

Another way that has the potential to increase the productivity of native chickens is to use betaine. Betaine has an effect as a methyl donor for methionine and its diverse physiological properties can improve the intestinal environment and increase the ability of feed absorption. Accumulation of betaine in cells may protect against osmotic stress. This can increase the utilization of amino acids for protein synthesis. Utilization of Betaine can improve performance (Ezzat *et al.* 2018).

Several studies such as the use of Guanidino-acetic Acid from the research by Khalil *et al.* (2021) show that a dose of 0.06% can reduce the FCR by 2.44% from 0 to 50 days of age and the use of Guanidino-acetic Acid at a dose of 0.12% can reduce the FCR by 3.15%–3.39% at the age of 10 to 42 days. According to Peng *et al.* (2023), the use of Guanidino-acetic Acid as much as 6 g/kg as a functional additive is effective in reducing intestinal injury in livestock experiencing heat stress. As for the use of Betaine from the research by Ratriyanto and Mentari (2018), it is known that the use of Betaine 0.1% can increase body weight gain.

One of the factors that influence the performance of the digestive organs is the quality of the feed consumed. The addition of GAA and Betaine can stimulate livestock growth and is thought to affect the health of the digestive tract. A healthy digestive tract is characterized by the development of the weight and length of the digestive organs. Optimal development of the digestive organs will maximize the function of the digestive system and nutrient absorption will increase.

Based on the background above, it is necessary to research to find out the effect of using a combination of GAA and Betaine on the weight and size of the digestive organs of native chickens. The use of this research is a source of information regarding the effect of the combination of Guanidino-acetic Acid (GAA) and Betaine on the weight and size of digestive organs.

2 MATERIALS AND METHODS

2.1 *Time and place of research*

Research on the use of Guanidino-acetic Acid (GAA) and Betaine on the weight and size of the digestive organs of native chicken was carried out from April to June 2023. The rearing and sampling process was carried out in closed-house mini cages at, the Feed Technology and Industry Laboratory, Faculty of Animal Science, Hasanuddin University Makassar.

2.2 *Research material*

The tools used in this research were analytical scales, feed containers, drinkers, incandescent lamps, brooms, shovels, hanging scales, scalpels, surgical scissors, rulers, measuring tapes, hand mixers, scissors, hand sprayers, jars for holding treated feed and feed mixing container. The material used in this research was 120 ULU native chickens produced by PT. Unggas Lestari Unggul, ABS BF commercial feed produced by PT. Japfa Comfeed Indonesia Tbk, GAA (CreAMINO®; Alzchem Group), betaine and litter.

2.3 *Research design*

The experimental design used is a Complete Randomized Design (CRD) with 4 treatments and 5 repetitions so that there are 20 observation plots with 120 native chickens, with 6 heads in each plot. The order of treatment is as follows: P0: (commercial ration), P1: (commercial ration + 0.06% GAA + 0,1% betaine), P2: (commercial ration + 0.12% GAA + 0.1% betaine) and P3: (commercial ration + 0.18% GAA + 0.1% betaine).

2.4 *Research procedure*

Chickens are reared using a mini closed house type cage of 20 plots using litter made from rice husks with a thickness of around 5 cm. A week before DOC is put into the cage, sanitation and disinfection of the cage is first carried out to kill and break the chain of development of microorganisms. The cage equipment (feeding and drinking containers) is previously washed using detergent and rinsed using water mixed with disinfectant. Next, whitewash the cage evenly to kill or reduce remaining bacteria, such as on the walls and floor of the cage. The cage is equipped with an incandescent lamp as a heater for the brooding phase with a temperature of 32–33°C and as a light at night.

This research used 120 ULU native chicken strains with mixed sex (unsexed). Maintenance starts at the age of 1 day (DOC) until the age of 70 days with a brooding phase for 14 days using a lamp as a heater. Disease control is carried out by implementing biosecurity in cages to reduce the risk of spreading disease, such as controlling traffic in and out of the cage. Carry out drum sanitation such as cleaning and disinfection to obtain a clean, hygienic and healthy environment.

Native chickens were placed randomly in cages that had been prepared by dividing them into 4 treatments and 5 replications, where each treatment consisted of 6 chickens. The feed used is commercial feed then GAA and betaine are added according to each treatment. Feeding and drinking water are provided individually ad libitum.

Sampling was carried out on 70-day-old chickens. Two chicken samples were taken at the unit experiment, then slaughtered and the digestive organs removed and separated according to the parameters to be measured. The parameters observed in this study were the digestive tract organs of ULU chickens, including proventriculus weight, ventriculus weight and weight and size of the small intestine (duodenum, jejunum and ileum). Organ weights are weighed using analytical scales by separating the organ to be observed from the digestive tract, then weighing is carried out, while measurements are carried out by separating each organ and measuring using a measuring tape.

Measurement of the length of the small intestine in the duodenum was carried out by measuring the distance from the base of the gizzard to the end of the pancreas. Measurement of the jejunum is carried out by measuring the distance from the endpoint of the duodenum to the dividing bulge or Meckel diverticulum. Ileum measurements are carried out by measuring the distance from the Meckel diverticulum to the cecum. Measurements are made using a measuring tape.

2.5 *Data analysis*

The data obtained were analysed using analysis of variance in a Completely Randomized Design with 4 treatments and 5 repetitions. Treatments that had a significant effect on the measured parameters were followed by the Duncan test (Gasperz 1991).

3 RESULTS AND DISCUSSION

Data from research on the effect of giving a combination of Guanidino-acetic Acid (GAA) and Betaine in feed on the weight and size of the digestive organs of ULU native chickens are presented in Table 1.

Table 1. Weight and size of the digestive organs of ULU native chickens.

Parameter	P0	P1	P2	P3
Proventriculus weight (g)	5.61 ± 0.34	5.56 ± 0.65	5.73 ± 0.43	5.21 ± 0.57
Ventriculus weight (g)	27.26 ± 1.42	29.48 ± 1.98	27.79 ± 3.46	28.05 ± 3.90
Duodenum weight (g)	7.36 ± 0.84	7.46 ± 0.69	7.83 ± 0.19	7.70 ± 1.07
Jejunum weight (g)	12.65 ± 0.93	12.73 ± 1.60	12.91 ± 0.71	12.78 ± 1.21
Ileum weight (g)	9.86 ± 0.50	10.04 ± 1.19	10.69 ± 1.58	10.21 ± 1.21
Duodenum length (cm)	26.30 ± 1.48	27.35 ± 2.59	27.20 ± 1.25	26.10 ± 1.08
Jejunum length (cm)	58.65 ± 4.06	59.55 ± 5.78	58.40 ± 5.41	56.30 ± 6.01
Ileum length (cm)	62.25 ± 3.61	62.40 ± 3.83	59.45 ± 4.61	59.30 ± 3.81

P0: (commercial ration), P1: (commercial ration + 0.06% GAA + 0,1% betaine), P2: (commercial ration + 0.12% GAA + 0.1% betaine) and P3: (commercial ration + 0.18% GAA + 0.1% betaine)

3.1 *Proventriculus weight*

Table 1 shows that the addition of GAA and betaine did not have a significant effect ($P > 0.05$) on the weight of the proventriculus of 10-week-old native chickens. The average proventriculus weight tended to be high in the P2 treatment (commercial ration + 0.12% GAA + 0.1% betaine) with a value of 5.73 g/head. The average proventriculus weight tended to be low in the P3 treatment (commercial ration + 0.18% GAA + 0.1% betaine) with a value of 5.21 g/head. The average proventriculus weight in this study was higher than the results of research conducted by Mistiani *et al.* (2020) where the proventriculus weight produced by administering burahol leaf extract in the ration ranges from 4.8–5.4 g/head.

The addition of GAA and betaine to commercial feed has not been able to influence the performance of the proventriculus in digesting feed which has an impact on the weight of the proventriculus. This is due to the protein content in the feed in this study ranging from 11.91–13.30% where the crude protein content cannot meet the protein needs of native chickens. According to Auza *et al.* (2023), the protein content in the ration which will be broken down with the help of the pepsinogen enzyme is one of the factors that influences the relative weight of the proventriculus organ.

3.2 *Ventriculus weight*

Table 1 shows that the addition of GAA and betaine did not have a significant effect ($P > 0.05$) on the weight of the ventricles of 10-week-old native chickens. The average ventricular weight tended to be high in treatment P1 (commercial rations + 0.06% GAA + 0.1% betaine) with a value of 29.48 g/head. The average ventricular weight tended to be low in the P0 treatment (commercial rations) with a value of 27.26 g/head. The average ventricular weight in this study was higher than the results of research conducted by Raham *et al.* (2022) where the ventricular weight produced by the substitution of *A. microphylla* in the rations ranged from 19.17–25.83 g/head.

The addition of GAA and betaine to the feed did not have a significant effect on the weight of the ventricles of 10-week-old native chickens, this was due to the crude fibre content being almost the same in each treatment so there was no difference in the size and weight of the ventricles. The crude fibre content in the feed which reaches 6.00% does not make the ventricular muscle contractions work hard to break down the fibrous feed particles so that the resulting weight does not show a significant difference. This is following research conducted by Auza *et al.* (2023) which provided feed with a crude fibre content of up to 5.1% which was not able to have a real effect on ventricular weight. According to Indiyani *et al.* (2023), the increase in ventricular weight is caused by the high crude fibre content.

The increase in ventricular weight can be caused by crude fibre content and can also be influenced by the amount of feed consumed. This is following the opinion of Winarti *et al.* (2019) who state that the size of the gizzard is determined by animal feed consumption, where the more feed consumed, the thicker and heavier the gizzard. According to Mistiani *et al.* (2020), The size of the ventricle weight is more influenced by the work activity of the ventricle and the type of feed given. This is also supported by the opinion of Maradon *et al.* (2015) who state that providing coarser feed will cause the gizzard to perform harder in digesting food, thereby causing the gizzard to increase in size.

3.3 *Duodenum weight*

Table 1 shows that the addition of GAA and betaine did not have a significant effect (P> 0.05) on the duodenal weight of 10-week-old native chickens. The average duodenal weight tended to be high in the P2 treatment (commercial ration + 0.12% GAA + 0.1% betaine) with a value of 7.83 g/head. The average duodenal weight tended to be low in the P0 treatment (commercial ration) with a value of 7.36 g/head. The average duodenal weight in this study was lower than the results of research conducted by Tahu *et al.* (2022) where duodenal weights treated with different forms of feed resulted in duodenal weights ranging from 11.3–11.6 g/head.

The addition of GAA and betaine in commercial feed has not been able to influence the development of the small intestine, allegedly because the GAA that enters the livestock's body is used for muscle formation. This is following the opinion of Noboa *et al.* (2018) who stated that chickens fed feed containing GAA will produce more ATP than chickens without GAA supplementation so that chickens have higher energy availability for muscle development. Research conducted by Melinda (2023) using ULU native chickens using GAA also showed a significant effect on the carcass weight of ULU native chickens with GAA supplementation. GAA has a positive effect on the metabolism and utilization of arginine, thereby increasing muscle growth and resulting in increased carcass. Portocarero and Braun (2021) stated that in skeletal muscle, creatine phosphate provides most of the phosphate groups that regenerate ATP and GTP used in ribosomal amino acids.

The increase in duodenal weight, which did not show a significant difference, was also influenced by the level of feed consumption which was relatively the same between treatments. These results are in line with research conducted by El-Faham *et al.* (2019) which stated that the addition of GAA up to 0.12% did not affect feed consumption. This makes GAA supplementation unable to affect duodenal weight. Harefa *et al.* (2022) also stated that higher and lower levels of ration consumption will affect the weight of the small intestine.

3.4 *Jejunum weight*

Table 1 shows that the addition of GAA and betaine did not have a significant effect ($P > 0.05$) on the weight of the jejunum of 10-week-old native chickens. The average weight of the jejunum tended to be high in the P2 treatment (commercial ration + 0.12% GAA + 0.1% betaine) with a value of 12.91 g/head. The average weight of the jejunum tended to be low in the P0 treatment (commercial ration) with a value of 12.65 g/head. The average weight of the jejunum in this study was higher than the results of research conducted by Aulia (2023) where the weight of the jejunum in chickens that are given fish meal-sweep on the feed ranges from 4–18.6 g/head.

The factor that caused the addition of GAA and betaine to feed did not have a significant effect on the weight of the jejunum of 10-week-old native chickens was that the nutritional content was almost the same between treatments. This makes the enzymatic activity in the digestive tract in digesting nutrients also the same, resulting in the same intestinal weight between treatments. This is the opinion of Azhar *et al.* (2022) who stated that changes in the mass and size of digestive tract organs can be influenced by enzymatic activity.

Jejunum weight can be influenced by the nutritional content in the diet such as crude fiber in the feed. This research used crude fibre ranging from 5.53–6.00% and was not able to have a significant effect on jejunum weight. This follows the opinion of Mistiani *et al.* (2020) who stated that high crude fibre feed ingredients in the ration significantly increased the weight of the small intestine. Silitonga *et al.* (2023) also stated that rations with high crude fibre content can strengthen, lengthen and thicken various digestive tracts.

3.5 *Ileum weight*

Table 1 shows that the addition of GAA and betaine did not have a significant effect ($P > 0.05$) on the ileum weight of 10-week-old native chickens. The average ileum weight tended to be high in the P2 treatment (commercial ration + 0.12% GAA + 0.1% betaine) with a value of 10.69 g/head. The average ileum weight tended to be low in the P0 treatment (commercial ration) with a value of 9.86 g/head. The average weight of the ileum in this study was not much different from the results of research conducted by Aulia (2023) where the weight of the ileum in chickens given broom fish meal in the feed ranged from 3.4–13.4 g/head.

The average ileum weight in this study ranged from 9.86 to 10.69 g/head. The addition of GAA and betaine at different levels was not able to have a real effect on ileum weight in each treatment. This also happened in research conducted by Delfani *et al.* (2023) which stated that there was no significant difference ($p > 0.05$) in the relative weight of ileum between experimental groups that used 1.8 g/kg GAA in the feed. This is thought to be because the nutrient content in feed with the addition of GAA and betaine at different levels has not been able to significantly influence the weight of the ileum.

The increase in ileum weight can be influenced by several factors such as the type of chicken used in research and chicken activities during rearing such as the tendency to move or the tendency not to move other than to consume food or drink, which also affects intestinal development. This is following the opinion of Ananda *et al.* (2022) who stated that several factors influence the development of the small intestine, namely race, gender, daily activities, environmental temperature, feed, health, feed additives and maintenance management.

3.6 *Duodenum length*

Table 1 shows that the addition of GAA and betaine did not have a significant effect ($P > 0.05$) on the duodenum length of 10 weeks native chickens. The average length of the duodenum tended to be high in treatment P1 (commercial ration + 0.06% GAA + 0.1% betaine) with a value of 27.35 cm. The average length of the duodenum tended to be low in the P3 treatment (commercial ration + 0.18% GAA + 0.1% betaine) with a value of 26.10 cm. The average length of the duodenum in this study was lower than the results of research conducted by Berliana *et al.* (2022) where the average length of the duodenum with the addition of multi enzymes in rations containing palm kernel meal ranged from 29.61–36.27 cm.

The addition of GAA and betaine to the feed did not have a significant effect on the duodenum length of 10-week-old ULU native chickens. The length of the duodenum is related to the weight and length of the villi, where the weight of the duodenum in this study did not show a significant difference between treatments so the length of the duodenum also did not show a significant difference between treatments. This follows the opinion of Satimah *et al.* (2019) who state that the length of the duodenum is closely related to the length of the villi and the relative weight of the duodenum, where the longer the intestinal villi, the wider the surface for nutrient absorption and the more optimal nutrient absorption, causing the duodenum to become heavier and long.

Guanidino-acetic Acid supplementation at a level of 0.06–0.18% in feed is the recommended standard for adding GAA. This is following the opinion of Asiriwardhana and Bertolo (2022) who stated that the optimal Guanidino-acetic Acid supplementation to increase productivity ranges between 0.6–1.2 g/kg in poultry and a dose of 0.6 g/kg is recommended as the minimum dose to increase productivity so that the effect of Guanidino-acetic Acid on livestock productivity depends on the dose given. According to the European Food Safety Authority (2009), a dose of 0.6-0.8 g/kg Guanidino-acetic Acid is considered a safe concentration as a feed additive to increase poultry productivity

3.7 *Jejunum length*

Table 1 shows that the addition of GAA and betaine did not have a significant effect ($P > 0.05$) on the jejunum length of 10-week-old native chickens. The average length of the jejunum tended to be high in treatment P1 (commercial ration + 0.06% GAA + 0.1% betaine) with a value of 59.55 cm. The average length of the jejunum tended to be low in the P3 treatment (commercial ration + 0.18% GAA + 0.1% betaine) with a value of 56.30 cm. The results of this study were higher than the results of research conducted by Rimbawanto *et al.* (2019) where the length of the jejunum with the administration of various types of acidifiers ranged from 36.21 to 43.42 cm.

The addition of GAA and betaine to feed did not have a significant effect on the jejunum length of 10-week-old native chickens. This is thought to be because the environmental conditions of the livestock are optimal condition so betaine and Guanidino-acetic Acid supplementation does not show its effectiveness, whereas betaine can work more effectively in the body when the chicken is in a condition exposed to stress such as heat stress or is in a sub-optimal condition. This follows the opinion of Ratriyanto and Mentari (2018) who state that betaine shows more effectiveness in sub-optimal conditions such as methionine deficiency and heat stress and according to Asiriwardhana & Bertolo (2022), Guanidino-acetic Acid can be considered as an additional feed to increase poultry productivity under heat stress.

Utilization of Guanidino-acetic Acid allows the availability of creatine as a result of the conversion of Guanidino-acetic Acid which is useful in repair and regeneration of epithelial cells. This is per the opinion of Hardiyanto (2022) who states that the availability of creatine as a result of conversion from GAA can increase the efficiency of energy utilization needed for repair and regeneration of intestinal epithelial cells. Biochemical processes at the tissue and cell level such as cell metabolism, cell motility and muscle contraction will be more efficient when the ratio of PCr to ATP increases. With the development of intestinal villi through GAA supplementation, the surface area for digestion and absorption of nutrients will increase, so it is hoped that livestock performance will also increase.

3.8 *Ileum length*

Table 1 shows that the addition of GAA and betaine did not have a significant effect ($P > 0.05$) on the ileum length of 10-week-old native chickens. The average length of the ileum tended to be high in treatment P1 (commercial ration + 0.06% GAA + 0.1% betaine) with a value of 62.40 cm. The average weight of the ileum tended to be low in the P3 treatment (commercial ration + 0.18% GAA + 0.1% betaine) with a value of 59.3 cm. The average length of the ileum in this study is not much different from the results of research conducted by Berliana *et al.* (2022) where the average length of the ileum with the addition of multi enzymes in rations containing palm kernel meal ranged from 61.89–67.27 cm.

The length of the ileum was not significantly different between treatments due to the influence of feeding which also did not make a significant difference to the live weight of ULU native chickens. This is because live weight is related to the length of the small intestine so that live weight tends to be the same resulting in intestinal length which tends to be the same. Berliana *et al.* (2022) stated that the length of the small intestine is very closely related to live weight and significantly, this means that the length and width of the small intestine correlate with the live weight of chickens.

Factors that can cause the development of the size of the ileum of 10-week-old native chickens are differences in the texture of the feed used in the research. Research conducted by Ananda *et al.* (2022) which used powdered feed was thought to result in the absorption of food substances in the ileum segment not being absorbed properly. However, each treatment in this study had the same feed texture so it did not have a real effect on the length of the ileum. This is in accordance with the opinion of Azhar *et al.* (2022) who stated that feed texture is one of the factors that influences changes in the morphology of the digestive tract.

4 CONCLUSION

The research that has been carried out, it can be concluded that the addition of a combination of Guanidino-acetic Acid (GAA) and betaine in feed has not yet affected the weight and size of the digestive organs of 10-week-old ULU native chickens.

AUTHORS' CONTRIBUTIONS

Sri Purwanti, Jasmal A. Syamsu, Nancy Lahay, Zaraswati Dwiyana, Abdul Alim Yamin, Raymundus Genty Laras, Sumiati conducted the investigation and validated the findings; Sri Purwanti, Jasmal A. Syamsu and Muh. Yusuf formal analysis and data curation; Abdul Alim Yamin, and Raymundus Genty Laras prepared the original draft; Sri Purwanti and Sumiati reviewed and edited the final manuscript; Marhamah Nadir provided project administration. All authors have read and agreed to the published version of the manuscript.

ACKNOWLEDGEMENTS

Thanks are expressed to the Hasanuddin University Community Service Institute (LPPM) for the funding provided through a Fundamental Research Grant with contract number: 00323/UN4.22/PT.01.03/2023 dated January 25 2023.

REFERENCES

Ananda, S., M. N. Hidayat, A. Qurniawan, H. I. Susanti, K. Asgaf. 2022. Penambahan temulawan (*Curcuma zanthorrhiza* Roxb) dan susu bubuk afkir pada level yang berbeda terhadap bobot relatif profil organ dalam broiler. *Jurnal Ilmu dan Industri Peternakan*. 8(1): 58–74. DOI:https://doi.org/10.24252/jiip.v8i1.28298

Asiriwardhana, M., R. F. Bertolo. 2022. Guanidinoacetic acid supplementation: a narrative review of its metabolism and effect in swine and poultry. *Frontiers in Animal Science*: 1–14. doi.org/10.3389/fanim.2022.972868

Aulia, A. 2023. Pemanfaatan tepung ikan sapu-sapu (*Pterygoplichths pardalis*) dalam ransum terhadap bobot dan ukuran organ pencernaan ayam broiler. *Skripsi*. Universitas Hasanuddin, Makassar.

Auza, F. A., R. Badaruddin, P. D. Isnaeni, A. B. Kimestri. 2023. Profil organ pencernaan, kualitas karkas dan potongan bagian karkas ayam broiler yang diberi tepung daun mengkudu (*Morinda citrifolia* Linn) fermentasi sebagai imbuhan pakan. *Jurnal Galung Tropika*. 12(1): 71–81. DOI: https://doi.org/10.23960/jrip.2022.6.2.110-117

Azhar, M., Rahmawati, U. Sara, M. Taufik. 2022. Respons organ saluran pencernaan dan morfologi usus halus ayam lokal dengan In-Ovo Feeding menggunakan L-Argine. *Jurnal Ilmu dan Industri Peternakan*. 8 (1): 1–10. DOI: https://doi.org/10.24252/jiip.v8i1.25667

Berliana, A. Azis, Sestilawarti, Yusrizal, Noferdiman. 2022. Penambahan multienzim dalam ransum yang mengandung bungkil inti sawit terhadap performa pertumbuhan dan morfometrik usus halus broiler. *Jurnal Ilmiah Ilmu-Ilmu Peternakan*. 25(1): 1–12. DOI: 10.22437/jiiip.v25i1.19188

Delfani, N., M. Daneshyar, P. Farhoomand, Y. A. Alijoo, S. Payvastegan, G. Najafi. 2023. Effect of arginine and guanidinoacetic acid with or without phenylalanine on ascites susceptibility in cold-stressed broilers fed canola meal-based died. *Journal of Animal Science and Technology*. 65(1): 69–95. doi: 10.5187/jast.2022.e68

El-Faham, A. I., A. G. Abdallah, M. H. S. El-Sanhoury, N. G. M. Ali, M. A. M. Abddelaziz, A. Y. M. Abdelhady, A. S. M. Arafa. 2019. Effect of graded levels of guanidine acetic acid in low protein broiler diets on performance and carcass parameters. *EJNF*. 22(2): 223–233. Doi: 10.21608/EJNF.2019.103502

European Food Safety Authority (EFSA). 2009. Safety and efficacy of guanidino acetic acid as a feed additive for chickens for fattening. *The EFSA Journal*. 7(3) 1–30. DOI: 10.2903/j.efsa.2009.988

Ezzat, W., A. A. Habeib, Y.S. Rizk, M. M. Beshara. 2018. Effects of betaine with different levels of guanidino acetic acid supplementation on productive and reproductive performance of local Mamourah strain during the summer season in Egypt. *Journal of Product*. 23(3): 691–715. DOI: 10.21608/JPD.2018.42601

Gaspersz, V. 1991. *Metode perancangan untuk ilmu-ilmu pertanian*. Bandung: Armico.

Hardiyanto, Y. 2022. *Performa, Kualitas Daging, Profil Usus Dan Profil Darah Ayam Broiler Yang Diberikan Asam Guanidino Asetat: Meta-Analisis.* Tesis. Sekolah Pascasarjana, Institut Pertanian Bogor.

Hardiyanto, Y., A. Jayanegara, R. Mutia, S. Nofyangtri. 2022. Performance, carcass traits, and relative organ weight of broiler supplemented by guanidinoacetic acid A meta-analysis. *Journal of Earth and Environmental Science*. 951: 1–6. DOI 10.1088/1755-1315/951/1/012030.

Harefa, F., B. W. I. Rahayu, P. Sambodo. 2022. Rumput kebar (*Biophytum petersanium*) dan ampas buah merah (Pandanus conoideus) pada profil usus halus broiler. *Prosiding Seminar Nasional*. Polbangtan Yogyakarta Magelang.

Indiyani, K. Kiramang, A. Mutmainna, A. H. Thahah. 2023. Pengaruh penambahan tepung daun pepaya (*Carica papaya* L.) pada pakan terhadap profil organ pencernaan ayam buras. *Jurnal Peternakan*. 7(2): 133–144. DOI: http://dx.doi.org/10.31604/jac.v7i2.10371

Khalil, S., N. Saenbungkhor, K. Kesnava, P. Sivapirunthep, R. Sitthigripong, S. Jumanee, C. Chaosap. 2021. Effects of guanidinoacetic acid supplementation on productive performance, pectoral myopathies, and meat quality of broiler chickens. *Journal of Animal*. 11: 1–19. DOI: 10.3390/ani11113180

Maradon, G. G., R. Sutrisna, Erwanto. 2015. Pengaruh ransum dengan kadar serat kasar berbeda terhadap organ dalam ayam jantan tipe medium umur 8 minggu. *Jurnal Ilmiah Peternakan Terpadu*. 3(2): 6–11. DOI: http://dx.doi.org/10.23960/jipt.v3i2.p%25p

Melinda, A. 2023. *Penambahan Guanidinoacetic Acid (GAA) dan Betaine terhadap Bobot dan Persentase Karkas Ayam Kampung ULU Fase Grower*. Skripsi. Fakultas Peternakan, Universitas Hasanuddin. Makassar.

Mistiani, S., K. A. Kamil, D. Rusmana. 2020. Pengaruh tingkat pemberian ekstrak daun burahol (*Stelechocarpus burahol*) dalam ransum terhadap bobot organ dalam ayam broiler. *Jurnal Nutrisi Ternak Tropis dan Ilmu Pakan*. 2(1): 42–50. DOI: https://doi.org/10.24198/jnttip.v2i1.26669

Noboa, H. A. C., E. O. O. Rondon, A. H. Sarsour, J. Barnes, P. Ferzola, M. R. Heilshorn, U. Braun. 2018. Performance, meat quality, and pectoral myopathies of broilers fed either corn or sorghum-based diets supplemented with guanidino acetic acid. *Journal of Poultry Science*. 97: 2479–2493. DOI: 10.3382/ps/pey096

Peng, X. Y., T. Xing, J. L. Li, L. Zhang, Y. Jiang, F. Gao. 2023. Guanidinoacetic acid supplementation improves intestinal morphology and mucosal barrier function of broilers subjected to chronic heat stress. *Journal of Animal Science*. 101(1): 1–11. DOI: 10.1093/jas/skac355

Portocarero, N., U. Braun. 2021. The physiological role of guanidinoacetic acid and its relationship with arginine in broiler chickens. *Poultry Science*. 100(7): 1–10. doi: 10.1016/j.psj.2021.101203

Rahma, W., R. Sutrisna, P. E. Santosa, F. Fathul. 2022. Pengaruh subtitusi A.Microphylla terhadap bobot karkas, persentase lemak abdomen, bobot gizzard dan panjang usus broiler. *Jurnal Riset dan Inovasi Peternakan*. 6(2): 110–117. DOI: 10.23960/jrip.2022.6.2.110-117

Ratriyanto, A., S. D. Mentari. 2018. Pertumbuhan dan efisiensi pakan ayam broiler betina yang diberi pakan mengandung metionin cukup dan disuplementasi betain. *Jurnal Ilmu-Ilmu Peternakan*. 28(3): 233–240. DOI:https://doi.org/10.21776/ub.-jiip.2018.028.03.06

Rimbawanto, E. A., N. Iriyanti dan B. Hartoyo. 2019. Bobot dan panjang usus halus serta bobot organ ayam broiler dengan pemberian berbagai jenis acidifier. Prosiding Seminar Nasional dan Call for Papers, Purwokerto 19–20 November 2019: Universitas Jenderal Soedirman.

Sasmito, E. D. N. 2022. *Karakteristik saluran pencernaan dan laju digesta ayam kampung fase grower yang diberi pakan kombinasi sumber protein. Skripsi.* Universitas Hasanuddin, Makassar.

Satimah, S., V. D. Yunianto, F. Wahyuno. 2019. Bobot relatif dan panjang usus halus ayam broiler yang diberi ransum menggunakan cangkang telur mikropartikel dengan suplementasi probiotik Lactobacillus sp. *Jurnal Sains Peternakan Indonesia*. 14(4): 396–402. doi.org/10.31186/jspi.id.14.4.396-403

Silitonga, L., S. Wibowo, I. Yuanita, S. Ma'rifah, N. Putriani. 2023. Pengaruh pemberian tepung singkong (*Manihot utillisima* Pohl.) fermentasi terhadap bobot karkas dan organ pencernaan ayam broiler. *Ziraa'ah*. 48(3): 395–405. DOI: http://dx.doi.org/10.31602/zmip.v48i3.11806.

Tahu, R. K. I., F. U. Atta, H. Nitbani. 2022. Pengaruh bentuk pakan (crumble dan pellet) terhadap pertumbuhan, berat karkas dan profil saluran pencernaan ayam broiler. *Jurnal Veteriner Nusantara*. 5(15): 1–10. DOI: https://doi.org/10.35508/jvn/vol5iss1pp143-153

Winarti, W., L. D. Mahfudz, D. Sunarti, S. Setyaningrum. 2019. Bobot proventrikulus, gizzard, sekum, rektum serta panjang sekum dan rektum ayam broiler akibat penambahan sinbiotik dari inulin ekstrak umbi gembili dan *Lactobacillus plantarum* dalam pakan. *Jurnal Ilmu Pertanian dan Peternakan*. 8(2): 301–314.

Technological Innovations in Tropical Livestock Development for Environmental Sustainability and Food Security – P. Dhian Isnaeni et al. (eds)
© 2025 The Author(s), ISBN 978-1-032-74373-8
Open Access: www.taylorfrancis.com, CC BY-NC-ND 4.0 license

Growth performance and nutrient digestibility characteristics of high tannin forage (*Calliandra calothyrsus* Meissn.) in Merino sheep receiving rumen microbe from Kaligesing goats

A. Bain*, Rahman, W. Kurniawan, A. Napirah, P.D. Isnaeni & F.M. Pancar
Department of Animal Science, Faculty of Animal Science, Universitas Halu Oleo, Kendari, Southeast Sulawesi, Indonesia

K.G. Wiryawan
Animal Science Faculty, IPB University, Bogor, Indonesia

B. Tangendjaja
Balai Penelitian Tenak, Bogor, Indonesia

ABSTRACT: This research aimed to evaluate the effectiveness of transferring rumen microbes from Kaligesing goats on changes in digestive characteristics and growth of Merino sheep fed with high-tannin forage, specifically Calliandra (*Calliandra calothyrsus* Meissn.). The study was based on previous research indicating that the rumen of Kaligesing goats harbours bacteria tolerant to tannins, demonstrated by their good performance when consuming Calliandra leaves containing high tannin. The experiment involved 18 Merino sheep (microbial recipients) and 2 Kaligesing goats as donors of tannin-tolerant rumen microbes. The study employed a randomized complete block design to test three treatments (transfer frequencies) with six replications for each treatment. The treatments consisted of T1 (no transfer of Kaligesing rumen microbes), T2 (one-time transfer of Kaligesing rumen microbes), and T3 (two-time transfer of Kaligesing rumen microbes) to recipient Merino sheep. The transfer of rumen microbes from Kaligesing goats was conducted by collecting rumen fluid through the goat's mouth. The diet used was 100% fresh Calliandra. Measured research parameters included nutrient intake (dry matter, organic matter, nitrogen intake), nitrogen retention, daily body weight gain, nutrient digestibility (dry matter, organic matter, and crude protein), total bacterial population, proteolytic bacteria, tannin-tolerant bacteria, total VFA content, rumen N-ammonia, and pH. The results indicated that the frequency of transferring rumen microbes from Kaligesing goats did not significantly affect consumption parameters, diet digestibility, daily weight gain, total VFA content, rumen N-ammonia, pH values, total bacterial population, and proteolytic bacteria of recipient Merino sheep. However, the tannin-tolerant bacteria population at 0 hours in Merino sheep treated with T2 (one-time transfer) and T3 (two-time transfer) was higher compared to Merino sheep without Kaligesing rumen microbe transfer (T1). In conclusion, transferring rumen microbes from Kaligesing goats twice resulted in better performance of tannin-tolerant bacteria populations in recipient Merino sheep. Meanwhile, growth performance, nutrient digestibility, fermentation characteristics, and microbial populations were relatively normal, indicating that Merino sheep in the study adapted well to consuming high-tannin Calliandra forage. Considering these findings, using Kaliandra as the sole diet component is not advisable, and alternative strategies to enhance microbial effectiveness should be explored.

Keywords: Merino sheep, Kaligesing Goat, microbe, Calliandra, tannin

*Corresponding Author: alibain67@uho.ac.id

DOI: 10.1201/9781003468943-18

1 INTRODUCTION

The current decline in the development of adult ruminant livestock farming is highly significant due to the increasing difficulty in obtaining nutritious feed with consistent productivity. This decline is attributed to the conversion of a substantial amount of agricultural land for other purposes such as industrial and residential development. Therefore, addressing this issue requires efforts to develop high-quality nutritious feed and high-yielding forages, with cultivation integrated into other agricultural subsectors. The intention is to optimize the land utilization system, making it more productive and efficient.

Kaliandra, with its various benefits, is a highly promising plant to be developed as a forage source for ruminant livestock. Apart from its high biomass production and nutritional quality compared to other leguminous tree plants, it also serves various purposes, such as being a pioneer plant, a conservation plant, a fuelwood source, a protective plant, or a live fence. With a planting density of 10.000 trees per hectare, a cutting height of 1 meter, and a cutting interval of 12 weeks, Kaliandra can yield 10 tons of forage per hectare, providing a sufficiently high protein intake for livestock (Tangendjaja *et al.* 1992). Kaliandra is also a type of plant that exhibits high tolerance to various soil topographies and climates in tropical regions. However, when utilizing Kaliandra as livestock feed, challenges arise due to its high tannin content. Excessive consumption of tannins by livestock can have negative impacts, such as reducing feed intake and digestibility, damaging various organs, especially the digestive and other body organs, inhibiting the function of digestive enzymes, and potentially poisoning rumen microbes (Makkar *et al.* 1995).

Observing this phenomenon, to maximize the utilization of Kaliandra as forage for ruminant livestock, there is a need to explore effective technologies to minimize the negative effects of tannins in forage when fed to livestock, especially ruminants. Various physical and chemical treatments to reduce the negative effects of tannins in Kaliandra have been conducted, both in vitro and in vivo. However, these efforts have not yielded effective and economical results when it comes to field implementation.

This research is conducted to examine the effectiveness of different frequencies and patterns of transferring Kaligesing goat rumen microbes on the digestive characteristics and growth of Merino sheep fed with forage containing fresh Kaliandra tannins and a mixed diet of dried Kaliandra with fresh elephant grass.

2 MATERIALS AND METHODS

2.1 *Material and type of treatments*

The study employed eighteen (18) Merino sheep to test 3 treatments (frequency of Kaligesing goat rumen fluid microbe transfer), with 2 Kaligesing goats as rumen fluid donor animals containing rumen microorganisms. The recipient Merino sheep and Kaligesing goats were fed 100% fresh Kaliandra leaves. The tested treatments consisted of: Treatment 1 (T1), which is the treatment without Kaligesing goat rumen microbe transfer; Treatment 2 (T2), which involves a single transfer of Kaligesing goat rumen microbe (during the first week); and Treatment 3 (T3), which includes two transfers of Kaligesing goat rumen microbe (during the first and second weeks) throughout the study. The research took place over 5 weeks, including the adaptation phase for experimental animals to the feed and experimental pens for 7 days, and the total collection phase, which involved sampling over 28 days related to the research parameters.

2.2 *Research procedure*

Eighteen (18) Merino sheep will be placed in metabolic cages to test three types of treatments (6 sheep for each treatment). Meanwhile, Kaligesing goats, serving as rumen microbe donors, will be placed in separate individual pens. Subsequently, over a period of 7 consecutive days, all experimental animals will be adapted to the metabolic cages and the experimental diet (100% fresh Kaliandra leaves) used. After the adaptation period, the experimental treatments will be applied as follows:

(i) Treatment one (T1): a treatment without Kaligesing goat rumen microbe transfer. Six (6) Merino sheep will be fed the experimental diet but will not receive any rumen microbe transfer.
(ii) Treatment two (T2): treatment with a single transfer of Kaligesing goat rumen microbe to six (6) Merino sheep (250 ml rumen fluid per sheep) at the beginning of the first week of the experiment.
(iii) Treatment three (T3): a treatment with two transfers of Kaligesing goat rumen microbe to six (6) Merino sheep (250 ml rumen fluid per sheep), conducted at the beginning of the first and second weeks of the study.

Sample collection and analysis for measuring experimental parameters will be conducted over a period of 4 weeks (28 days). The research is designed in a simple completely randomized design to test 3 types of treatments, each replicated six (6) times. The observed parameters include daily weight gain, dry matter intake (g/kgBW0.75/day), nutrient digestibility (%), nitrogen retention (g/kgBW0.75/day) (Mumo and Allison 1960), rumen fermentation characteristics, such as pH, N-ammonia content, total VFA content (General Laboratory Procedure 1966), total bacterial populations consist of proteolytic bacteria and tannin tolerant bacteria populations (Ogimoto and Imai 1980). Additionally, blood plasma mineral levels will be measured using the Atomic Absorption Spectrophotometer procedur

3 RESULT AND DISCUSSION

3.1 *Feed consumption, nitrogen retention and body weight gain*

All text, figures, tables, etc. should fit exactly in the type area of 15 × 24 cm (5.91" × 9.52"). All The influence of different frequencies of Kaligesing goat rumen microbe transfer on nutrient consumption, dietary nitrogen retention, and Merino sheep weight gain is presented in Table 1.

Table 1. Average nutrient consumption, nitrogen retention and body weight gain.

	Frequency of Kaligesing Goat Rumen Microbe Transfer			
Parameters	T1	T2	T3	Significance
DMI (gDM/kgBW$^{0.75}$/day)	42.58 ± 6.32	42.06 ± 8.36	43.79 ± 3.30	0.21
OMI (gBO/kgBW$^{0.75}$/day)	41.22 ± 5.75	40.87 ± 7.81	42.29 ± 3.18	0.18
NI (gN/kgBW$^{0.75}$/day)	4.39 ± 0.35	4.41 ± 0.64	20 ± 0.47	0.23
CPI (gCP/kgBW$^{0.75}$/day)	27.42 ± 2.66	27.55 ± 3.99	26.23 ± 2.92	0.31
N Retention (gN/day)	41.93 ± 5.59	45.18 ± 9.95	42.31 ± 9.18	0.17
Weight gain/sheep/day (g)	0.83 ± 3.86	3.87 ± 4.73	4.29 ± 3.56	0.09

Description: DMI = Dry Matter Intake, OMI = Organic Matter Intake, CPI = Crude Protein Intake, NI = Nitrogen Intake.

The data in Table 1 indicate that the different frequencies of Kaligesing goat rumen fluid transfer did not have a significant effect on the consumption of nutrients, nitrogen retention, and weight gain of Merino sheep consuming 100% fresh Kaliandra forage. The intake of dry matter (DM), organic matter (OM), and crude protein (CP) were lower than the ARC (1980) standards, which are dry matter intake at approximately 54.43 gDM/kgBW0.75/day and crude protein intake at approximately 28.6 gCP/BW0.75/day for sheep with an average body weight of 40 kg. The lower levels of nutrient consumption, nitrogen retention, and weight gain obtained in this experiment are likely due to the tannins in the 100% fresh Kaliandra forage, which reach 10% (Tangendjaja *et al.* 1992), causing negative effects on the digestion process of the experimental Merino sheep in general.

The negative impact of tannins seems to occur from the moment the tannin-containing feed enters the oral digestion, affecting the epithelial cells of the mouth and subsequently the rumen and post-rumen digestion (small intestine). The nature of tannins binding to the epithelial cells of the mouth reduces the palatability of the feed, leading to decreased livestock appetite. As Makkar and Bucker (1995) suggested, the consumption of feed containing tannins drastically decreases due to the astringent taste it causes upon entering oral digestion (mastication). In rumen digestion, the negative effects of tannins occur because of their toxicity to rumen microbes, resulting in a decrease in microbial growth and fermentative activity. Furthermore, tannins' ability to bind to components of nutrients and enzymes in the digestive tract lowers the degradation rate of feed fractions by enzymes in the rumen and post-rumen digestion. The low livestock consumption is a form of compensation by the animals for slow rumen emptying and post-rumen digestive tract. This can be understood because the rumen of ruminant animals is voluminous, and hunger stimuli highly depend on the rate of rumen emptying and post-rumen digestive tract. The implication of this occurrence is evident in the limited availability of nutrients for the animals, leading to low weight gain in the experimental livestock.

Meanwhile, the inoculation of tannin-tolerant rumen microbes from Kaligesing goats, expected to play a fermentative role, has proven to be insufficient in improving the composition of recipient sheep's rumen microbes to reduce the negative effects of tannins. The ineffectiveness of the microbe transfer treatment may also be attributed to the stable condition of the Merino sheep rumen, with an average age of 2 years. Therefore, the transfer of tannin-tolerant microbes from 250 ml of Kaligesing goat rumen fluid to each recipient Merino sheep appears to be inadequate in effectively influencing the rumen microbial composition of the recipient livestock. This is primarily related to the competitive ability of these microbes, which subsequently results in the low activity of microbes in the rumen of the recipient sheep in digesting Kaliandra feed containing high tannin levels.

Based on the above results, it seems that to optimize the benefits of Kaliandra feed, it is not advisable to use it as a sole ration. This is likely because using Kaliandra as a sole feed (100%), aside from its unbalanced nutritional components, may also result in tannin concentrations reaching levels intolerable by the rumen microbes and the digestive tract of the experimental sheep. As a consequence, it could have detrimental effects on the growth of the livestock.

3.2 *Nutrients digestibility*

The presentation of the influence of the frequency of Kaligesing goat rumen microbe transfer on the digestibility of nutrients in recipient Merino sheep can be observed in Table 2.

Table 2. Average digestibility of dry matter, organic matter, and crude protein in merino sheep fed fresh kaliandra forage.

	Frequency of Kaligesing Goat Rumen Microbe Transfer			
Parameters	T1	T2	T3	Significance
Digestibility of DM (%)	57.05 ± 4.63	58.20 ± 5.13	62.39 ± 5.84	0.21
Digestibility of OM (%)	59.31 ± 4.45	61.83 ± 4.49	64.13 ± 5.72	0.27
Digestibility of CP (%)	63.53 ± 8.76	64.93 ± 15.11	71.60 ± 6.74	0.41

As seen in Table 2, different frequencies of rumen microbe transfer have not shown significant differences in the digestibility of dry matter, organic matter, and crude protein in Merino sheep consuming 100% fresh Kaliandra forage.

The digestibility of nutrients in the recipient Merino sheep, which did not exhibit significant differences among the three given treatments, seems to be still influenced by the inability of the transferred tannin-tolerant rumen microbes from Kaligesing goats to break the complex bonds between tannins and the nutritional components of the consumed Kaliandra forage. This is because the concentration of tannins in 100% fresh Kaliandra forage is intolerable and toxic to rumen microbes, hindering their growth and fermentative activities. The binding of tannins with the nutritional components and enzymes continues in post-rumen digestion, resulting in the wastage of nutrients such as proteins, carbohydrates, vitamins, and minerals through faeces. Additionally, the tannins' property of damaging the mucosal epithelial layer of the small intestine and possibly other vital organ tissues seems to be a cause of impaired absorption and metabolism of nutrients in the animal's body tissues, leading to a serious disturbance. This occurrence will undoubtedly have implications for the low synthesis of the animal's body tissues.

The subsequent implications reveal the low growth rate (daily weight gain) of the recipient livestock in this experiment. Besides the fact that the animals are relatively old (approximately 2 years), at such an age, the growth curve of Merino sheep has already reached a level of stagnation. Therefore, even if provided with a high-quality and balanced diet, it will not be effective enough to elicit a positive growth response.

Based on the measurement results of the parameters mentioned above, it seems necessary to consider not providing Kaliandra as the sole component in the diet of the sheep. Additionally, another possible alternative to enhance the effectiveness of the inoculated Kaligesing goat rumen microbes in the recipient livestock should be explored. It is advisable to strive for a population of tannin-tolerant microbes that can reach 108 per millilitre of rumen fluid, as recommended by Syahrir (1988). This is intended so that with such a microbial population, it is expected to comprise bacteria that can adapt and effectively compete to digest nutrients bound by tannins in Kaliandra forage.

3.3 *Rumen microbial population and its metabolic products*

The values of nutrient consumption and digestibility, as well as the weight gain, which showed no significant differences among the treatments in this experiment, are also reflected in the phenomenon of rumen bacterial population parameters and their metabolic products (Table 3).

In Table 3, it can be observed that the different frequencies of Kaligesing goat rumen fluid transfer did not have a significant effect on the dynamics of the total bacterial population and proteolytic bacteria in the rumen of recipient sheep at the 0-hour and 4-hour periods, except for the tannin-tolerant bacterial population at the 0-hour period. The inoculation of Kaligesing goat rumen microbes through fresh rumen fluid tends to increase the population of tannin-tolerant bacteria in the recipient sheep's rumen. However, this inoculation effect did not consistently impact the population of tannin-tolerant bacteria at the 4-hour period (after the animals were fed Kaliandra forage). Thus, the effect of the different frequencies of Kaligesing goat rumen microbe transfer on the changes in the population of tannin-tolerant bacteria in the rumen of recipient Merino sheep at the 0-hour period cannot be conclusively considered effective. This is evident from the inability of these bacteria to maintain their population after the sheep consumed tannins-containing forage.

The total bacterial population, proteolytic bacteria, and tannin-tolerant bacteria at the 4-hour period (after the animals consumed 100% Kaliandra) showed no significant differences among the three tested treatments. This might be due to the inoculated bacterial population not reaching an optimal proportion to tolerate the tannin concentration in the 100% fresh Kaliandra forage consumed by the livestock. Additionally, it is suspected that

Table 3. Bacterial population, pH Level, N-Ammonia, and Total VFA in the Rumen fluid of Merino Sheep Fed Fresh Kaliandra Forage.

	Frequency of Kaligesing Goat Rumen Microbe Transfer			
Parameters	T1	T2	T3	Significance
Bacterial Population (Log x)				
Total Bacteria				
- 0 Hour Period	9.17 ± 0.49	9.19 ± 0.91	9.50 ± 0.88	0.63
- 4 Hour Period	10.02 ± 0.41	9.84 ± 0.95	10.02 ± 0.72	0.82
Proteolytic Bacteria				
- 0 Hour Period	9.05 ± 0.46	8.82 ± 0.84	9.44 ± 0.86	0.43
- 4 Hour Period	8.99 ± 0.94	9.39 ± 1.01	9.60 ± 0.89	0.65
Tannin-Tolerant Bacteria				
- 0 Hour Period	**6.73 ± 0.05[a]**	**7.33 ± 0.04[b]**	**7.50 ± 0.47[b]**	**0.03**
- 4 Hour Period	7.099 ± 0.59	7.831 ± 0.68	7.400 ± 2.08	0.28
Rumen pH				
- 0 Hour Period	6.73 ± 0.04	7.0443 ± 0.08	6.99 ± 0.37	0.47
- 4 Hour Period	6.93 ± 0.20	6.86 ± 0.09	7.02 ± 0.38	0.26
Rumen N-Ammonia (mm)				
- 0 Hour Period	8.82 ± 1.86	8.08 ± 2.48	7.68 ± 2.687	0.36
- 4 Hour Period	8.45 ± 3.44	7.17 ± 0.98	7.10 ± 0.45	0.21
Total VFA				
- 0 Hour Period	204.03 ± 55.57	334.44 ± 63.13	222.02 + 61.64	0.07
- 4 Hour Period	246.37 ± 149.22	288.77 ± 67.38	315.89 ± 31.03	0.14

Note: Values with different superscripts in the same row indicate a significant difference.

the tannin concentration has poisoned the rumen microbes, hindering their growth and activity to thrive and carry out their fermentative activities optimally.

The suboptimal transfer of Kaligesing goat rumen microbes regarding the dynamics of rumen microbial populations also has implications for its metabolic products, such as Volatile Fatty Acids (VFA). This results in inadequate energy availability for the sheep. This phenomenon can be understood because VFA production heavily depends on the degradation activity of fibre in the feed by rumen microbes. According to Arora (1986), VFAs, as the major energy supplier for ruminant animals, are the primary products of the fermentation process by rumen microbes, and their production rate is highly determined by the complex interaction between the population and activity of rumen microbes and feed factors (Hvelplund 1991).

Quantitatively, the total rumen VFA level (reaching 325.89 mm) obtained in this experiment sufficiently ensures the availability of energy for the sheep. However, in reality, it fails to provide optimum contributions to the growth of the experimental livestock. This could be due to tannin hindering the growth and activity of rumen papillae, thus impeding the absorption and metabolism of VFAs on the papillae of the reticulorumen wall. The inhibitory effect of tannin on papillae growth and activity is more evident in the observations of the size of the reticulum, rumen, and omasum papillae in the second stage of the experiment.

Apart from the parameters mentioned above, it seems that other metabolic parameters such as rumen fluid ammonia levels and pH also did not show significant differences among the treatments, indicating that the transfer of Kaligesing goat rumen fluid did not have distinct effects. Although considering the average pH values (6.73–7.04) with ammonia levels ranging from 7.10 to 8.82 mm, it falls within the ideal range for supporting bacterial fermentation processes in the rumen. Despite being often used as an indicator in evaluating protein availability in the diet of ruminant livestock (Orskov and Ryle 1990), adequate ammonia availability in the rumen is crucial. Preston and Leng (1987) stated that the ammonia level in rumen fluid supporting microbial growth and activity should fall within the range of 2.94-14.7 mm/ml rumen fluid with a pH range of 6.2–7.0.

The tendency for a decrease in rumen ammonia levels at both the 0-hour and 4-hour periods, alongside an increase in the frequency of Kaligesing goat rumen fluid transfer, might signify the utilization of ammonia by rumen bacteria. This tendency aligns with the increased frequency of Kaligesing goat rumen fluid transfer in this experiment. As stated by Preston and Leng (1987), the loss of rumen ammonia is, in part, due to its utilization by rumen microbes as a nitrogen source in de novo.

4 CONCLUSION

The different frequencies of Kaligesing goat rumen microbe transfer did not significantly affect nutrient consumption, nitrogen retention, and weight gain in Merino sheep consuming 100% fresh Kaliandra forage. Transferring rumen microbes from Kaligesing goats twice resulted in better performance of tannin-tolerant bacteria populations in recipient Merino sheep. Meanwhile, growth performance, nutrient digestibility, fermentation characteristics, and microbial populations were relatively normal, indicating that Merino sheep in the study adapted well to consuming high-tannin Calliandra forage.

The low levels of nutrient consumption and weight gain were attributed to the tannins in Kaliandra, negatively impacting the digestive process. Despite the inoculation of tannin-tolerant microbes, it proved insufficient to counteract the effects of tannins. Rumen microbial population dynamics and metabolic products, including volatile fatty acids (VFA), were suboptimal, leading to insufficient energy availability for the sheep. Additionally, rumen fluid parameters such as ammonia levels and pH did not show significant differences among treatments, suggesting that Kaligesing goat rumen fluid transfer had limited effects. Considering these findings, using Kaliandra as the sole diet component is not advisable, and alternative strategies to enhance microbial effectiveness should be explored

REFERENCES

ARC (Agricultural Research Council). 1985. *The nutrient requirements of ruminant livestock.* London: ARC.

Arora, S.P. 1986. *Microbial digestion in ruminants.* Yogyakarta: Gajah Mada University Press.

General Laboratory Procedures. 1966. *Department of Dairy Science University of Wisconsin Madison.* USA.

Hvelplund, T., 1991. Volatile fatty acids and protein production in the rumen. In: J.P. Jounal (Editor). *Rumen Microbial Metabolism and Ruminant Digestion.* INRA, Paris.

Makkar, H.P.S, M. Blummel, M., Beucker. 1995. In vitro Effects of and Interactions Between Tannins and Saponins and Fate of Tannins in the Rumen. *J.Sci. Food Agric.* 69.481–491.

Makkar, H.P.S. and Becker, K. 1995. Degradation of condensed tannins by rumen microbes exposed to Quebracho Tannin (QT) in rumen simulation technique (RUSITEC) and effects of QT on fermentative processes in the RUSITEC. *J. Sci. Food Agric.* Vol 69: 495–500.

Mumo, H.N. and J.C. Alison, 1960. *Mammalian protein metabolism* (Vol. 1). London: Academy Press.

Ogimoto, K and Imani, S. 1980. *Atlas of rumen microbiology*. Tokyo: Japan Scientific Societies Press.

Orskov, E.R. and Ryle, M. 1990. *Energy nutrition in ruminant*. London: Elsevier Appl. Sci..

Preston, T.R. and Leng, R.A. 1987. *Matching ruminant production system with available resources in the tropics.* Armidale: Penambul Book.

Syahrir, S. 1998. *Testing tannin tolerant bacteria and its inoculation effects on livestock fed with Kaliandra (Calliandra calothyrsus) forage*. Bogor: Graduate School of Bogor Agricultural Institute.

Tangendjaja, B., E. Wina, T. Ibrahim dan B. Palmer, 1992. *Kaliandra (Calliandra calothyrsus) and its utilization.* Livestock Research Institute Ciawi, and The Australian Centre for International Agricultural Research.

Wiryawan, K.G. 2000. Uji bakteri toleran tanin dan pengaruh inokulasinya terhadap mikroba rumen ternak kambing berpakan kaliandra (Calliandara calothyrsus). *Media Peternakan*, Vol.23. No 2. Hal.53–60

Technological Innovations in Tropical Livestock Development for Environmental Sustainability and Food Security – P. Dhian Isnaeni et al. (eds)

Utilization of water hyacinth, palm fronds and fermented sago dregs with the addition of digestive enzyme for the growth of young male Aceh cattle

Z.M. Gaznur*
Department of Animal Husbandry, Faculty of Agriculture, Syiah Kuala University, Indonesia
The Animal Husbandry Field Laboratory, Syiah Kuala University, Indonesia

W. Fatmala
Department of Animal Husbandry, Faculty of Agriculture, Syiah Kuala University, Indonesia

S. Wajizah
Department of Animal Husbandry, Faculty of Agriculture, Syiah Kuala University, Indonesia
The Animal Husbandry Field Laboratory, Syiah Kuala University, Indonesia

Mahmudi
Department of Animal Husbandry, Faculty of Agriculture, Syiah Kuala University, Indonesia

ABSTRACT: This research was carried out at the Animal Husbandry Field Laboratory of Syiah Kuala University, Rukoh, Syiah Kuala, Banda Aceh. The time for conducting the research is from 26 June 2022 to 13 April 2023. The material used in this research is 4 young male Acehnese cattle aged 1.5 years with an average body weight of 170 kg. The experimental design used was a 4 × 4 Latin Square Design (RBSL) with a length of each period of 21 days and an adaptation period of 7 days. The feed treatments for this study were: P0 (100% basal feed), P1 (80% basal feed + 20% fermented feed + 0.03% digestive enzyme), P2 (65% basal feed + 35% fermented feed + 0 digestive enzyme, 02%), and P3 (Basal Feed 50% + Fermented Feed 50% + digestive enzyme 0.01%). The research parameters observed consisted of daily body weight gain, feed consumption and feed conversion of young male Acehnese cattle.

Keywords: Aceh Cattle, Dygestive Enzyme, Daily Body Weight Gain, Feed Consumption and Feed Convertion Ratio

1 INTRODUCTION

Indonesia has rich and potential genetic resources for national beef cattle, which have been used as a source of food, meat, labor, energy and fertilizer (Awa *et al.* 2022). Efforts to maintain local livestock resources are important to achieve sustainable food security for millions of people. Aceh cattle (*Bos Indicus*) is one of Indonesia's local cattle which has a geographical distribution in Aceh Province. Acehnese cattle are spread throughout the Aceh region and are in demand as beef cattle. Some Aceh cattle are also used as a means of transportation (Putra *et al.* 2014).

The main problem with the low productivity of Aceh cattle is that farmers find it difficult to provide continuous forage, both in quality and quantity. This is mainly due to the lack of land use for planting forage and breeders are still very dependent on natural forage. Efforts that can be made to increase the productivity of Aceh cattle are by improving feed quality.

*Corresponding Author: zikrimaulina@usk.ac.id

 DOI: 10.1201/9781003468943-19

To overcome difficulties in providing animal feed, agricultural/plantation waste and water weed plants can be used as partial replacements for forage. Potential plant waste that is often found in the Aceh region is palm fronds and sago dregs. Apart from agricultural/plantation waste, aquatic weeds can also be used as alternative feed ingredients for livestock. Water hyacinth is one of the aquatic weeds that has been widely studied as animal feed.

Water hyacinth (*Eichornia crassipes*) has nutritional content that can be used as an alternative feed ingredient for livestock because it contains carotenoid pigments, especially β-carotene and xanthophyll pigments (Viomalini *et al.* 2020). However, the use of water hyacinth as a feed ingredient has several disadvantages, including too high air content, relatively low crude protein and nitrogen-free extract (NFE), and high crude fiber. Oil palm fronds and leaves can be used as cattle feed to replace grass as a forage source, because they have high levels of crude fiber (CF). The level of dry matter digestibility of palm fronds only reaches 45%. To be utilized optimally, palm fronds must be processed first (Nurhaita *et al.* 2019).

Sago starch is a source of carbohydrates which can be used as an energy source for microorganisms in the fermentation process. The carbohydrates contained in sago dregs are 65.7%, lignin 21%, cellulose 20% (Syadik *et al.* 2021). The nutritional content of sago dregs consists of 86.40% dry matter, 1% crude protein, 20.3% crude fiber, 1.8% crude fat, 71.3% NFE and 50.1% TDN (Sisriyenni *et al.* 2017). Optimizing the use of palm fronds, sago dregs and water hyacinth can be done using fermentation technology to improve their nutritional quality. The addition of digestive enzymes to the ration functions to increase rumen microbial activity and increase the digestibility of feed ingredients. Providing fermented feed with the addition of digestive enzyme is expected to improve the growth performance of aceh cattle.

2 MATERIALS AND METHODS

2.1 *Place and time of research*

This research was carried out at the Animal Husbandry Field Laboratory of Syiah Kuala University, Rukoh, Syiah Kuala, Banda Aceh. The research implementation time is from June 26 2022 to April 13 2023.

2.2 *Research materials and tools*

The material used in this research was 4 young male Acehnese cattle aged 1.5 years with an average body weight of 170 kg.

2.3 *Research materials and tools*

The materials used in this research include mixed grass consisting of field grass and elephant grass, palm fronds, sago dregs, water hyacinth, and digestive enzyme.

2.4 *Research methods*

The experimental design used was a 4 × 4 Latin Square Design with a length of each period of 21 days and an adaptation period of 7 days. The research feed treatments are listed in Table 1 below.

Table 1. The research feed treatments.

	Cattle			
Period	A	B	C	D
I	P0	P1	P2	P3
II	P2	P3	P0	P1
III	P3	P2	P1	P0
IV	P1	P0	P3	P2

Information:
P0: Basal Feed (100%)
P1: Basal Feed (80%) + Fermented Feed (20%) + Digestive Enzyme (0.03%)
P2: Basal Feed (65%) + Fermented Feed (35%) + Digestive Enzyme (0.02%)
P3: Basal Feed (50%) + Fermented Feed (50%) + Digestive Enzyme (0.01%)

The statistical model for the Latin Square Design is as follows:

$$Yijk = \mu + \alpha i + \beta j + \tau(k) + \in ij(k)$$

Information:
Yijk : Observation results on the ith line, jth lane, kth treatment
μ : General middle value
αi : Influence of the ith row
βj : Influence of the jth lane
τ(k) : Effect of the kth Treatment
ϵij(k) : Error on the ith line, jth lane for the kth treatment.

2.5 *Research procedure*

2.5.1 *Preparation of basal feed*

The basal feed used in this study consisted of forage. The types of forage used in this research were elephant grass (*Pennisetum Purpureum*) and field grass. The nutritional content of the grass used is presented in Table 2 below:

Table 2. Nutrient content of basal feed.

Material	Crude Protein (%)	Total Digestible Nutrients (%)	Crude Fiber (%)	Dry Matter (%)	Ash (%)	Crude Fat (%)	Nitrogen-free Extract (%)
Elephant Grass	6.20	67.68	32.60	20.30	12.50	2.10	41.80
Field Grass	6.70	56.20	34.20	35.40	9.70	1.80	47.60

Source: Laboratory of Feed Science and Technology, Faculty of Agriculture, Syiah Kuala University, 2023

Table 3. Nutritional content of fermented feed.

Material	Crude Protein (%)	Total Digestible Nutrients (%)	Crude Fiber (%)	Dry Matter (%)	Ash (%)	Crude Fat (%)	Nitrogen-free Extract (%)
Fermented Feed	14.50	63.75	20.05	38.21	16.76	0.23	48.,46

Source: Laboratory of Feed Science and Technology, Faculty of Agriculture, Syiah Kuala University, 2023

Table 4. Ration composition based on dry ingredients.

Material	P0	P1	P2	P3
		(%)		
Field Grass	10	15	15	15
Elephant Grass	90	65	50	35
Fermented Feed	0	20	35	50
Total	100	100	100	100

(*continued*)

Table 4. Continued

Material	P0	P1 (Kg)	P2	P3
Field Grass	0.45	0.68	0.68	0.68
Elephant Grass	4.05	2.93	2.25	1.58
Fermented Feed	0.00	0.90	1.58	2.25
Total	4.50	4.50	4.50	4.50

Table 5. Ration composition based on as fed and nutrient content of treated feed.

Material	P0	P1 (Kg)	P2	P3
Field Grass	1.27	1.91	1.91	1.91
Elephant Grass	19.77	14.28	10.98	7.69
Fermented Feed	0.00	2.36	4.12	5.89
Total	21.04	18.54	17.01	15.48
Component	**P0**	**P1 (%)**	**P2**	**P3**
Crude Protein	10.78	11.20	11.70	12.19
Total Digestibel Nutrients	65.06	64.11	63.76	63.42
Coarse Fiber	31.82	29.65	27.93	26.20
Dry Ingridients	21.98	26.27	28.93	31.59
Crude Fat	2.36	1.89	1.56	1.23
Ekstract Material Without Nitrogen	42.40	44.02	45.01	46.01

2.5.2 *Preparation of fermented feed*

The treatment feed used in this research was made using a fermentation process with a composition of ingredients consisting of 15% water hyacinth, 10% palm fronds, 48% sago dregs, 10% rice bran, 17% fine corn and several additional ingredients such as molasses 200 ml/100kg of ingredients, premix 200 gr/100kg of material, bioresik 25g/100kg of material and water 2 liters/100kg of material. These ingredients are mixed and then put into a fermentation container in the form of a drum.

2.6 *Research parameters*

The research parameters observed consisted of daily body weight gain, feed consumption and feed conversion of young male Aceh cattle.

3 RESULTS AND DISCUSSION

3.1 *Daily body weight gain of Aceh cattle*

Body weight gain is the increase in body weight achieved by an animal during a certain period. The average total body weight gain of Acehnese cattle obtained in this study is presented in Figure 1 below.

The results of the study showed that giving water hyacinth, palm fronds and fermented sago dregs with the addition of digestive enzymes in different percentages had no significant effect (P>0.05) on the increase in body weight of young male Aceh cattle, with an average ranging from 297.6–476. 19 gr. Although not statistically different, livestock that received 35% fermented feed with the addition of 0.02% digestive enzyme tended to show the highest

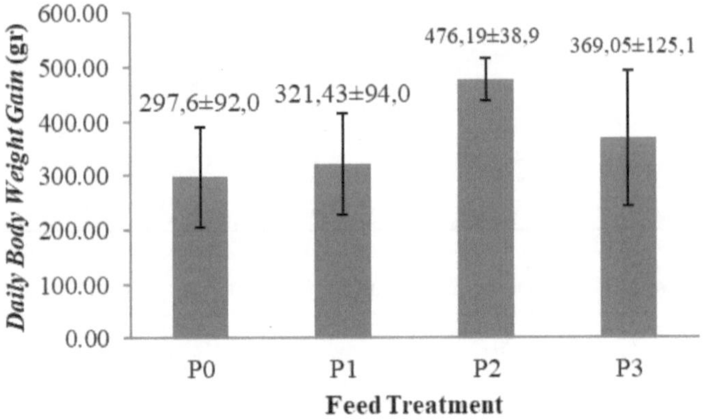

Figure 1. Daily body weight gain of Aceh cattle.

weight gain (476.19 gr), while livestock that were only given basal feed in the form of field grass and elephant grass had lowest weight gain (297.6 gr). The feed fermentation process can increase nutritional value, increase aroma and taste (palatability) and digestibility value (Thaaril 2018).

The weight gain of Acehnese cattle in this study was much lower than the standard daily weight gain of Acehnese cattle at BPTU-HPT Indrapuri which reached 0.7 kg (Putra *et al.* 2014). This is thought to be due to the poor nutritional quality of the ration and the seeds used were not selected so that they could not achieve optimal weight gain. However, the results of this study are relatively better than previous research which obtained an average increase in body weight of male Acehnese cattle given the substitution of elephant grass with fermented water hyacinth ranging from 0.26–0.46kg (Marbawi *et al.* 2016).

3.2 *Acehnese cattle feed consumption*

Feed consumption is the amount of feed consumed by cattle to meet basic living and production needs to stimulate livestock productivity. There are several factors that can influence feed consumption in cattle, namely: condition of the livestock, environment and level of palatability of the feed. The calculation of feed consumption in research is the difference between the amount of feed given and the remaining feed for 24 hours. Acehnese cattle feed consumption in this study can be seen in Figure 2 below.

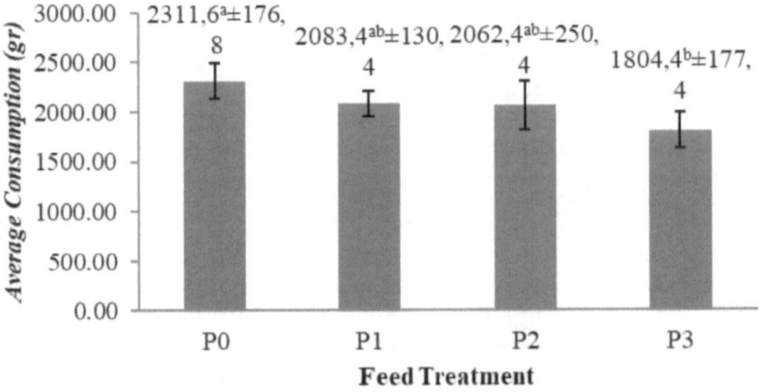

Figure 2. Feed consumption of Aceh cattle.

The results of variance analysis showed that water hyacinth, palm fronds and fermented sago dregs added with digestive enzyme had a significant effect ($P<0.05$) on feed consumption of young male Aceh cattle both based on treatment ration, livestock and treatment period. The highest dry matter consumption was obtained in treatment P0 which was only given basal feed in the form of field grass and elephant grass. Grass is generally more palatable than feedstuffs originating from agricultural/plantation waste, because the forage is usually eaten by livestock, especially if they are not old (Effendi *et al.* 2021).

3.3 *Aceh cattle feed conversion*

Feed conversion is a comparison between the amount of feed consumed at a certain time and the production produced (weight gain) in the same period (Budiarta *et al.* 2014). The lower the feed conversion value, the better. The feed conversion for Aceh cattle in this study is presented in Figure below.

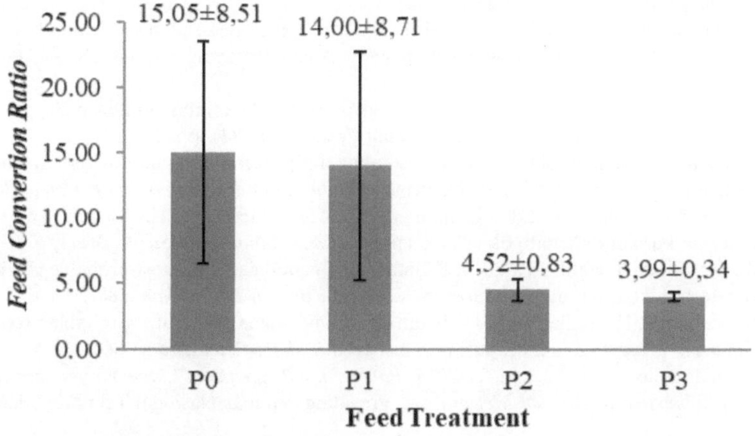

Figure 3. Feed conversion ratio of Aceh cattle.

In this study, the best feed conversion was found in the P2 and P3 treatments, namely 4.52 and 3.99 respectively, much better than previous research which reported that the feed conversion value for beef cattle was 12.86–15.86 (Adiwinarti *et al.* 2013). There are several factors that can influence the feed conversion value, namely environment, temperature, feed quality, genetic ability and energy level of fermented feed.

The addition of digestive enzymes is usually done on feed ingredients that are high in crude fiber and have low digestibility, so that it can increase the use of these feed ingredients. The use of digestive enzymes in feed rations can increase growth and efficiency in ration use (Berliana *et al.* 2022). Giving digestive enzymes to ruminants is less useful because the ruminant digestive system involves rumen microorganisms which produce enzymes in the fermentation and degradation of fiber feed, in contrast to poultry which requires digestive enzymes to assist in the digestion and energy absorption of the ration given so as to increase the rate of ration consumption to maximize achievements in poultry production (Allaily *et al.* 2022).

4 CONCLUSIONS

Addition of water hyacinth, palm fronds and fermented sago dregs with the addition of digestive enzyme did not have a significant effect on daily body weight gain and feed conversion, but had a significant effect on feed consumption. The percentage of giving fermented feed of 50% as a substitute for forage gives the best results with the lowest conversion value, indicating more efficient use of feed nutrients.

REFERENCES

Adiwinarti, R., Kusuma, I. P. & Lestari, S. C. M., 2013. Penampilan produksi sapi po dan pfh jantan yang mendapat pakan konsentrat dan hay rumput gajah. *Sains Peternakan*, 8(1), pp. 1–7.

Allaily., Septian , A. W. & Daud , M., 2022. Analisis usaha pemeliharaan ayam broiler dengan penambahan probiotik dan enzim pencernaan dalam ransum fermentasi. *Jurnal Ilmiah Peternakan Terpadu*, 10(2), pp. 124–132.

Awa, S. R. L. A., Kaka, A. & Pati, D. U., 2022. Struktur populasi sapi sumba ongole di kelurahan lambunapu kecamatan kambera kabupaten sumba timur. *Manokwari*, e ISSN : 2774–1982, pp. 473–474.

Berliana, Aziz, A., Sestilawarti, Yusrizal, and Noferdiman. 2022. Penambahan multienzim dalam ransum yang mengandung bungkil inti sawit terhadap performapertumbuhan dan morfometrik usus halus broiler. *Jurnal Ilmiah Ilmu-Ilmu Peternakan*, 25(1), pp. 1–12.

Budiarta, D. H., Sudjarwo, E. & Cholis, N., 2014. Pengaruh kepadatan kandang terhadap konsumsi pakan, pertambahan bobot badan dan konversi pakan pada Ayam Pedaging. *Jurnal Ternak Tropika*, 15(2), pp. 31–35.

Effendi, R. A., D. & Rachmawati, J., 2021. Perbedaan tingkat palatabilitas domba pada pakan hasil fermentasi dan rumput segar. *Jurnal Keguruan dan ilmu Pendidikan*, 2(3), pp. 243–250.

Marbawi, Mahyuddin & Rachmadi, D., 2016. Analisis ekonomi pengemukan sapi aceh jantan yang diberikan substitusi rumput gajah dengan eceng gondok fermentasi. *Jurnal Ilmiah Mahasiswa Pertanian Unsyiah*, 1(1).

Nurhaita, Definiati, N. & Feni, R., 2019. Pemanfaatan pakan komplit berbasis limbah sawit untuk usaha penggemukan sapi kurban di kelompok ternak sumber rezeki. *Sinar Sang Surya*, 3(1), pp. 1–7.

Putra, W. P. B., Sumadi & Hartatik , T., 2014. Estimasi nilai pemuliaan dan most probable producing ability produksi sapi aceh di kecamatan indrapuri provinsi Aceh. *Buletin Peternakan*, 38(1).

Putra, W. P. B., Sumadi & Hartatik , T., 2014. Estimasi nilai pemuliaan dan most probable producing ability produksi sapi aceh di kecamatan indrapuri provinsi aceh. *Buletin Peternakan*, 38(1).

Sisriyenni, D., Simanjuntak, A. & Adelina, T., 2017. *Potensi dan Penggunaan Limbah Sagu Fermentasi sebagai Pakan Sapi di Kabupaten Kepulauan Meranti*. s.l., Prosiding Seminar Nasional Teknologi Peternakan dan Veteriner.

Thaariq, S. M. H., 2018. Pengaruh Pakan Fermentasi terhadap Kadar Protein Kadar Air dan Kadar Lemak Daging Ayam Lokal Pedaging Unggul (Alpu). *BIOnatural*, 5(1), pp. 12–20.

Viomalini, S. D. E. & Nugrahini, Y. L. R. E., 2020. *Pemanfaatan Eceng Gondok (eichornia crassipes) sebagai Pakan Alternatif untuk Meningkatkan Average Daily Again, Konsumsi serta Tingkat Kecernaan pada Ternak Ruminansia*. E-ISSN : 2615–7721, 4(1).

Technological Innovations in Tropical Livestock Development for Environmental Sustainability and Food Security – P. Dhian Isnaeni et al. (eds)

Cashew nut shell nutrient profile (*Annacardium occidentale*) as a potential feed source

H. Has*, A. Bain, T. Saili & W. Kurniawan
Department of Animal Science, Faculty of Animal Science, Universitas Halu Oleo, Kendari, Southeast Sulawesi, Indonesia

Sahidin
Pharmacy Study Program, Universitas Halu Oleo, Kendari, Southeast Sulawesi, Indonesia

ABSTRACT: Cashew shell is one of the wastes from cashew processing, cashew shell contains active compounds that can be used as antibiotics, besides that cashew shell has nutrient content that can still be used as animal feed. The use of cashew shells in animal feed either as an additive or feed ingredient is expected to add information about the utilization of cashew shells. This research was conducted by using cashew shells from Lombe Sub-district, Central Buton District, Southeast Sulawesi. The cashew shell used is the epidermis and outer shell of the cashew. The method used to determine the nutrient content of cashew shell samples is the nutrient analysis proximate method, the variables seen are the content of dry matter, organic matter, ash content, crude protein, crude fat, crude fibre, and non-nitrogen extract. The data obtained were analyzed descriptively. The results showed that the protein content and ash content of the epidermis were higher than the outer shell while the fat content, crude fibre and non-nitrogen extract of the outer shell were higher than the cashew epidermis. Cashew shell has the potential to be used as animal feed based on its nutrient content.

Keywords: nutrient content, cashew shell, animal feed

1 INTRODUCTION

The cashew plant is one of the mainstay commodities in eastern Indonesia, especially on the island of Sulawesi. The result of cashew plants is cashew seeds, cashew seeds are further processed to get cashew nuts and leave cashew shells. The increasingly massive cashew processing industry increases the amount of cashew shell waste produced. Cashew nut shell (CNS), an agricultural waste generated from cashew nut processing plants, is proven to be one of the renewable raw materials that has many benefits. This food waste also has significant potential to be used as a feedstock for the production of fuels and value-added chemical products, as well as potential use as an animal feed ingredient due to its abundance. The part of cashew that is most often processed is the true fruit or nut because cashew nuts have a high selling value because of their delicious taste. These cashew nuts contain fat, protein, carbohydrates, and various minerals. The fat content is what causes the delicious flavour of cashew nuts. However, in the processing of cashew nuts, the shells of these nuts are discarded and not used anymore. Cashew seeds consist of 70% seed coat and 30% seed meat (Simpen 2008). The cashew nut shell is a waste produced in the postharvest cashew nut shelling industry. Cashew nut shells until now have not

*Corresponding Author: hamdan_has@uho.ac.id

DOI: 10.1201/9781003468943-20

been maximally utilized, most of which are still wasted. In addition to cashew shells, another byproduct is the epidermis shell. This part has quite useful potential, it can be used as an ingredient for animal feed which has a fairly high nutritional value (Muljohardjo 1990).

The utilization of cashew shells in the field of animal husbandry in addition to being used as an additive for antibacterial can also be used as animal feed, parts of cashew shells such as the epidermis and outer shell can be used as animal feed because they still contain nutrients that are important for livestock. The utilization of cashew shells in the context of animal feed is a promising innovation in improving the health and productivity of livestock. Cashew shells contain several nutrients that have the potential to add value to livestock rations. The high fibre content in cashew shells can play a role in improving the health of the animal's digestive tract, reducing the risk of digestive disorders, and supporting the growth of good microflora in the digestive system. In addition, antioxidants and bioactive compounds in cashew shells can protect against free radicals and stimulate the immune system of livestock. By utilizing cashew shells as a component of animal feed, we not only reduce agricultural waste but also provide nutritious feed alternatives for livestock. Information on the nutrient content of cashew shells is very important in their utilization as animal feed.

2 MATERIAL AND METHOD

This research is a chemical test as a nutrient evaluation method conducted at the Nutrition and Feed Laboratory of the Faculty of Animal Husbandry, Halu Oleo University. This study used cashew shells (*Anacardium occidentale*) from the cashew nut industry processing, cashews were obtained from Lombe District, Central Buton Regency, Southeast Sulawesi Province. At first, cashew shells were sorted from various impurities (remaining shell, leaves, stems and other impurities) then cleaned by washing and then dried by drying in the sun for two days to reduce water content, then dried using an oven at 60 degrees for two days. The dried cashew shell was then ground to reduce its size to facilitate the analysis of its nutrient content.

The cashew shell was then put into the oven at 105 degrees Celsius for two days, then weighed to obtain the dry matter content and then continued with other proximate analyses such as ash content, crude protein content, fat content, crude fibre and non-nitrogen extract. Materials used in this study include H_2SO_4, Kjeldhal catalyst, Na-thiosulfate, sodium hydroxide, boric acid, indicator mix, HCl 0.02 N, petroleum ether, NaOH, acetone and cashew shell. Measurement of nutrient content in the feed was analyzed using the proximate analysis method. Proximate analysis is a chemical analysis that classifies components in feed ingredients based on their chemical composition and function (Mikdarullah 2020).

3 RESULTS AND DISCUSSION

The results showed that the nutrient content of the proximate analysis process shows that the nutrient content of the rind and shell has a considerable difference, as seen in Table 1 the nutrient content is quite varied except for the dry matter which is relatively the same.

Table 1. Nutrient content analysis of cashew nut shell.

Nutrient content	Dry matter (%)	Ash (%)	Crude Protein (%)	Fat (%)	Crude Fiber (%)	Non-Nitrogen Extract
Cashew nut epidermis	82.21	5.20	13.94	4.540	4.63	68.98
Cashew nutshell	81.30	3.10	6.10	35.40	23.55	73.50

Cashew nut is an ingredient that contains quite high nutrients but the shell has a quite different content, the protein content in the epidermis is 13.94%, this figure is high when compared to other feed ingredients from waste. The shell is 6.1% which is relatively low but still in the reasonable category when compared to other waste-derived feed ingredients. Feed from waste generally contains low protein so its utilization is still rarely used. Harianto (2008) reported that the cashew epidermis has a crude protein of 16.94%. Cashew shell protein content of 6.23% and ash content of 1.2%. (Ocheja *et al.* 2013). Crude protein is the amount of nitrogen content contained in the material multiplied by 6.25 (Brasileiro *et al.* 2012). Protein acts as the main substance for the formation of cells in the body and becomes energy reserves when carbohydrates and fats are reduced (Ashar 2016).

The results showed that the fat content of the epidermis was relatively low at about 4.54% while the shell was 40.4% which was classified as very high, indicating that the shell contains a very high amount of oil. the fat content of the epidermis is 4.54% (Harianto 2008). the oil in the cashew shell contains a lot of fatty acids (Botutihe *et al.* 2016). The testa is a thin layer that protects the cashew seed and weighs about 12% of the cashew seed. Cashew nut testa has a high nutrient content but has not been utilized as a feed ingredient, is still a residual material or as fuel (Muljohardjo 1990). The nutrient content of cashew seed testa is moisture content 8.1%; mineral content 1.8%; fibre 11%; protein 7.6%; carbohydrate 59.2%; fat 12.3%.

The results of the analysis of crude fibre showed that the crude fibre content of the shell was 35.4% which was classified as high. Feed ingredients that can be used as a source of crude fibre are materials that have a crude fibre content of more than 18% or a cell wall component content of 38% (Yaman 2019). The crude fibre content of cashew seed shells is 23.05% ADF 1.95 and NDF 26.30% (Ocheja *et al.* 2015).

Feed ingredients that contain more than 20% protein with less than 18% SK can be classified as protein-source feed ingredients (Tilman *et al.* 1991). Therefore, its use in rations, especially for monogastric livestock, needs to be combined with other feed ingredients.

4 CONCLUSION

Cashew shells contain nutrients that can be utilized by livestock, the content of cashew epidermis contains high protein, low fat and crude fibre, while the shell tends to have low protein, high fat and crude fibre.

REFERENCES

Azhar M. (2016). *Biomolekul Sel Karbohidrat,Protein dan Ezim. In [Book]. UNP Press.*

Botutihe SIR, J Abidjulu, PVY Yamlean. 2016. Analisis kadar asam lemak esensial pada kulit biji jambu mete (*Annacardium occidentale* L.) PHARMACON. *Jurnal Ilmiah Farmasi* 5(4)

Brasileiro, O. L, Cavalheiro, JMO., Prado, J de, S., Anjos, A. G. dos, & Cavalheiri, T. T. B. (2012). Determination of the chemical composition and functional properties of shrimp waste protein concentrate and lyophilized flour. *Ciência e Agrotecnologia*, 36(2), 189–194.

Harianto D. 2008, *Pengaruh Penggunaan Kulit Ari Biji Mete(Anacardium occidentale) dalam ransum terhadap penampilan produksi domba lokal jantan. Fakultas Pertanian Universitas Sebelas Maret Surakarta.*

Mikdarullah, M., Nugraha, A., & Khazaidan, K. (2020). Analisis proksimat tepung ikan dari beberapa lokasi yang berbeda. *Buletin Teknik Litkayasa Akuakultur*, 18(2), 133.

Muljohardjo, M. 1990. *Jambu Mete dan Teknologi Pengolahannya (Anacardium occidentale L.)* Liberty. Yogyakarta.

Ocheja, OJ, AO Aduku, JA Ayoade and BC Lalabe. Effect of steaming and soaking on the chemical composition of cashew nutshell. *Pakistan Journal of nutrition* 12(7):683–687.

Ocheja, OJ, BC Lablabe, HGE Oguche and GO Usman. 2015. Vitamin composition and fibre fractions of cashew nut shell. *Pakistan Journal of nutrition* 14(5):252–254

Simpen, IN. 2008. Isolasi *cashew nut shell liquid* dari kulit biji jambu mete (*Anacardium occidentale* L.) dan kajian beberapa sifat fisiko-kimianya. *J. Kimia* 2:71–76.

Tillman AD., H Hartadi, S Reksohadiprodjo, S Prawirokusumo, S Labdosoekojo. 1991. *Ilmu makanan ternak dasar*. Gadjah Mada University Press. Yogyakarta.

Yaman, A. (2019). *Teknologi Penanganan, Pengolahan Limbah Ternak Hasil Samping Peternakan. Syiah Kuala University Press.*

Technological Innovations in Tropical Livestock Development for Environmental Sustainability and Food Security – P. Dhian Isnaeni et al. (eds)
© 2025 The Author(s), ISBN 978-1-032-74373-8

Prevalence of gastrointestinal parasites of beef cattle in Polewali Mandar district

N.S. Said*
N.S. Said Publishers, Sains Veteriner, Faculty of Veterinary Medicine, Airlangga University, Surabaya, Indonesia
Faculty of Animal Science and Fishery, Sulawesi Barat University, Majene, Indonesia

D.U. Fahrodi
Faculty of Animal Science and Fishery, Sulawesi Barat University, Majene, Indonesia

ABSTRACT: This research aims to determine and measure the incidence of gastrointestinal parasite infections in beef cattle in Polewali Mandar Regency. This research used samples of beef cattle feces from four sub-districts that have the largest population of beef cattle in Polewali Mandar Regency, namely Campalagian, Mapilli, Wonomuliyo, and Luyo sub-districts with a total sample of 98 samples. The data obtained was then analyzed descriptively. The results of an examination of 98 samples of beef cattle feces in this study found that 58 samples were positively infected with gastrointestinal parasites with an infection incidence rate of 59.18%. In microscopic identification of worm eggs, several types of endoparasites were found with the following disease incidence rates, namely nematode class worms, *Haemonchus sp.* (28.57%), *Trichostrongylus sp.* (13.27%), *Bunostomum sp.* (28.57%), *Oesophagostomums sp.* (1.02%), *Strongyloides sp.* (18.37%) and *Ascaris sp.* (2.04%), the cestoda class, namely *Taenia sp.* (12.24%), *Moniezia sp.* (14.29%) and *Diphyllobothrium sp.* (3.06%) and the trematode class, namely *Paramphistomum sp.* (16.33%) and *Fasciola sp.* (1.02%) there are also protozoan parasites, namely *Eimeria sp.* (27.55%).

Keywords: Gastrointestinal parasites, Beef cattle, Polewali Mandar

1 INTRODUCTION

The population of beef cattle in West Sulawesi Province is currently entirely growing, with the population in 2021 reaching 115,199 heads, Polewali Mandar Regency has the highest population of beef cattle, namely 35,683 heads (BPS 2021). Most cattle farms in Polewali Mandar Regency still operate cattle farming as a side business with a traditional rearing system. Cattle are kept in open fields and given grass forage. Feeding like this allows livestock to contract parasites in the digestive tract easily. It is very likely that there are worm eggs and protozoan oocysts in the grass eaten by cows, worm eggs and protozoan oocysts are carried by snails and attached to damp grass (Almuhardi *et al.* 2022).

One of the diseases always a problem in Indonesia is digestive tract parasitic diseases or gastrointestinal parasites. The types of parasites that often infest the digestive tract are worms in the Trematoda, Cestoda, and Nematoda classes, as well as protozoa. Losses due to digestive tract worm disease include weight loss, decreased meat quality, skin, offal, fat productivity, and milk production in livestock. Worms infect the digestive tract, decreasing

*Corresponding Author: nursaidah@unsulbar.ac.id

 DOI: 10.1201/9781003468943-21

nutrient absorption and causing growth delays so that cow production performance decreases (Susilo *et al.* 2020).

Gastrointestinal parasitic infections in cattle can cause losses to farmers and reduce the economic value of beef. The Directorate General of Animal Husbandry (2018) stated that Indonesian cattle suffer losses yearly due to gastrointestinal parasite infections reaching 4 billion Rupiah annually. The life cycle of gastrointestinal parasites is direct, and they can live without an intermediate host, so their presence is always found infecting ruminant livestock, especially cattle. Gastrointestinal parasitic infections cause weight loss in livestock and can cause death or decreased production, resulting in reduced productivity and performance of cattle (Mensah *et al.* 2018).

Data from the Agriculture and Food Service of Polewali Mandar Regency shows that there were 203 cases of worms in 2020 and 192 in 2021. This is because the parasites found in the cow's digestive tract will affect the nutritional intake that enters the body. Based on this background, researchers are interested in researching the prevalence of gastrointestinal parasites in beef cattle in Polewali Mandar Regency.

2 MATERIALS AND METHODS

The sample used in this research was beef cattle feces collected from people's farms in the sub-district of Polewali Mandar district, which has the largest population of beef cattle, namely Campalagian, Mapilli, Wonomuliyo, and Luyo sub-districts with a total sample size of 98 samples.

Sampling is done by collecting fresh feces from beef cattle, each ± 10 grams, through rectal palpation. For cows that do not allow feces to be collected by rectal palpation, samples are taken from fresh feces that have just been defecated. Next, the feces are collected in a plastic container and given information about the district of origin, sample number, age, and gender. The sample is stored in cold conditions to prevent the eggs from hatching, the sample is sent to the laboratory for further examination.

The methods used to examine gastrointestinal parasites are the floating concentration and sedimentation methods. The floating method begins by taking a feces sample of ± 2 grams and putting it in a beaker, then adding distilled water up to 10 ml and stirring until homogeneous. Filter using ¾ of the tube volume, then homogenize using a vortex, then place it in a centrifuge and centrifuge at 1,500 rpm for 3 minutes. Next, separate the supernatant from the sediment, add saturated NaCl to ¾ of the tube volume, stir until homogeneous, put it back into the centrifugator, and centrifuge at 1,500 rpm for 3 minutes. After centrifuging, place the centrifuge tube on a rack in an upright position, then drop saturated NaCl using a Pasteur pipette until it forms a convex shape on the surface of the tube and then slowly cover it using a cover glass, leave for 2 minutes so that worm eggs and oocysts from protozoa float on the surface. Slowly move the cover glass over the object glass and identify it using a microscope with a 40x magnification objective. Identification using the sediment method is done by discarding ½ the sample solution in the centrifuge tube used for the floating method. Next, add one drop of 1% methylene blue, then homogenize using a vortex. Then, take one drop of the sample solution, place it on the object glass, and cover it with a cover glass. Examine using a microscope with 40x objective magnification. Identifying gastrointestinal parasites refers to the parasitology book by Taylor *et al.* (2016). The research data obtained were analyzed descriptively.

3 RESULTS AND DISCUSSION

The results of identifying 98 samples of beef cattle feces showed 58 samples that were positive for infection with gastrointestinal parasites. Based on gender, there were 16 feces samples from male beef cattle infected with gastrointestinal parasites with a disease incidence rate of 43.24%. In comparison, 42 samples from feces from female beef cattle were infected with gastrointestinal parasites, with a prevalence of 68.85% (Table 1).

Table 1. Prevalence of gastrointestinal endoparasites in beef cattle in Polewali Mandar Regency based on sex.

Gender	Number of Samples	Positive	Prevalence (%)
Male	37	16	43.24
Female	61	42	68.85
Total Prevalence	98	58	59.18

Table 1 shows that female beef cattle are more susceptible to infection with gastrointestinal parasites than male beef cattle. The results of this study are different from research by Paramitha *et al.* (2017), which showed that the level of digestive tract worm infestation in male beef cattle was higher, namely 83% (10/12) when compared to female beef cattle, namely 69% (20 /29). This could be caused by the purpose of keeping male beef cattle different from females; breeders at the research location keep male beef cattle until they are mature for sale or as sacrificial animals and can also be used for traditional events, in contrast to female beef cattle whose maintenance tends to be longer because they are used as meat cattle. as broodstock and will continue to be kept as long as they are still producing so there is a risk of being infected again even though treatment has been carried out. The unstable condition of immunity in female cows during pregnancy, giving birth, and lactation also influences the high level of helminthiasis infection (Inbaraj *et al.* 2022).

Based on the age of beef cattle, calves (<6 months) have more potential to be infected with gastrointestinal parasites than those aged above, namely 6–24 months and >24 months. Based on identification results in beef cattle feces samples, the prevalence of gastrointestinal parasites at calf age (<6 months) reached 68.75%, at young age (6–24 months) reached 67.44%, and at adult age (>24 months) reached 46.15% (Table 2).

Table 2. Prevalence of gastrointestinal endoparasites in beef cattle in Polewali Mandar Regency based on age.

Age	Number of samples	Positive	Prevalence (%)
Calves (<6 months)	16	11	68.75
Young (6–24 months)	43	29	67.44
Adult (>24 months)	39	18	46.15
Total Prevalence	98	58	59.18

Based on the results obtained, it is known that gastrointestinal parasites can infest beef cattle in all age groups, but young beef cattle are more susceptible to infestation. This proves that the incidence of gastrointestinal parasitic diseases will decrease as the age of the livestock increases. This research is on research results from Paramitha *et al.* (2017) that cows less than one year old have a higher incidence of gastrointestinal parasite infections than adults. The high prevalence of gastrointestinal parasites at a young age can be associated with developing the body's defense system. In contrast, in adulthood, the body's defense system is more active and more resistant to parasite infections. This is by Grencis *et al.* (2014) opinion that the animal's body's defense system against parasites will only be actively formed at the age of 5–8 months. Apart from increasing age, routine administration of worm medicine will also affect the prevalence of gastrointestinal parasites in livestock. Putri *et al.* (2022) research results show that administering worm medicines such as albendazole and ivermectin effectively treats worm infections in the digestive tract and can reduce EPG values by up to 75–95%.

The microscopic examination of fecal samples found that 43 beef cattle feces had infection with more than one gastrointestinal parasite, and 15 feces samples were identified with only one gastrointestinal parasite. Most infections with more than one parasite species occur between worm parasites and protozoan parasites. Based on morphological identification, the parasite eggs found came from nematode class worm eggs, namely Haemonchus sp., Trichostrongylus sp., Bunostomum sp., Oesophagostomums sp., Strongyloides sp. and Ascaris sp., cestoda class, namely Taenia sp., Moniezia sp. and Diphyllobothrium sp. and the trematode class, namely Paramphistomum sp. and Fasciola sp. There are also protozoan parasites, namely Eimeria sp.. The prevalence of types of gastrointestinal parasites in beef cattle in Polewali Mandar district can be seen in Table 3.

Table 3. Prevalence of digestive tract endoparasites in beef cattle in Polewali Mandar Regency.

Types of parasites	Positive	Prevalence (%)
Nematodes		
- *Haemonchus sp.*	28	28.57
- *Trichostrongylus sp.*	13	13.27
- *Bunostomum sp.*	28	28.57
- *Oesophagostomums sp.*	1	1.02
- *Strongyloides sp.*	18	18.37
- *Ascaris sp.*	2	2.04
Cestoda		
- *Taenia sp.*	12	12.24
- *Moniezia sp.*	14	14.29
- *Diphyllobothrium sp.*	3	3.06
Trematodes		
- *Paramphistomum sp.*	16	16.33
- *Fasciola sp.*	1	1.02
Protozoa		
- *Eimeria sp.*	27	27.55
Overall prevalence	58	59.18

Based on the results of identifying gastrointestinal parasites in beef cattle feces samples, worm eggs from the nematode class have the most species with the highest prevalence rate. The highest prevalence of nematode classes comes from the Haemonchus sp. and Bunostomum sp (28.57% each), a strongyloid group characterized by the formation of eggs containing 4 to 16 cells clustered together resembling grapes. Environmental factors can contribute to the high prevalence of strongyloid nematode class worms because poor sanitary conditions in the cage will facilitate the development of worm eggs and larvae. After all, the strongyloid class has a direct life cycle without an intermediary host; the eggs will hatch in the soil so that poor sanitation will increase the chances of infection. Apart from that, the semi-intensive rearing system is also a supporting factor in the occurrence of gastrointestinal parasite infections because beef cattle are grazed in the exact location without rotation so that infected cattle will excrete feces containing nematode eggs and then hatch into infective larvae in the grazing area at any time. Healthy cattle can ingest it. Setiawan *et al.* (2022) explained that small breeders whose rearing systems use semi-intensive care by allowing livestock to find their food, some of which are not even kept in cages at all, cause livestock to be more easily infested by worm-carrying vectors and contaminated with worm eggs. The next factor is the grazing area. For livestock that are kept semi-intensive, the farmer will choose a grazing area that the farmer considers sufficient to meet the livestock's needs. However, the cows are left to find food to meet their needs, so the quality and quantity are not guaranteed. Lack of food causes livestock to experience malnutrition, making cows more susceptible to parasitic worm infestation (Purwanta *et al.* 2006).

The cestode classes identified from beef cattle feces samples were the worm species Moniezia sp., Taenia sp., and Diphyllobotrium sp., with the highest prevalence in the Moniezia sp species. Namely 14.29%. Moniezia sp. includes a type of tapeworm with a length of up to 200cm and a width of 1.5cm with triangular (Moniezia expansa) and quadrangular (Moniezia benedeni) egg shapes. The Moniezia expansa species is more often found infecting sheep and goats but can also infect cattle (Taylor *et al.* 2016). Infected cattle can come from grass feed that is not sterile and contains worm larvae. Apart from that, the age of the cow also influences the susceptibility to worm infections. Young cattle are more susceptible to worm infections. The reason is that young cattle's immune system is not as strong as adult cattle. One way to overcome this is by administering a vaccine to introduce antigens into the cow's body (Mafruchati 2020).

Worm eggs from the trematode class were also found in feces samples from beef cattle, namely Paramphistomum sp. (16.33%) and Fasciola sp. (1.02%). The life cycle of the worm Paramphistomum sp. requires an intermediary host, namely snails (Lymnea rubiginosa); this type of snail lives very well in rice fields, so if beef cattle are grazed in rice fields, it will allow them to be infected with Paramphistomum sp. worms. According to Darmin *et al.* (2016), snails live in environments with good vegetation and water, such as around rice fields, lakes, rivers, swamps, and ponds.

The results of identifying gastrointestinal parasites, apart from worm eggs, also found the presence of oocysts from protozoan parasites. One type of protozoa is identified: oocysts from Eimeria sp. (27.55%). Beef cattle rearing patterns, gender, type of livestock, age, environmental conditions, economic status, and breeder education can be factors causing Eimeria sp infection. (Baihaqi *et al.* 2015). Traditional rearing patterns without separation between the mother cage and her offspring will increase the chances of transmission of Eimeria sp.

The immune status of livestock is one of the intrinsic factors in the degree of gastrointestinal parasite infection. Beef cattle with good immunity will inhibit parasite activity in the digestive tract. The pathogenic effect of gastrointestinal parasites will decrease if the animal's immune system is good, this is due to the existence of a complex mechanism between specific and non-specific body defense systems. The mucosal lining of the digestive tract of young beef cattle is the first line of defense in the event of endoparasite investment. Goblet cells will secrete mucin, and epithelial cells will secrete galectin to bind carbohydrates found on the surface of the parasite's body (Grencis *et al.* 2014). Colostrum also affects endoparasites' manifestation in beef calves' digestive tract because it can stimulate the immune response when infection occurs.

Gastrointestinal parasite infections can cause significant losses to livestock by looking at clinical symptoms such as decreased appetite, diarrhea, anemia, dirty and dull fur, decreased body weight, and slow growth in young cattle. Some general disease prevention, according to Subekti *et al.* (2011), includes reducing the source of infection with therapeutic measures, monitoring water sanitation, food, the condition of rubbish housing, and eradicating intermediate hosts.

REFERENCES

Almuhardi, I., Saputra, F., & Kustiati, K. (2022). Prevalensi Helminthiasis pada sapi potong di Kecamatan singkawang tengah, kota singkawang. *Biologica Samudra*, 4(2), 105–115.

Baihaqi, H. U., Oka, I. B. M., & Dwinata, I. M. (2015). Prevalensi dan identifikasi nematoda saluran pencernaan kerbau lumpur di kecamatan sambelia, lombok timur, NTB. *Indonesia Medicus Veterinus*, 4(1), 1–8.

Darmin, S., Yuliza, P. F., & Sirupang, M. (2016). Prevalensi paramphistomiasis pada sapi bali di kecamatan libureng kabupaten bone. *JIIP*, 2(2):149–161.

Grencis, R. K., Humphreys, N. E., & Bancroft, A. J. (2014). Immunity to gastrointestinal nematodes: mechanisms and myths. *Immunological reviews*, 260(1), 183–205.

Inbaraj, S., Sejian, V., & Ramasamy, S. (2022). Role of environmental stressor-host immune system–pathogen interactions in development of infectious disease in farm animals. *Biological Rhythm Research*, 53(5), 707–724.

Mafruchati, M. (2020). Moniezia, Sp is found inside cow intestines slowing down the growth of the cattle. *Systematic Reviews in Pharmacy*, 11(11).

Mensah, G. T., Bosompem, K. M., Ayeh-Kumi, P. F., Brown, C. A., & Niampoma, S. (2018). Parasitic load of cattle faecal matter from selected farms in Kpong and its health implications. *Ghana Journal of Science*, 58, 35–39.

Paramitha, R. P., Ernawati, R., & Koesdarto, S. (2017). Prevalensi helminthiasis saluran pencernaan melalui pemeriksaan feses pada sapi di lokasi pembuangan akhir (LPA) Kecamatan benowo surabaya. *Journal of Parasite Science. (J. Parasite Sci.)* 1(1).

Purwanta, Ismaya, N.R.P., dan Burhan. 2006. Penyakit cacing hati (Fascioliasis) pada sapi bali di perusahaan daerah rumah potong hewan (RPH) Kota makassar. *Jurnal Agrisistem* 2(2): 63—69.

Putri, R. R., Ningrum, A. L. Y., Septiyani, E., & Kholik, K. (2022). Efektifitas pemberian albendazol dan ivermectin terhadap cacing saluran pencernaan sapi bali. *Jurnal Ilmu dan Teknologi Peternakan*, 10(2): 59–63

Setiawan, A., Candra, A. A., & Zairiful, Z. (2022). Tingkat kejadian kecacingan sapi potong pada peternakan rakyat di kabupaten mesuji. *PETERPAN (Jurnal Peternakan Terapan)*, 4(2), 33–37.

Subekti, S., S. Mumpuni, S. Koesdarto dan Kusnoto. 2011. Ilmu penyakit helminth veteriner. *Buku Ajar Fakultas Kedokteran Hewan Universitas Airlangga*. Surabaya.

Susilo, H., Abdillah, N. A., & Amelia, K. R. (2020). Identifikasi telur cacing parasit pada feses hewan ternak di propinsi banten. biodidaktika: *Jurnal Biologi dan Pembelajarannya*, 15(2).

Taylor M.A, Coop R.L. & Wall R.L., (2016). *Veterinary Parasitology*, 4th Ed. Oxford. Blackwell Publishing. *Hlm*. 259–803.

Technological Innovations in Tropical Livestock Development for Environmental Sustainability and Food Security – P. Dhian Isnaeni et al. (eds)
© 2025 The Author(s), ISBN 978-1-032-74373-8
Open Access: www.taylorfrancis.com, CC BY-NC-ND 4.0 license

Use of Moringa Leaf flour *(Moringa oleifera)* fermented with *Neurospora crassa* on broiler carcass quality

Y. Fenita*, U. Santoso, Kususiyah, Nurmeiliasari, R. Damayanti & A. Rizky
Departement of Animal Husbandry, Faculty of Agriculture, Bengkulu University, Indonesia

ABSTRACT: The research aims to evaluate Moringa leaf flour (*Moringa oleifera*) fermentation (MOF) with *Neurospora crassa* on broiler carcass quality. The design used was a Completely Randomized Design (CRD), four treatments, and five replications, each replication using eight broilers. P0: control (without (MOF), P1: using 5% (MOF), P2: using 10% (MOF), P3: using 15% (MOF). Variables observed included carcass color, carcass weight, percentage of carcass weight, meat-bone ratio, cooking loss, and drip loss. Data were analyzed using ANOVA (*analysis of variance*). (MOF) had a significant effect (P<0.05) on carcass color, carcass weight, and percentage of carcass weight but had no significant effect (P>0.05) on meat-bone *ratio, cooking loss,* and drip *loss*. In conclusion, using (MOF) levels of 10% and 15% improves carcass color but can reduce carcass weight. In comparison, levels of 5%–15% reduce the percentage of carcass weight without affecting the meat-bone ratio, cooking loss, and drip loss of broiler meat aged 35 days.

Keywords: Broiler, Carcass Quality, Moringa Leaves

1 INTRODUCTION

Protein is an important element required for poultry's growth and feed efficiency of poultry. One of the local feed ingredients with high protein and active substance content and sufficient availability is moringa (*Moringa oleifera*). Moringa is a plant that can reach 10 meters in height and has soft and brittle stems, with leaves the size of a fingertip, which are oval and compound (Suriawiria 2005). Rahmawati (2020) stated that the nutrition in Moringa leaves, especially the high protein content, makes Moringa leaf flour a substitute source of protein rather than an additional feed (feed supplement) at a low level. Using Moringa leaf flour as a protein source has been reported to be able to replace soybean meal. Moringa leaves have weaknesses such as low protein digestibility caused by high fiber, anti-nutrient content, and unbalanced amino acids (Gadzirayi *et al.* 2012). Putri (2022) stated that using Moringa leaves with the addition of Aspergillus *niger* in the ration on broiler carcass quality does not decrease the cooking *loss* of broiler meat. Manihuruk (2018) stated that feeding feed containing fermented Moringa leaf flour with a 5% dose of EM4 showed the best increase in carcass weight compared to other groups. However, treatment with a dose of 10% can reduce broiler carcass weight. It is necessary to research the use of Moringa leaf flour (*Moringa oleifera*) fermentation with *Neurospora crassa* on broiler carcass quality. This study aims to evaluate the use of Moringa leaf flour (*Moringa oleifera*) fermentation with *Neurospora crassa* on broiler carcass quality.

*Corresponding Author: yosifenita@gmail.com

 DOI: 10.1201/9781003468943-22

2 MATERIALS AND METHODS

2.1 *Chicken and feed*

DOC are reared together in brooding cages of 200 animals until they are 14 days old with a commercial diet (BR 1). At the age of 15 days, 160 chickens were selected for treatment. The production of fermented moringa leaf flour ((MOF) used 1 kg of moringa leaf flour with 800 ml of water, and then the moringa leaf flour was steamed with a steamer for 30 minutes. The fermentation used 1% *Neurospora crassa.*

2.2 *Research procedure*

This research used a completely randomized design (CRD) with four treatment levels and five replications. A sample of 160 broilers was distributed into experimental plots randomly. The dietary treatment was applied for 21 days starting at the age of 15 days. The research treatments are P0: Ration without (MOF) *Neurospora crassa.* P1: Ration contains 5% (MOF) *Neurospora crassa.* P2: Ration contains 10% (MOF) *Neurospora crassa.* P3: Ration contains 15% (MOF) *Neurospora crassa*

Sampling was carried out when the broilers were 35 days old. Two animals were taken from each cage plot based on the average body weight of the treatment. Before slaughtering, broilers are fasted for 12 hours to empty the digestive tract and then weighed. Variables measured are: 1. Carcass color is measured by comparing the chest color of the carcass with the standard color according to the DSM broiler color fan. 2. Carcass weight is the weight of the chicken after deducting non-carcass components, namely the head, feet, feathers, blood and all stomach contents. Carcass weight was measured by weighing the broiler carcass. 3. Carcass percentage was measured by weighing live weight and broiler carcass weight. 4. MBR measurements were carried out on all carcasses obtained. MBR is measured by dividing the weight of meat by the weight of bones. 5. Data Cooking loss obtained by taking a meat sample from the left breast with a size of 2 × 2 cm then placing it in heat-resistant plastic and weighing it. The weight lost during cooking is called cooking loss. The lost water content is calculated based on the percentage of sample weight lost during cooking to the initial weight of the sample. Once the water temperature reaches 80°C, the sample is put in water bath for 20 minutes, then the sample is removed and drained on glass for 15 minutes. 6. Drip Loss; Testing drip loss carried out in four stages, namely the sampling stage, sample weighing, storage in the freezer, and measurement. The meat sample was cut from the left side of the chest with a size of 2 × 2 cm and put in freezer. After 72 hours, the samples were thawing (left at room temperature for 60 minutes) and then weighed again.

All variable data were analyzed using ANOVA (Analysis of Variance). When the treatment has a significant effect ($P<0.05$), it is tested by using Duncan's Multi Range Test (DMRT) to see differences between treatments.

3 RESULTS AND DISCUSSION

3.1 *Broiler carcass quality*

The results of research on the use of fermented Moringa leaves (*Moringa oleifera*) 5%, 10%, and 15% in the ration on carcass color, carcass weight, percentage of carcass weight, meat bone ratio, cooking loss, and drip loss presented in Table 1.

3.2 *Carcass color, carcass weight, and carcass weight percentage*

The use of Moringa leaf flour up to 15% had a significant effect ($P<0.05$) on broiler carcass color. Further test results show that P0 is not significantly different from P1 but is

Table 1. Average carcass color, carcass weight, percentage of carcass weight, *meat-bone ratio*, *cooking loss*, *drip loss*.

Variable	Treatment				P
	P0	P1	P2	P3	
Carcass Color	102.40±0.52[a]	102.50±0.71[a]	103.50±0.53[b]	104.30±0.67[c]	0.00
Carcass Weight	1,131.44±63.5[b]	1,088.65±61.08[ab]	1,060.65±45.60[a]	1,060.83±75.09[a]	0.049
Carcass percentage	72.76±2.81[b]	69.08±3.16[a]	66.94±3.34[a]	67.33±5.20[a]	0.005
Meat Bone Ratio	3.01±0.08	2.95±0.11	3.03±0.38	3.03±0.31	0.183
Cooking Loss	34.02±3.17	33.40±3.88	35.35±5.89	34.11±2.56	0.754
Drip Loss	4.62±2.17	5.97±2.34	4.11±1.72	4.31±2.26	0.224

Note: P0: Control ration without TDKF; P1: Use of 5% TDKF; P2: Use of 10% TDKF; P3: Use of 15% TDKF: P<0.05 (significant effect) and P>0.05 (no significant effect).
Different superskips on the same line have a significant effect (P<0.05).

significantly lower than P2 and P3. The average broiler carcass color scores were P0(102.40), P1(102.50), P2(103.50), and P3(104.30). The use of TDKF levels of 10% and 15% can improve broiler carcass color. According to Krisnadi (2015) Moringa leaves contain *β*-carotene affect carcass color. According to Samudra and Arief (2008), pigments obtained from feed will accumulate in the tissue, then be absorbed in the blood and circulated throughout the body, which will then have a pigmentation effect on the skin color of the carcass. The (MOF) had a significant effect (P<0.05) on carcass weight. Further test results showed that P0 is not significantly different from P1, but is higher than P2 and P3. The average carcass weight ranges from P0(1131.44 g), P1(1088.65 g), P2(1060.65 g), P3(1060.83 g). The use of 10% and 15% TDKF reduced broiler carcass weight. According to Lesson and Summer (2005), the carcass weight produced by a chicken will be proportional to the live weight. The results of analysis of variations in live weight showed that live weight before slaughter had no significant effect, but the use of 10% and 15% TDKF reduced carcass weight. The results of analysis of variance showed that the use of TDKF had a significant effect (P<0.05) on the percentage of carcass weight. Further test results show that P0 is significantly different from P1, P2, and P3, while the difference between P1, P2, and P3 is not significant. Average carcass weight percentages P0(72.76%), P1(69.08%), P2(66.94%), and P3(67.33%). TTDKF use at the level of 5% -15% reduced the percentage of carcass weight. The percentage decrease in carcass weight was respectively P1 (3.68%), P2 (5.82%), and P3 (5.43%). The results of this research's carcass weight percentage are still within the standard value of carcass weight percentage, namely 66.94–72.76%. Nirwana (2011) stated that a carcass percentage of 67–75% is the percentage of broilers that have high growth. According to Soeparno (2015), generally, the broiler carcass percentage ranges from 65–72%. Fenita *et al.* (2011) stated that the percentage of carcass weight in 42-day-old broilers given noni fruit juice ranged from 58.04–60.36%.

3.3 *Meat Bone Ratio (MBR), cooking loss and drip loss*

The results of the analysis of variance show that the use of TDKF has no significant effect (P>0.05) on MBR (meat bone ratio). Average MBR P0(3.01), P1(2.95), P2(3.03), P3(3.03). The TDKF treatment did not affect MBR. According to Soetan and Oyewole (2009), tannin in Moringa leaves forms complex compounds that broilers cannot digest. Putri (2022) stated that giving Moringa leaf flour as a substitute for soybean meal did not affect MBR, allegedly due to factors such as the feed ration consumed and the protein content in the feed. Moringa leaf flour fermented feed rations cannot affect the metabolism of muscle formation in broilers because of the anti-nutrient content, which inhibits protein breakdown and nutrient absorption. Tannin is an antinutrient that inhibits protein absorption in broilers. The results of the analysis of variance indicate the use of TDKF *has* no significant effect (P>0.05) on cooking loss. To the track cooking loss respectively P0 (34.02), P1(33.40), P2(35.35), and P3 (34.11). A 15 % TDKF did not decrease the cooking loss of broiler meat. Suradi's research results (2006) show that the pH value of the meat influences the value of cooking loss. The higher the pH value decreases; the more protein is damaged so that the protein's ability to bind water is lost. Fenita *et al.* (2011) show that cooking loss in 42-day-old broilers it ranges from 15.71% –17.09%. The average cooking loss in this study ranged from 33.40%–35.35%. Banes *et al.* (2017) stated that cooking loss in broilers aged 35 days ranges between 21,40%–33,19%. The results of the analysis of variance showed that the use of TDKF had no significant effect (P>0.05). drip loss. TDKF at the level of 5%–15% does not *reduce drip loss i*n broiler meat. Putri (2022) stated that fermented Moringa leaf flour given with *Aspergillus niger* up to the level of 15% in the ration does not reduce drip loss of broiler meat because of its high protein content. It can bind water. The research results of Nurkhasanah (2015) reported that drip loss in broiler chickens aged 35 days ranged between 5.22–5.72%. Banes *et al.* (2017) drip loss in broiler chickens aged 35 days, ranging from 3.39–5.74%. The results of this study were still normal, with an average *drip loss of* 4.11–5.97%. So, from the research results, the use of TDKF can be used in broiler feed at a level of 5–15% without having a negative impact on the drip loss of broilers. Santoso (2014) stated that the water-binding capacity of meat is influenced by meat protein. High meat protein increases the water binding ability so that the liquid that comes out during thawing is less. From an economic point of view, a low drip loss will provide an advantage because the weight and nutritional content of the meat is not lost much.

4 CONCLUSIONS

Based on the results of this research, it can be concluded that the use of fermented Moringa leaf flour *Neurospora crassa* levels of 10% and 15% improve carcass color, but reduce carcass weight. In contrast,e levels of 5%-15% can reduce the percentage of carcass weight without affecting MBR, cooking loss, and drip loss.

REFERENCES

Banes, S. S., Kususiyah and Y. Fenita. 2017. Effect of katuk leaf extract (*Sauropus androgynus*) fermentation on broiler carcass quality. *Indonesian Journal of Animal Science*, 12(2): 199–208.

Fenita, Y., Warnoto and A. Nopis. 2011. The effect of giving noni fruit water (*Morinda citrifolia*) on broiler chicken carcass quality. *Indonesian Journal of Animal Science*, 6(2): 142–150.

Gadzirayi, C. T., B. Masamha, J. F. Mupangwa, S. dan Washaya. 2012. Performance of broiler chickens. Fed on mature Moringa oleifera leaf meal as a protein supplement to soybean meal. *Int. J. poult. Sci.*, 11(1):5–10.

Krisnadi, A. D. 2015. Super nutritional moringa. *Indonesian Moringa Plant Information and Development Center, Non-Governmental Organization–Environmental Care Media.*

Leeson, S. dan Summer, J. D. 2009. *Broiler Breeder Production*. Inggris: Nottingham University Press.

Manihuruk, F. M, Ismail, Rastina, Razali, M. Sabri, Zuhrawzti, and M.. Jalaludin. 2018. Effect of Fermentation*Moringa leaf* (*Moringa oleifera*) powder in Feed To Increase Broiler Carcass Weight. Banda Aceh, *Jurnal Medika Veterina*.

Nirvana. 2011. Providing various forms of rations made from local raw materials on the percentage of carcass weight, carcass fat and abdominal fat in broilers. Thesis. Hasanuddin University Faculty of Animal Husbandry. *Makassar*.

Nurkhasanah, B. 2015. Effect of katu leaf extract supplementation (*Sauropus androgynus*) and turmeric powder (*Curcuma domestica*) on the carcass quality of broiler chickens fed low protein feed. Thesis. Faculty of Agriculture, Bengkulu University, Bengkulu.

Putri, A. E. 2022. The effect of using Moringa leaf flour (*Moringa oleifera*) fermentation in the diet on broiler carcass quality. Department of Animal Husbandry. Bengkulu University. *Bengkulu.*

Rahmawati. D. 2020. Carcass weight and carcass parts of male laying hens *(Gallus gallus domesticus l.)* after administering Moringa leaf flour *(Moringa oleifera)* as a feed additive. journal of tropical biology. Diponegoro University, *Semarang.*

Samudera, R and Arief, H. 2008. Skin color, abdominal fat, and carcass fat of Alabio ducks (*Anas plathyrhincos* Borneo) male as a result of giving Azolla in the ration. *Anima Productions.* 10(3): 164–167.

Santoso, U. 2014. *Multi-Efficacy Plant Katuk.* Publishing Agency for the Faculty of Agriculture (BPFP) Bengkulu University, Bengkulu.

Sjofjan, O, dan Ardyati, T. 2011. Extracellular amylase activity of amylolytic bacteria isolated from quail's (*Coturnix japonica*) intestinal tract in corn flour medium. *International Journal of Poultry Science*, 10(5), 411–415.

Soeparno. 2015. *Meat Science and Technology. Fifth Printing.* Gadjah Mada University Press, Yogyakarta

Soetan, K. O dan Oyewole, O. E. 2009. The need for adequate processing to reduce the anti-nutritional factors in plants used as human food and animal feeds : A review. *Afriacan jounal food dan veteriner.* Bogor.

Suradi, K. 2006. Changes in the physical properties of post mortem broiler chicken meat during room temperature storage. *JITV*, 6(1): 23–27.

Suriawiria, U. 2005. *Basic Microbiology.* Jakarta (ID): Papas Sinar Sinanti

Technological Innovations in Tropical Livestock Development for Environmental Sustainability and Food Security – P. Dhian Isnaeni et al. (eds)

The effects of *Phyllanthus niruni* (Meniran) extracts on anti-inflammatory activity in raw 264.7 macrophage cells

L. Purnamasari*
Department of Animal Husbandry, Faculty of Agriculture, University of Jember, Jember, Indonesia
School of Animal Life Convergence Science, Hankyong National University, Anseong-si, South Korea

H. Khasanah
Department of Animal Husbandry, Faculty of Agriculture, University of Jember, Jember, Indonesia

S.G. Hwang, I.S. Nam & J.K. Yi
School of Animal Life Convergence Science, Hankyong National University, Anseong-si, South Korea

J.F.d. Cruz
Department of Basic Veterinary Science, College of Veterinary Medicine, University of the Philippines, Los Banos, Philippines

N. Pratiwi
Research Innovation Agency of the Republic of Indonesia (BRIN) Cibinong Sciences Center, Cibinong, Bogor, Indonesia

ABSTRACT: *Phyllanthus niruri* (meniran) is well known as an Indonesian traditional medicine due to its antioxidant properties to treat several infectious diseases. Meniran extract is a potential candidate for feed additives to substitute antibiotics. However, the biological activity of meniran has remained to be fully elucidated. The present study aimed to evaluate the anti-inflammatory effects of a meniran extract (ME) on lipopolysaccharide-induced RAW264.7 macrophage cells and were investigated via DPPH radical scavenging assay, CCK-8 assay, NO-assay, and RT-PCR analysis. LPS-induced RAW264.7 macrophage cells were grown in RPMI media containing 10% FBS, and 1% penicillin-streptomycin and then were cultured with ME (25, 50, 100, 200, and 400 ppm). ME showed an anti-inflammatory by increasing cell proliferation and was not toxic up to 400 ppm ($P < 0.05$). The ME activity suppressed the production of nitric oxide (NO) and the mRNA expression of inducible NO synthase. It also decreases the production of the pro-inflammatory cytokine's interleukin-6, Nuclear factor-κB, and tumor necrosis factor-α in mRNA expression. These results suggest that ME has anti-inflammatory properties that can be used to prevent or cure inflammatory diseases and potential candidate for feed additives to substitute antibiotics.

Keywords: meniran, anti-inflammatory, feed additives, Raw 264.7 Cells, Macrophage Cell

1 INTRODUCTION

Antibiotics have been used at sub-therapeutic levels to encourage growth and minimize morbidity and mortality throughout the animals' life cycle (Reddy *et al.* 2020). However, usage has been banned in the European Union since January 2006 because it is feared that it

*Corresponding Author: listyap.faperta@unej.ac.id

DOI: 10.1201/9781003468943-23

will cause antibiotic residue. The encouraged use of plant secondary metabolites or natural herbal extracts as feed additives to substitute antibiotics has been deeply studied.

Plant secondary metabolites are an exceedingly large group of compounds with small molecular weights that play important roles as antioxidants, antibacterials, antifungals, antivirals, anti-inflammatory and anticancer activities (Alhazmi *et al.* 2021; Rodríguez-Yoldi 2021). *Phyllanthus niruri* (meniran) is well known as an Indonesian traditional medicine due to its bioactive compounds and antioxidant properties to treat several infectious diseases. Meniran contains lignans and flavonoid compounds as antioxidants to increase the immune system (Purwitasari *et al.* 2023). Meniran as a medical drink is often used to boost the immune system in Indonesian traditional medication (Tjandrawinata *et al.* 2017).

The RAW 264.7 cells are monocyte/macrophage-like cells, derived from BALB/c mice. These cells are described as an appropriate model for macrophages (Taciak *et al.* 2018). Macrophages are versatile cells that play many roles in both innate and specific immune responses. Although most of the beneficial effects of meniran could be related to immunomodulatory activities, the validity of the anti-inflammatory effect has not been scientifically investigated so far. Therefore, the research aimed to investigate the latent anti-inflammatory ability of meniran aqueous and ethanol extract on RAW 264.7 cells.

2 MATERIAL AND METHODS

2.1 *Reagents*

Folin–Ciocalteu reagent and gallic acid were purchased from Sigma-Aldrich. Sodium carbonate (Na2CO3) was from VWR Life Science. DPPH reagent from Gibco and quercetin from Sigma-Aldrich. Raw cells 264.7 were obtained from the Korean Cell Bank (Korea). Cell growth mediums are Roswell Park Memorial Institute (RPMI) 1640 from Gibco, penicillin/streptomycin (P/S) from Lonza, and Fetal Bovine Serum (FBS) from Biowest. To investigate the effect of different concentrations of meniran extract on Raw cells 264.7, a proliferation assay was performed using CCK-8 assay (Biomax). Production of NO by Lipopolysaccharide (LPS, Sigma-Aldrich)-activated Raw 264.7 cells was measured by using Griess reagent (Sigma-Aldrich). RNA was extracted using RNAiso Plus Takara Shuzo Co. cDNA was synthesized using a Maxime PCR premix kit (i-Taq) from iNtRON Biotechnology.

2.2 *Plant extraction*

Meniran leaves (*Phyllantus niruni*) were dried and crushed into a powder. The powder (50 g) was soaked in 500 ml distilled water for aqueous extraction and then shaken at 90°C for 4 h in a water bath. For ethanol extraction, the powder (50 g) was extracted in 500 mL of 80% ethanol for 24 h stirring, filtering then extracted under compact pressure using a rotary evaporator. Subsequently, the filtered mixture was stored in a freezer to make small ice blocks and the plant extract was obtained by using a freeze-drying machine. All extracts were kept at 4°C until the tests were performed.

2.3 *Total phenolic compound (TPC) assay*

TPC was determined using Folin–Ciocalteu reagent using gallic acid as a standard. 10 μL of extract solution (1 mg/mL) was added in a test tube, followed by 0.5 mL of 1:10 Folin–Ciocalteu reagent. The mixture was incubated at room temperature for 5 min. Then, 0.35 mL of 115 mg/mL sodium carbonate (Na2CO3) was added and mixed thoroughly. The mixture was then allowed to stand at room temperature for 2h. Absorbance readings were taken spectrophotometrically at 765 nm and all determinations were done in triplicate. The total phenolic content was expressed as milligrams of gallic acid equivalent to grams of dried plant material.

2.4 *2,2-Diphenyl-1-picrylhydrazyl (DPPH) assay*

The DPPH assay was determined to show herbal free radical scavenging activity. Meniran extracts and the reference standard (Quercetin) were prepared as stock solutions, and a series of dilutions with varying concentrations were tested. 50 μL of samples/standards were loaded, followed by 150 μL DPPH reagent. The mixtures were then mixed vigorously and incubated in the dark at room temperature for 30 min, and the absorbance was measured spectrophotometrically at 517 nm. The percentage of DPPH free radical scavenging activity was calculated as:

$$Scavenging\ ability\ (\%) = 1 - \frac{OD\ of\ sample}{OD\ of\ control} \times 100$$

2.5 *Cell viability assay*

Raw cells were grown in a 10 mL RPMI-1640 medium containing 10% fetal Bovine Serum, 1% penicillin/streptomycin, and incubated at 37°C under 5% CO2. The medium will be replaced every 2 days. For the cell proliferation experiment, Raw cells 264.7 were seeded in a 96-well plate at a density of $(1\times10)^5$ per ml and incubated for 6 hours. Cells were then treated with different media preparation concentrations of meniran extract (25, 50, 100, 200, and 400 ppm) with 1 μg/mL of lipopolysaccharide (LPS) for 24 and 48 hours. After each time frame, the media was removed, and fresh media was added with CCK-8 reagent to quantify cell proliferation activity. Optical Density was measured under 450 nm. The percentage of cell proliferation was computed concerning the control.

2.6 *Nitric oxide assay*

Production of NO by LPS-activated Raw cells 264.7 was measured by using a Griess reagent. Raw cells 264.7 were incubated at 5 × 104 cells/well in 96 well plates for 24 h at 37 ° C and 5% CO2. Then the cells were treated with various concentrations in the presence of LPS (1 μg/mL). After 24 h treatment, 50 μl of supernatant was mixed with 50 μl Griess reagent and incubated for 30 minutes. Optical Density was measured under 540 nm. The percentage of nitric oxide was computed concerning the control.

2.7 *Reverse transcription-polymerase chain reaction (RT-PCR)*

Confluent cultures of Raw cells 264.7 in 6-well plates were induced as previously described for 2 days. According to the manufacturer's instructions, total RNA was extracted from Raw cells 264.7 pellets using 500 μL RNAiso Plus. cDNA was synthesized from 1 μg of total RNA in a 20 μl reaction using Maxime RT Premix Kit. PCR reactions consisted of an initial denaturation cycle at 95°C for 5 minutes, followed by 30 amplification cycles at 95°C for 40 seconds, followed by annealing for 40 seconds (temperature ranging from 56–62) and extension at 72°C for 1 minute. Sequences of the primers used for PCR amplification are shown Table 1.

Table 1. Sequences of the primers used for PCR amplification of Raw cells 264.7.

Primer		
β-actin	forward	5'-CACCCCAGCCATGTACGT-3'
	Reverse	3'-GTCCAGACGCAGGATGGC-5'
iNOS	forward	5'-GCTCTACACCTCCAATGTGACC-3'
	Reverse	3'-CTGCCGAGATTTGAGCCTCATG-5'
IL-6	forward	5'-TACTCGGCAAACCTAGTGCG-3'
	Reverse	3'-GTGTCCCAACATTCATATTGTCAGT-5'
NFk-B	forward	5'-CGCAAAAGGACCTACGAGAC-3'
	Reverse	3'-TGGGGGAAAACTCATCAAG-5'
TNF-α	forward	5'-GTCTTGGCCGAGGACTAAGG-3'
	Reverse	3'-GTCTTGGCCGAGGACTAAGG-5'

2.8 *Statistical analysis*

All quantitative data are representative of at least three independent experiments and the results were expressed as means ± standard deviation. Differences between means were evaluated using a one-way ANOVA test followed by Duncan's Multiple Range Test (DMRT). Differences were considered significant at $P < 0.05$ using SPSS 24 software package

3 RESULT AND DISCUSSION

The murine macrophage cell line, RAW 264.7, was a macrophage-like, Abelson leukemia virus-transformed cell line derived from BALB/c mice. This cell line is a commonly used model of mouse macrophages for the study of cellular responses and bioactivity to microbes and other natural products (Merly & Smith 2017).

3.1 *Total phenolic compound*

Phenolic compounds in plants are responsible for antioxidant activity. Total phenolic compounds (TPC) are one of the important parameters of total antioxidant capacity and are widely used for the evaluation of the antioxidant properties of plants (Molole *et al.* 2022). The whole extracts of meniran leaves were analyzed for total phenolic content (Table 2.).

Table 2. The total phenolic compound of meniran leaves extract.

Item	Total phenolic compounds
MEE	1226.10 mg GAE/g
MAE	1130.45 mg GAE/g

MEE = Meniran ethanol extract, MAE = Meniran aquoues extract

The higher phenolic content results from meniran ethanol extract. Previous studies reported ethanol is the most suitable solvent that can be used for the extraction of phenolic compounds from plant sources (Brglez *et al.* 2016; Lohvina *et al.* 2022; Venkatesan *et al.* 2019). The polarity of the ethanol is more consistent for the extraction of polar components like phospholipids, polysaccharides, and lipoproteins (El Mannoubi 2023), which may be the most dominant components of meniran leaves. Plants are rich in secondary metabolites and bioactive compounds that provide protective actions to prevent or cure disease (Gil-Martin *et al.* 2022). The presence of phenolic content shows that the extract has an advantage for medical treatment. The extraction process is a crucial stage that has a decisive effect on the reliability of the results (Gościnna *et al.* 2021). The total phenol produced from plant extract is influenced by various factors, including drying method, particle size, plant form, and solvent type (Shi *et al.* 2022). Different plant material requires different solvent types for the maximum extraction of phenolic compounds.

3.2 *2,2-Diphenyl-1-picrylhydrazyl (DPPH) assay*

The hydroxyl groups in plant extracts are responsible for facilitating free radical scavenging and phenolic molecules are responsible for deactivating free radicals based on their ability to donate hydrogen atoms to free radicals (Shresta & Dhillion 2006). Phenolic compounds and flavonoids are well known for their free radical scavenging (antioxidant) activities

(Dirar *et al.* 2019). The DPPH assay is widely used to evaluate the radical scavenging ability of plants with a simple and acceptable technique (Aryal *et al.* 2019). The scavenging ability from MAE and MEE is shown in Figure 1.

Meniran aqueous extract has a low scavenging ability below 50% up to 400 ppm. However, at concentrations of 800 ppm MAE scavenging ability is quite high at 60%. Interestingly, the concentration of 1000 ppm between MAE and MEE has the same ability to neutralize oxidants (DPPH) by 95%. In contrast to extracts using ethanol, with a concentration under 100 ppm, the scavenging ability is under 20% but starting at 200 ppm the scavenging ability is above 55%.

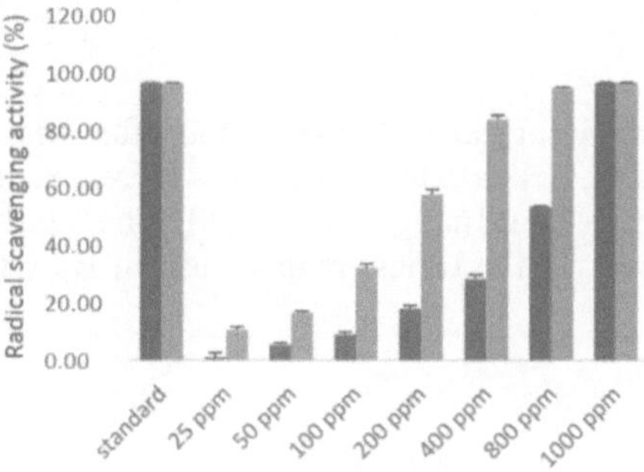

Figure 1. Scavenging ability (%) of aqueous and ethanol meniran extract. MAE = meniran aqueous extract; MEE = meniran ethanol extract. Standard = ascorbic acid.

The capability of scavenging ability supported by the bioactive compound of its extract. Bioactive phytochemicals are antioxidants, to which available evidence attributes some of the therapeutic benefits of the diet (Amarowicz & Pegg 2019). DPPH scavenging activity were highly correlated with total phenolic content. A previous study reported ethanol extract of plant leaves had the strongest antioxidant activity as well as the highest phenolic content compared to other solvents such as methanol and aqueous (Hikmawati *et al.* 2021; Lohvina *et al.* 2022).

3.3 *Cell proliferation (%)*

The result of the DPPH assay was used for evaluating the cytotoxicity in Raw Cells 264.7 cells via CCK-8 assay as shown in Figure 2. MEE was chosen to evaluate cell proliferation with concentrations 25, 50, 100, 200, and 400 ppm.

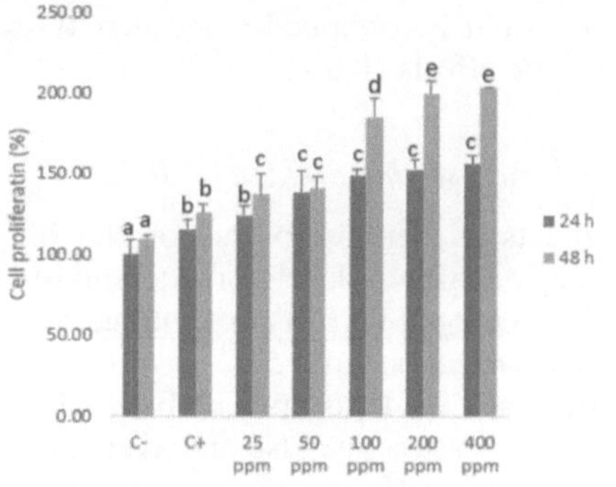

Figure 2. Cell proliferation (%) of ethanol meniran extract. C- = control negative (without lipopolysaccharide); C+ = control positive (with lipopolysaccharide).

Treatment with different concentrations (25–400ppm) for 24 hours and 48 h was able to stimulate the proliferation of raw cells 264.7 without any toxicity occurring. At the 48-hour treatment doses of 200 and 400 ppm began to show a stagnant in proliferation but still higher than the control. Meniran extract was found to stimulate raw 264.7 cell and not toxic effectively.

Macrophages play a crucial role in protecting the body via the swallowing and digestion of foreign substances and contribute to host defense mechanisms as a part of the innate immune system (Kim *et al.* 2023). Phyllanthus species provide important medicinal properties specially, the lignans and tannins that exhibit diverse biological and pharmacological effects including immunomodulatory activities (Jantan *et al.* 2019).

3.4 *Nitric oxide (%)*

Inflammation is a complex biological response to harmful stimuli such as infections and injuries. During inflammation, activated macrophages secrete excessive inflammatory mediators, such as nitric oxide (NO) (Huang *et al.* 2018). The synthesis of the inflammatory mediator NO was performed via the Griess reagent test in Raw Cells 264.7 cells shown in Figure 3.

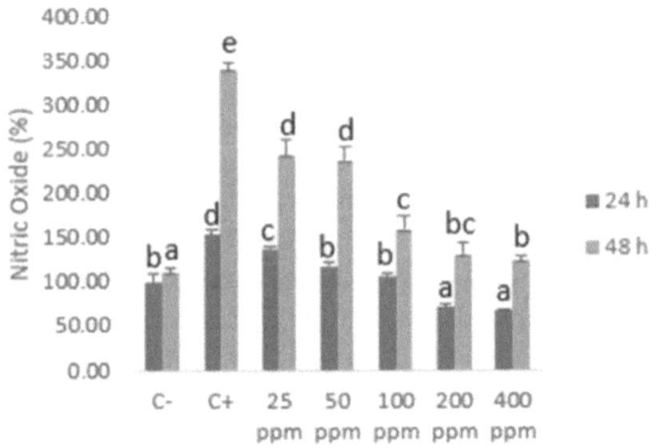

Figure 3. Nitric oxide (%) of ethanol meniran extract. C- = control negative (without lipopolysaccharide); C+ = control positive (with lipopolysaccharide).

The results indicated that the concentration of meniran extract suppressed the production of nitric oxide (NO) in LPS-stimulated Raw 264.7 cells. Flavonoids and lignans as well as some amounts of volatile oil could be obtained from alcohol extraction and they showed anti-inflammatory and antibiotic effects (Kim *et al.* 2019).

3.5 *Reverse transcription-polymerase chain reaction (RT-PCR)*

To further investigate the effects of meniran extract on the LPS-induced RAW 264.7 cell inflammation model, the relative mRNA levels of interleukin-6 (IL6), Nuclear factor-κB (NFκB), and tumor necrosis factor-α (TNF-α), and inducible NO synthase (iNOS) were determined by Real-Time PCR (Figures 4 and 5).

Proinflammatory cytokines such as IL-6 and TNF-α, which play crucial roles in the development of inflammatory diseases, are also involved in innate immunity and autoimmune diseases (Hirano 2020). The ME activity suppressed the production of nitric oxide (NO) and the mRNA expression of iNOS. It also decreases the production of the proinflammatory cytokine's IL-6, NFκB, and TNF-α in mRNA expression.

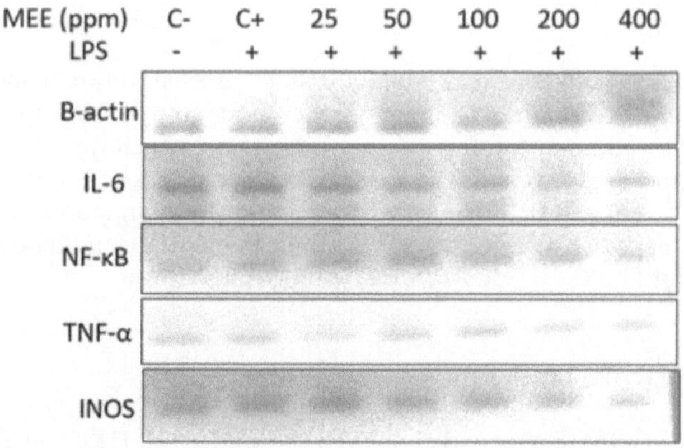

Figure 4. Effect of meniran ethanol extract on the mRNA expression of inflammatory and immunomodulatory genes in LPS-stimulated Raw 264.7 cells.

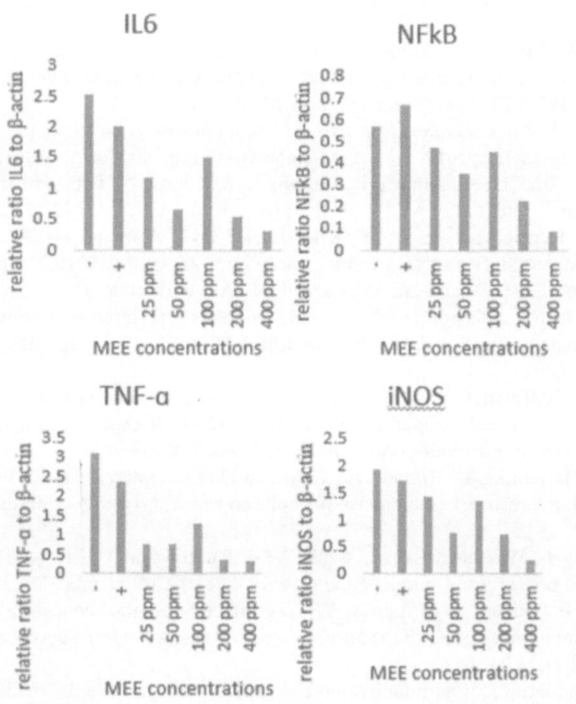

Figure 5. Relative value of mRNA expression of inflammatory and immunomodulatory genes in LPS-stimulated Raw 264.7 cells.

Inflammatory mediators and cytokines are responsible for the pathogenesis of a vast number of diseases (Hwang *et al.* 2017). The noxious agent has ability to induced inflammation via transcription and translation of inflammatory biomarkers such as iNOS, IL-6, NFκB, and TNF-α (Tambewagh *et al.* 2017). Our findings show that meniran extract exhibits potential anti-inflammatory activities due to the decreasing level of pro-inflammatory cytokines.

4 CONCLUSION

Both *P. niruri* (meniran) aqueous and ethanol extract showed antioxidant activity however ethanolic extract showed high scavenging activity in comparison to aqueous extract. Meniran extract showed an anti-inflammatory by increasing cell proliferation and was not toxic up to 400 ppm ($P < 0.05$). and suppressed the production of INOS, IL-6, NFkB, and TNF-α. These results suggest that meniran extract has anti-inflammatory properties that can be used to prevent or cure inflammatory diseases and potential candidate for feed additives to substitute antibiotics.

AUTHORS' CONTRIBUTIONS

LP, HK, JFC, and SGH designed and conceived the study. LP, HK, and JFC experimented with the study. LP, SGH, ISN, and JKL performed the statistical analysis. LP, HK, NP, and JFC drafted the manuscript. All authors read and approved the final manuscript.

REFERENCES

Alhazmi H. A., Najmi A., Javed S. A., Sultana S., Al Bratty M. & Makeen H.A., *et al.* Medicinal plants and isolated molecules demonstrating immunomodulation activity as potential alternative therapies for viral diseases including COVID-19. *Front Immunol.* 2021;12(May):1–24.

Amarowicz R. & Pegg R. B. *Natural antioxidants of plant origin [Internet].* 1st ed. Vol. 90, *Advances in Food and Nutrition Research.* Elsevier Inc.; 2019. 1–81 p. Available from: http://dx.doi.org/10.1016/bs.afnr.2019.02.011

Aryal S., Baniya M. K., Danekhu K., Kunwar P., Gurung R. & Koirala N. Total Phenolic content, Flavonoid content and antioxidant potential of wild vegetables from western Nepal. *Plants.* 2019;8(4).

Brglez Mojzer E., Knez Hrnčič M., Škerget M., Knez Ž. & Bren U. Polyphenols: Extraction methods, antioxidative action, bioavailability and anticarcinogenic effects. *Molecules.* 2016;21(7).

Dirar A. I., Alsaadi D. H. M., Wada M., Mohamed M. A., Watanabe T. & Devkota H. P. Effects of extraction solvents on total phenolic and flavonoid contents and biological activities of extracts from Sudanese medicinal plants. *South African J Bot [Internet].* 2019;120:261–7. Available from: https://doi.org/10.1016/j.sajb.2018.07.003

El Mannoubi I. Impact of different solvents on extraction yield, phenolic composition, in vitro antioxidant and antibacterial activities of deseeded Opuntia stricta fruit. *J Umm Al-Qura Univ Appl Sci [Internet*]. 2023;9 (2):176–84. Available from: https://doi.org/10.1007/s43994-023-00031-y

Gil-Martín E., Forbes-Hernández T., Romero A., Cianciosi D., Giampieri F., & Battino M. Influence of the extraction method on the recovery of bioactive phenolic compounds from food industry by-products. *Food Chem.* 2022;378.

Gościnna K., Pobereżny J., Wszelaczyńska E., Szulc W. & Rutkowska B. Effects of drying and extraction methods on bioactive properties of plums. *Food Control.* 2021;122(November 2020).

Hikmawanti N. P. E., Fatmawati S. & Asri A. W. The effect of ethanol concentrations as the extraction solvent on antioxidant activity of Katuk (Sauropus androgynus (L.) Merr.) leaves extracts. *IOP Conf Ser Earth Environ Sci.* 2021;755(1):0–7.

Hirano T. IL-6 in inflammation, autoimmunity and cancer. *Int. Immun.* 2020;33(3):127–148. Available from: https://doi.org/10.1093/intimm/dxaa078.

Huang C., Li W., Zhang Q., Chen L., Chen W. & Zhang H., *et al.* Anti-inflammatory activities of Guang-Pheretima extract in lipopolysaccharide-stimulated RAW 264.7 murine macrophages. *BMC Complement Altern Med.* 2018;18(1):1–11.

Hwang K. A., Hwang Y. J., & Song J. Aster yomena extract ameliorates pro-inflammatory immune response by suppressing NF-κB activation in RAW 264.7 cells. *J Chinese Med Assoc [Internet].* 2018;81(2):102–10. Available from: https://doi.org/10.1016/j.jcma.2017.06.017

Jantan I., Haque M. A., Ilangkovan M. & Arshad L. An insight into the modulatory effects and mechanisms of action of phyllanthus species and their bioactive metabolites on the immune system. *Front Pharmacol.* 2019;10(JULY):1–19.

Kim J. W., Kim J. H., Kim C. Y., Jeong J. S., Ko J. W., Kim T. W. Green tea extract improves cyclophosphamide-induced immunosuppression in mouse spleen and enhances the immune activity of RAW 264.7 cells. *Heliyon [Internet]*. 2023;9(11):e22062. Available from: https://doi.org/10.1016/j.heliyon.2023.e22062

Kim S., Jo E. S., Kim N. Y., Hwang K. W., Park S. Y. Immune-enhancing screening of fourteen plants on murine macrophage RAW 264.7 cells. *Trop J Pharm Res*. 2019;18(1):85–92.

Lohvina H., Sándor M., Wink M. Effect of ethanol solvents on total phenolic content and antioxidant properties of seed extracts of fenugreek (Trigonella foenum-graecum l.) varieties and determination of phenolic composition by hplc-esi-ms. *Diversity*. 2022;14(1).

Merly L. & Smith S. L. Murine RAW 264.7 cell line as an immune target: are we missing something?. *Immunopharmacol Immunotoxicol*. 2017;39(2):55–8.

Molole G. J., Gure A., Abdissa N. Determination of total phenolic content and antioxidant activity of Commiphora mollis (Oliv.) *Engl. resin. BMC Chem [Internet]*. 2022;16(1):1–11. Available from: https://doi.org/10.1186/s13065-022-00841-x

Purwitasari N., Siswodihardjo S., Alhoot M. A., Agil M. Pharmacological Potential of Some Indonesian Medicinal Plants as Promising Options for COVID-19 During the Pandemic Era: A Literature Review. *J Med Chem Sci*. 2023;6(6): 2735–49.

Reddy P. R. K., Elghandour M. M. M. Y., Salem A. Z. M., Yasaswini D., Reddy P. P. R., Reddy A. N., et al. Plant secondary metabolites as feed additives in calves for antimicrobial stewardship. *Anim Feed Sci Technol [Internet]*. 2020;264(January):114469. Available from: https://doi.org/10.1016/j.anifeedsci.2020.114469

Rodríguez-Yoldi M. J. Anti-inflammatory and antioxidant properties of plant extracts. *Antioxidants*. 2021;10(6):7–10.

Shi L., Zhao W., Yang Z., Subbiah V., Suleria H. A. R. Extraction and characterization of phenolic compounds and their potential antioxidant activities. *Environ Sci Pollut Res [Internet]*. 2022;29(54):81112–29. Available from: https://doi.org/10.1007/s11356-022-23337-6

Shrestha P. M., Dhillion S. S. Diversity and traditional knowledge concerning wild food species in a locally managed forest in Nepal. *Agrofor Syst*. 2006;66(1):55–63.

Taciak B., Białasek M., Braniewska A., Sas Z., Sawicka P., Kiraga Ł, et al. Evaluation of phenotypic and functional stability of RAW 264.7 cell line through serial passages. *PLoS ONE*. 2018;13(6):1–13.

Tambewagh U. U., Kandhare A. D., Honmore V. S., Kadam P. P., Khedkar V. M., Bodhankar S. L., et al. Anti-inflammatory and antioxidant potential of Guaianolide isolated from Cyathocline purpurea: Role of COX-2 inhibition. *Int Immunopharmacol [Internet]*. 2017;52(August):110–8. Available from: http://dx.doi.org/10.1016/j.intimp.2017.09.001

Tjandrawinata R. R., Susanto L. W., Nofiarny D. The use of phyllanthus niruri L. as an immunomodulator for the treatment of infectious diseases in clinical settings. *Asian Pacific J Trop Dis*. 2017;7(3):132–40.

Venkatesan T., Choi Y. W., Kim Y. K. Impact of Different Extraction Solvents on Phenolic Content and Antioxidant Potential of Pinus densiflora Bark Extract. *Biomed Res Int*. 2019;2019.

Technological Innovations in Tropical Livestock Development for Environmental Sustainability and Food Security – P. Dhian Isnaeni et al. (eds)
© 2025 The Author(s), ISBN 978-1-032-74373-8
Open Access: www.taylorfrancis.com, CC BY-NC-ND 4.0 license

The effect of *Andrographis paniculata* leaf extract on macroscopic and microscopic features of the kidneys in mice (*Mus musculus*) infected with *Salmonella typhi*

F.A. Auza, P.D. Isnaeni*, M.A. Pagala, F.M. Pancar, M. Rusdin, A.B. Kimestri & A.B. Pratiwi
Department of Animal Husbandry, Faculty of Animal Husbandry, Halu Oleo University, Indonesia

ABSTRACT: This study aimed to analyze the macroscopic and microscopic features of the kidneys of mice infected by *Salmonella typhi* bacteria treated with *Andrographis paniculata* leaf extract. The treatment groups consisted of control negative (uninfected, untreated mice), control positive (infected, untreated mice), APC_1 (infected, 200mg/kg BW AP), APC_2 (infected, 300mg/kg BW AP), and APC_3 (infected, 400mg/kg BW AP). The results of statistical tests in this study showed there was a significant difference ($p<0.05$) in the body weight of mice, but the relative weight of mice kidney organs did not show a significant difference ($p>0.05$). The results of the study of the macroscopic features given *A. paniculata* leaf extract found no abnormalities, such as bleeding spots, in all treatments, while microscopic findings found damage to kidney organ tissue in positive controls, APC_2 and APC_3 in the form of mild tubular necrosis, mild and moderate interstitial nephritis with some bowman's capsules atrophied.

Keywords: Andrographis paniculata, macroscopic feature, microscopic feature, kidney

1 INTRODUCTION

Indonesia has a diverse biodiversity. Some plants have been widely used by the community in various ways including for treatment as traditional medicine. Currently, herbal plants are starting to be used by the people of Indonesia, with considerations regarding milder side effects, easily available ingredients, and cheaper prices. Many studies have been conducted on herbal plants, especially their efficacy in the form of single extracts. One of them is *Andrographis paniculata* which is used as a medicinal plant, including the use of medicinal plants as phytobiotics. Phytobiotics are feed additives derived from plant-derived products used in animal feed which aim to improve the performance of the livestock. Active substances derived from medicinal plants are generally found in the form of secondary metabolites.

Andrographis paniculata is known as an herb plant that contains the active substance andrographolide which has immunomodulatory, antibacterial, anti-inflammatory, anti-viral and antioxidant properties (Vetvicka & Vannucci 2021). *Andrographis paniculata* is one of the plants that has been researched by the researchers Nugrahani *et al.* (2019) stated that the administration of *A. paniculata* leaf extract was able to reduce the level of necrosis of rat renal tubular cells induced by toxic doses of gentamicin. This shows the antioxidant function of the extract to reduce tissue damage due to free radicals (Windisch *et al.* 2008).

*Corresponding Author: purnaningdhian@uho.ac.id

 DOI: 10.1201/9781003468943-24

One of the most important organs in the observation of toxicity, the process of elimination of toxic substances from the body and is associated with other structures to facilitate urine output. High blood flow to the kidneys and increased concentration of excreted products followed by reabsorption of water from the tubular fluid are the main factors involved in sensitizing the kidneys to toxic substances (Hodgson 2004). Administration of phytobiotics at inappropriate doses may cause side effects. If kidney damage occurs, it will cause reduced kidney function (Tuominen *et al.* 2001). *Andrographolide* compounds can prevent inflammation that can occur due to hypertension in both blood vessels and kidneys. Changes in the weight of organs are an indicator of changes in the cells of the organ due to exposure to chemical compounds (Michael *et al.* 2007; Sellers *et al.* 2007).

In general, research related to the use of herbs and medicines is carried out on experimental animals, one of which is mice. Mice are one of the experimental animals that are easy to obtain, maintain, and can be used to test a drug or the phytochemical content of an herb. In this context, it is necessary to study the extract of *A. paniculata* leaves on the macroscopic and microscopic picture of the kidneys in mice with different various doses infected with *Salmonella typhi.*

2 MATERIAL AND RESEARCH METHODOLOGY

2.1 *Preparation of A. paniculata leaf extract*

A. paniculata flour was made by drying the leaves using sunlight and continued with an oven at 50°C until the moisture content reached 10–18%, then ground into flour. Extraction of *A. paniculata* leaves was carried out by maceration method using 96% ethanol for 48 hours with a ratio of flour to ethanol 1: 5, the macerate was then evaporated using an evaporator at 40°C for 6 hours until a thick extract was obtained (Susanti *et al.* 2014).

2.2 *Experimental design and treatment stages*

The study was conducted in a laboratory under controlled conditions. Forty adult female mice were grouped into five treatment groups consisted of: control negative/C- (uninfected and untreated mice), control positive/C+ (Salmonella-infected, untreated mice), AP_1 (*Salmonella*-infected, treated with 200 mg/kg BW AP), AP_2 (Salmonella-infected, treated with 200 mg/kg BW AP), and AP_3 (*Salmonella*-infected, treated with 400 mg/kg BW AP). The mice were reared for a total of 30 days. The first 7 days, the mice were on adapting period and were not treated.

The AP was given by oral gauge according to the groups for 21 days after adaptation. On day 22, the C+, AP_1, AP_2, and AP_3 groups were infected with 10^6 CFU (colony forming unit) of *Salmonella typhi* orally. Mice were given food and water *ad libitum*. The volume of extract solution administered was 0.2 ml/mice.

2.3 *Measurement*

2.3.1 *The relative weight of organ*

Mice maintenance was carried out for 30 days, at the end of the study, weighing was previously carried out to determine the final body weight, then continued to take mice organs at 48 hours post-infection. Kidney organs that have been taken are cleaned and then weighed with analytical scales. The data obtained were calculated using the following formula (Incharoen 2013).

$$\text{The relative weight of organ} = \frac{\text{Weight of organ}}{\text{Live weight}} \times 100\%$$

2.3.2 *Histopathology of Kidney tissue*

The euthanized mice were necropsied and the kidneys were removed. The kidneys were then placed in 10% formalin solution and histopathological preparations were made using HE (hematoxylin and eosin) staining. The condition of the kidney tissues was examined under a microscope at 100x magnification (Prahanarendra 2015).

2.4 *Statistical analysis*

Data were analyzed using analysis of variances (ANOVA) according to a completely randomized design. The significant effects of treatments were further determined using Duncan's Multiple Range Test at a 5% level of significance (Steel RGD 1991), while the analysis of macroscopic and microscopic images of the kidneys was carried out descriptively.

3 RESULT AND DISCUSSION

3.1 *Final body weight and macroscopic feature of kidney*

Kidney is an important organ in the elimination of waste products derived from endogenous metabolism and xenobiotic metabolism (Hodgson 2004). The final body weight and kidney organ weight in female mice after administration of Andrographis leaf extract are presented in Table 1.

Table 1. Final body weight, relative organ weights and macroscopic features of kidney organs of mice after given of different doses of *A. paniculata* leaf extracts.

	Treatments					
Parameter	Control (+)	Control (-)	APC_1	APC_2	APC_3	P-Value
Final body weight (g)	30.21 ± 3.38^{ab}	27.50 ± 1.10^{b}	25.83 ± 1.59^{a}	25.00 ± 0.82^{a}	24.50 ± 3.67^{a}	0.029
Relative organ weight (%)	0.42±0.95	1.84±0.28	1.98±0.15	1.87±0.07	1.86±0.05	0.487
Macroscopic change	Normal	Normal	Normal	Normal	Normal	

Note: Different superscripts in the same line showed significant differences (*p<0.05*) control negative (uninfected, untreated mice), control positive (infected, untreated mice), APC_1 (infected, 200mg/kg BW AP), APC_2 (infected, 300mg/kg BW AP), and APC_3 (infected, 400mg/kg BW AP).

The given of ethanol extract of A. paniculate leaves on minute body weight gain is shown in Table 1. The results of variance analysis showed that the final body weight of mice showed significant differences ($p<0.05$) between the negative control group with a dose of 200 mg/kg BW (APC_1), 300 mg/kg BW (APC_2) and a dose of 400 mg/kg BW. The body weight of mice decreased as the dose of ethanol extract of *A. paniculata* leaves increased. The decrease in mice body weight is thought to be because *A. paniculate* leaves contain quite diverse active substances, including andrographolid, diterpenoids, flavonoids which can cause a bitter taste that can reduce food consumption and absorption so that there is a change in body weight in mice. This is in line with research (Ranti *et al.* 2013) that flavonoid extract can reduce rat body weight by 7.85%. The mechanism of action of flavonoids is to inhibit FAS (*Fatty acid synthase*) by blocking *acetyl*-CoA and *malonyl*-CoA which are substrates of *acyl-transferases* that have the potential to inhibit genes that play a role in adipogenesis, thereby reducing the amount of adipose tissue (Jeyakumar *et al.* 2005). The active compounds contained in *A. paniculata* leaf extract can trigger weight loss in mice.

The results of the ANOVA test showed that the relative weight of the kidney organs did not show a significant effect ($p>0.05$), which means that there was no decrease or increase in the weight of the kidney organs, in this case still within the normal range. This is thought to be because the administration of ethanol extract of *A. paniculata* leaves at doses of 200, 300 and 400 mg/kg BW is able to suppress the effects of damage caused by hypercholesterolemia so as not to cause changes in kidney weight. Ethanol extract of *A. paniculata* leaves is able to influence or suppress the adverse effects of hypercholesterolemia. Free radicals that increase in hypercholesterolemia conditions can attack cell macromolecules so that they can cause necrosis and cell degeneration (Wresdiyati *et al.* 2011).

Macroscopic conditions were observed visually to determine the presence or absence of changes in size, changes in colour, and changes in organ shape in the control group with the treatment group. Based on the macroscopic data of the kidney organs of female mice for 48 hours after treatment and until the 22nd day there were no changes in each treatment group. This is in accordance with (Rahayu 2022) which states that the oral given of ethanolic extract of land kale in female mice does not change the shape and size of the kidney organs.

3.2 *Microscopic features of kidney*

The microscopic features of mice treated with *A. paniculata* and infected with *Salmonella typhi* orally with a bacterial concentration of 1×10^6 CFU (*Colony Forming Unit*) is presented in the following picture.

Control positive

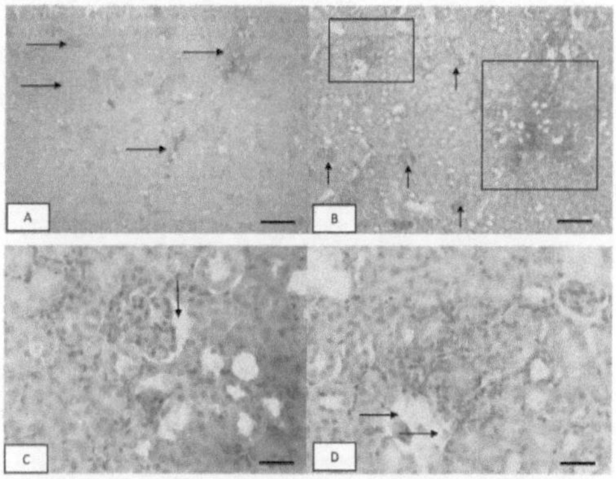

Figure 1. Histopathological features of the kidneys of control positive mice infected with *Salmonella typhi.* (A) mononuclear inflammatory cells (→), (B) glomerular atrophy (↑) and MN cell infiltration (□), (C) glomerular tube and bowman space dilation (↓), (D) karyolitic (→) (H&E staining)

Control negative

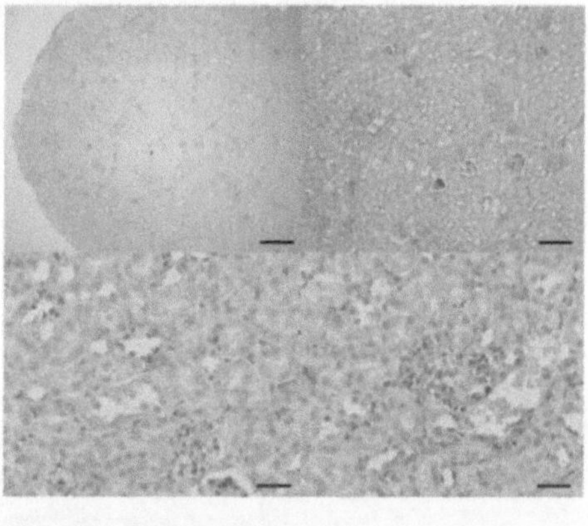

Figure 2. The histopathological picture of the kidneys of the control negative mice appeared normal (H&E staining).

The positive control without *A. paniculata* extract showed that the kidney organs of mice had interstitial nephritis characterized by the appearance of several points of hypercellular clusters containing mononuclear (MN) and slightly polymorphonuclear (PMN) type inflammatory cells and the accumulation of mononuclear inflammatory cells in the interstitial cells. The renal tubules had mild necrosis with some bowman's capsules atrophied. The proliferation of inflammatory cells is indicative of the body's defense reaction to foreign bodies (Mittrücker *et al.* 2000).

The microscopic features of the kidneys of mice in the negative control (Figure. 2) showed no changes. The tubule and glomerular areas looked normal, no necrosis or changes in the glomerulus were observed and the interstitial space was relatively normal. The results of this study are supported by (Windhartono *et al.* 2013) that the structure of the kidney tissue is normal as the cells appear normal.

Figure 3 shows that in the APC_1 treatment with *Salmonella typhi* infection 1×10^6 CFU and given *A. paniculata* extract at a dose of 200 mg/kg body weight, the kidneys did not experience significant changes, there was no accumulation of inflammatory cells in the interstitial tubules. Tubules, glomerulus and bowman's capsule did not experience significant changes after infection.

The given of 300 mg/kg BW of *A. paniculata* extract (Figure. 4) showed mild tubular necrosis and interstitial nephritis. Tubular necrosis was characterized by karyolitic of the tubules and lysis of the epithelium. Interstitial nephritis is characterized by mononuclear inflammatory cell infiltration in the interstitial area. This is the result of morphological damage, which is characterized by inflammation and is thought to occur with increasing doses of *A. paniculata* extract. According to Confer and Panciera (1995), that the damage is often caused by immune complex deposition, thrombosis, embolism, and viral infection of the glomerular components.

APC_1

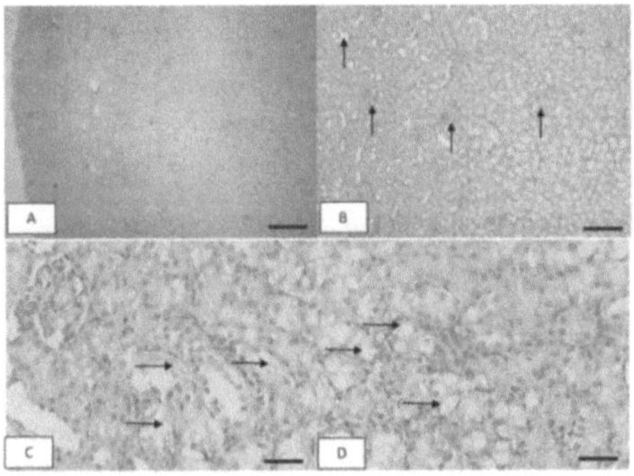

Figure 3. (A) The tubule area appears normal, (B) glomerular capillaries appear congested (↓). (C) no necrosis or changes in the glomerulus were observed. (D) the intertitial space is relatively normal (H&E staining).

APC_2

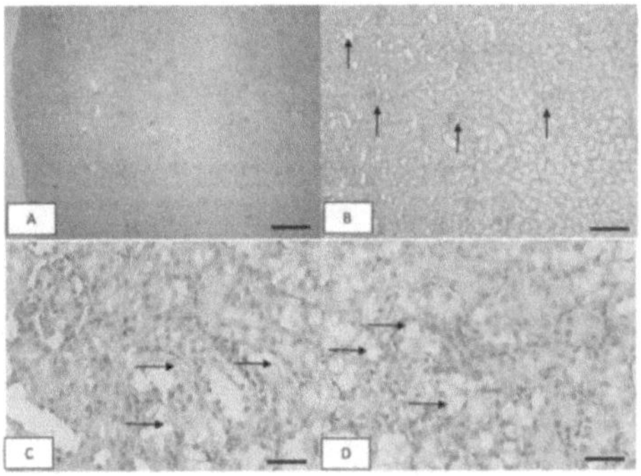

Figure 4. (A) and (B). mononuclear inflammatory cells (↑), (C) and (D) karyolysis (→) (H&E staining).

APC_3

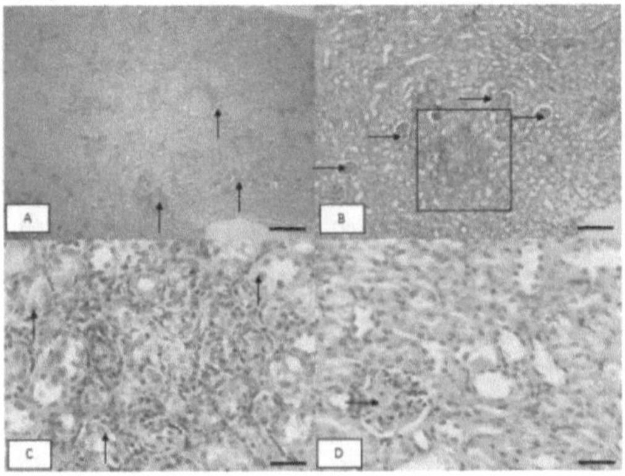

Figure 5. (A) mononuclear inflammatory cells (↑), (B) glomerular atrophy (→) and accumulation of MN inflammatory cells (□), (C) karyolysis (↑), (D) epithelial detachment (→) (H&E staining).

The APC_3 treatment, given 400 mg/kg BW of *A. paniculata* extract (Figure 5), showed moderate interstitial nephritis, mild glomerulonephritis, and renal tubular necrosis. Interstitial nephritis showed infiltration of mononuclear inflammatory cells around the glomerulus which was multifocal, most of the glomerular tuft appeared atrophied which was characterized by shrinkage of glomerular size and dilation of bowman space. Tubular necrosis was mild with karyolitic of the tubular epithelium and detachment of the tubules into the lumen.

4 CONCLUSION

The given of *A. paniculata* leaf extract decreased the body weight of mice as the dose given increased and infected with *Salmonella typhi* by 24.50 g. In contrast, the macroscopic picture of the relative weight of the kidney organs did not show significant changes in shape within the normal range. The microscopic picture of mice given *A. paniculata* extract and infected with *Salmonella typhi* perorally with a bacterial concentration of 1×10^6 CFU (*Colony Forming Unit*) pathology changes in each treatment, with the best results in the APC_1 treatment (200 mg/kg BW) with normal-looking kidneys.

ACKNOWLEDGEMENT

The authors would like to thank Halu Oleo University for funding this research, as well as the staff of the veterinary anatomical pathology laboratory of Brawijaya University who assisted in our experiment.

REFERENCES

Confer A. W., & Panciera R. J. (1995). Thomson's special veterinary pathology. *Edisi ke-2*. Edited : Carlton WW dan McGavin MD. Mosby.

Hodgson. E. (2004). Toxicology of the nervous system. In *Lu's Basic Toxicology: Fundamentals, Target Organs, and Risk Assessment*, Seventh Edition. https://doi.org/10.4324/9781315391700-21

Incharoen, T. (2013). Histological adaptations of the gastrointestinal tract of broilers fed diets containing insoluble fiber from rice hull meal. *American Journal of Animal and Veterinary Sciences*, 8(2), 79–88. https://doi.org/10.3844/ajavsp.2013.79.88

Jeyakumar, S. M., Vajreswari, A., Sesikeran, B., & Giridharan, N. V. (2005). Vitamin A supplementation induces adipose tissue loss through apoptosis in lean but not in obese rats of the WNIN/Ob strain. *Journal of Molecular Endocrinology*, 35(2), 391–398. https://doi.org/10.1677/jme.1.01838

Michael, B., Yano, B., Sellers, R. S., Perry, R., Morton, D., Roome, N., Johnson, J. K., Schafer, K., & Pitsch , S. (2007). Evaluation of organ weights for rodent and non-rodent toxicity studies: a review of regulatory guidelines and a survey of current practices. *Toxicologic Pathology*, 35(5), 742–750. https://doi.org/10.1080/01926230701595292

Mittrücker, H.-W., Raupach, B., Köhler, A., & Kaufmann, S. H. E. (2000). Cutting Edge: Role of B Lymphocytes in Protective Immunity Against Salmonella typhimurium Infection. *The Journal of Immunology*, 164(4), 1648–1652. https://doi.org/10.4049/jimmunol.164.4.1648

Nugrahani, A. D., Nangoi, L., Meles, D. K., V. T. Widiyatno, Hamid, I. S., & Santoso, K. P. (2019). *The Effect of Leaves Extract of Sambiloto (Andrographis paniculata) on Renal Histopathologi Features Induced by Gentamicin In White Rats (Rattus norvegicus)*. 8(1), 29–34..

Prahanarendra, G. (2015). Gambaran Histologi Organ Ginjal, Hepar, dan Pankreas tikus sprague dawley dengan Pewarnaan He Dengan fiksasi 3 minggu. *Studi Awal Histoteknik*, 1–69.

Rahayu, T. (2022). *Uji Toksisitas Akut Ekstrak Etanolik Kangkung Darat (Ipomoea reptans, Poir) Terstandar Secara Oral Pada Mencit Betina Galur DDY*.

Ranti, G. C., Fatimawali, & Wehantouw, F. (2013). Uji efektivitas ekstrak flavonoid dan steroid dari gedi (abelmoschus manihot) sebagai anti obesitas dan hipolipidemik pada tikus putih jantan galur wistar. *PHARMACON Jurnal Ilmiah Farmasi-UNSRAT*, 2(02), 34–38.

RJ., C. A. dan P. (1995). *Thomson's Special Veterinary PathologyNo Title* (Carlton & W. dan M. M. Mosby. (eds.); *ke*-2).

Sellers, R. S., Morton, D., Michael, B., Roome, N., Johnson, J. K., Yano, B. L., Perry, R., & Schafer, K. (2007). Society of toxicologic pathology position paper: organ weight recommendations for toxicology studies. *Toxicologic Pathology*, 35(5), 751–755. https://doi.org/10.1080/01926230701595300

Susanti, P. N. M., Warditiani, N. K., Laksmiani, N. P. L., Widjaja, I. N. K., Rismayanti, A. A. M. I., & Wirasuta, I. M. A. G. (2014). perbandingan metode ekstraksi maserasi dan refluks terhadap rendemen andrografolid dari herba sambiloto. Universitas Udayana, 29–32.

Steel RGD, T. J. (1991). *Procedure of Statistic*..Terjemahan. Edisi ke-2. PT. Gramedia, *Jakarta*.

Tuominen, T., Jämsä, T., Oksanen, J., Tuukkanen, J., Gao, T. J., Lindholm, T. S., & Jalovaara, P. (2001). Composite implant composed of hydroxyapatite and bone morphogenetic protein in the healing of a canine ulnar defect. *In Annales Chirurgiae et Gynaecologiae* (Vol. 90, Issue1).

Vetvicka, V., & Vannucci, L. (2021). Biological properties of andrographolide, an active ingredient of Andrographis Paniculata: a narrative review. *Annals of Translational Medicine*, 9(14), 1186–1186. https://doi.org/10.21037/atm-20-7830

Windhartono, Kamal, Z., & Sasmito E. (2013). Pengaruh Infusa Wortel (Daucus Carota L.) Terhadap histopatologi ginjal tikus jantan yang diinduksi uranium. *Jurnal Kedokteran YARSI*, 21(1), 33–40. https://www.neliti.com/id/publications/105215/

Windisch, W., Schedle, K., Plitzner, C., & Kroismayr, A. (2008). Use of phytogenic products as feed additives for swine and poultry. *Journal of Animal Science*, 86(14), E140–E148. https://doi.org/10.2527/jas.2007-0459

Wresdiyati, T., Hartanta, A. B., & Astawan, M. (2011). Tepung rumput laut (eucheuma cottonii) menaikkan level superoksida dismutase (sod). *Jurnal Veteriner*, 12(2), 126–135.

Technological Innovations in Tropical Livestock Development for Environmental Sustainability and Food Security – P. Dhian Isnaeni et al. (eds)

Optimizing fermented corn straw for increasing *Peranakan etawa* goat livestock production

D. Zulkarnain*, L.O.M. Munadi & N. Sandiah
Department of Animal Science, Faculty of Animal Science, Universitas Halu Oleo, Kendari, Southeast Sulawesi, Indonesia

R. Astarika
Faculty of Science and Technology, UPBJJ Universitas Terbuka, Kendari, Southeast Sulawesi, Indonesia

Kamari
Postgraduate Animal Science, Universitas Halu Oleo, Kendari, Southeast Sulawesi, Indonesia

ABSTRACT: The productivity of *Peranakan etawa* goats can reach its peak when adequately supplied with feed, both in terms of quantity and nutritional quality. This research was conducted from October 2022 to January 2023 in Wonua Raya Village, Kolaka Regency, to enhance the productivity of *Peranakan etawa* goats. The study involved 12 *Peranakan etawa* goats, each at least 6 months old with an average weight of approximately 10–12 kg. The feed materials used were Gamal leaves, corn straw, and agricultural waste. The study employed a Completely Randomized Design (CRD) with 4 treatments and 3 replications. Data from surveys and in vitro digestibility were analyzed using one-way ANOVA and further tested with the Duncan test using SPSS version 22 software. The findings indicate that using corn straw waste through fermentation with EM-4 inoculum improved the corn straw's chemical, physical, and digestibility qualities. Furthermore, incorporating a blend of fermented corn straw and Gamal leaves at a level of 30% in the *Peranakan etawa* goat's diet resulted in enhanced feed consumption, weight gain, and improved feed conversion efficiency in the livestock. In conclusion, using corn straw waste through fermentation with EM-4 inoculum enhanced the corn straw's chemical, physical, and digestibility qualities. Furthermore, including the fermented corn straw mixture with Gamal leaves at 30% in the diet of *Peranakan etawa* goats resulted in increased feed consumption, weight gain, and feed conversion efficiency in the livestock.

Keywords: Peranakan etawa, Corn Straw, Fermentation, Productivity

1 INTRODUCTION

Peranakan etawa goat farming management is closely related to five main aspects of livestock operations: selection of breeding stock, feed provision, barn management, disease control, and maintenance management. These five aspects are very important controls in achieving success in the livestock business (Mogiye *et al.* 2020). Goats, as livestock that are very efficient in utilizing natural resources, especially plants that grow on marginal land, have superior economic value in terms of care. In addition, adult female *Peranakan etawa*

*Corresponding Author: deki.zulkarnain@uho.ac.id

DOI: 10.1201/9781003468943-25

goats can reach a live weight of around 35 kg, while male goats have a body weight of around 40 kg. They have characteristic downward-hanging ears with a length of around 18–19 cm and a body height ranging from 75–100 cm. This makes *Peranakan etawa* goats an excellent choice in efforts to reduce poverty in rural areas, especially in tropical regions. The productivity of *Peranakan etawa* goats can achieve optimal performance if supported by the availability of sufficient feed (Mudawamah *et al.* 2021), both in terms of quantity and nutritional quality (Gong *et al.* 2020).

Corn is not only used for human consumption but can also be used as a source of animal feed. Apart from the seeds, which are rich in vegetable protein and carbohydrates, other parts such as leaves, cobs, husks, and corn bran can be used as animal feed components, either directly or after undergoing processing using special technology. Corn plants produce corn products such as flour and oil and produce processed waste such as corn straw. Each corn plant produces waste around 50% of the total biomass produced (Amna *et al.* 2021).

The use of corn straw (*Zea mays*) as an animal feed ingredient has been widely adopted in several countries, such as China, Taiwan, and various regions in Indonesia, including Bali, North Sumatra, Toraja (South Sulawesi), and Papua. Usually, corn straw is used as feed for pigs, cattle, and goats. Regarding nutritional composition, corn straw has a dry matter content of 24.03%, obtained after the corn straw undergoes a drying process before being converted into silage. The crude protein content in corn straw silage is around 7.93%. Corn plants' soil, especially at the young fruit stage, has a dry matter nutrient content of around 26%, total digestible nutrients of around 65%, crude protein of 8%, and crude fiber of around 26% (Trisnadewi *et al.* 2017).

Peranakan etawa goat farming is one of the mainstays of agriculture in Kolaka Regency, especially in Toari District. The goat population in this area reaches 5,985 heads. This advantage is supported by its geographical characteristics, located in a coastal area with undulating land contours and adequate rainfall for plant growth. The latest data from the Statistics Agency for 2023 records that corn production in Kolaka Regency reached 10,033 tons. This is one of the beneficial factors in providing feed for livestock.

Considering the high production and area of corn plantations in Kolaka Regency, it is clear that this will produce waste that is not fully utilized. This waste is corn straw, which can still be used as feed for goats. However, to increase the digestibility of corn waste, additional steps are needed, one of which is implementing fermentation technology.

2 RESEARCH METHODS

2.1 *Study location*

This study was conducted from October 2022 to January 2023 in Wonua Raya Village, Toari District, Kolaka Regency. The research also involved laboratory facilities, namely the Animal Food Nutrition Laboratory, Faculty of Animal Science, Halu Oleo University, Kendari, and the Animal Food Chemistry Laboratory, Department of Animal Food Nutrition, Hasanuddin University, Makassar.

2.2 *Research materials*

2.2.1 *Tools and materials*

Making hay from corn straw uses corn straw as raw material from agricultural residues mixed with EM4 inoculum. The tools used in this research are feed containers made from partitioned boards, tools for the fermentation process, including machetes, drums, shovels, plastic containers, digital scales with a capacity of 100 kg, equipment for writing and recording data, and a stage cage.

2.2.2 *Livestock and feed*

The study included 12 *Peranakan etawa* goats, each weighing approximately 10–12 kg on average, and all were at least 6 months old. The feed components comprised Gamal leaves, corn straw, and agricultural by-products from farmers' harvests. Gamal leaves are used as basic feed for livestock in fresh form. Before being given to experimental livestock, corn straw undergoes a fermentation process with the help of EM4 inoculum. The feeding process in this study involved mixing fresh Gamal leaves with corn straw hay that had been fermented using EM4, with comparisons according to the research design.

2.3 *Research design*

This research used a Completely Randomized Design (CRD) method with the application of 4 treatments and 3 replications. Each replication involved 3 male *Peranakan etawa* goats, so 12 goats were used in this study. The feed consisted of fresh Gamal leaves as basic feed for *Peranakan etawa* goats, while the research treatment involved corn straw that had undergone a fermentation process. The treatment composition in this study was as follows:

R0 = Control feed (Gamal Leaves)
R1 = 90% Gamal leaves and bran + 10% fermented corn straw
R2 = 80% Gamal leaves and bran + 20% fermented corn straw
R3 = 70% Gamal leaves and bran + 30% fermented corn straw

The mathematical model of Completely Randomized Design (CRD) is as follows:

$$Yij = \mu + \sigma i + \sum ij$$

Information:

Yij = Treatment observation data to –i, repeat to –j
i = Treatment
j = Test (1, 2, 3)
μ = General average or general middle value
σi = Effect of feeding to –j
$\sum$ij = Experimental error treatment to-i and repeat to –j

2.4 *Data treatment and collection*

2.4.1 *Livestock adaptations*

The experimental animals underwent an adaptation period of 2 weeks to adapt well to the cage environment and type of feed given during the study to consume it efficiently.

2.4.2 *Data retrieval*

The data collection process in the research was carried out in two stages. The first stage involved measuring the potential of corn straw waste in Toari District, Kolaka Regency, and in vitro digestibility analysis of the treated feed used during this research. The second stage of this research involved measuring the performance of *Peranakan etawa* goats fed corn straw that had undergone a fermentation process.

2.5 *Research variable*

The variables observed in the research included (1) Potential corn straw waste, (2) In Vitro digestibility of fermented corn straw and Gamal leaves, and (3) Production performance of *Peranakan etawa* goats, including feed consumption, weight gain, and feed conversion.

2.6 *Data analysis*

Data obtained from surveys related to the potential of corn straw waste were analyzed using a tabulation process, and this research applied qualitative descriptive analysis. Data related to in vitro digestibility and production performance were analyzed by statistical methods using ANOVA based on a completely randomized design with a unidirectional pattern. If there is a significant difference between treatments, a further test using the Duncan test is carried out. For statistical data analysis, SPSS version 22 software was used.

3 RESULTS AND DISCUSSION

3.1 *Potential of corn straw waste*

The government has implemented an agricultural acceleration program, including expanding land for food crops. This is in line with efforts to support the development of agricultural agribusiness and improve the community economy, which is the main pillar of the national economic system. In expanding food crops, corn straw has great potential to meet forage needs, especially for ruminants (Elly *et al.* 2020). Corn straw, which consists of young stems and leaves, also known as corn husks and corn cobs, is a waste from the corn plant that can be used as animal feed. Even though breeders have used it as forage for livestock, its use has not yet reached its optimal potential.

Husks are generally called the skin or wrapping of corn cobs and have various functions. Besides its role as animal feed, husks also protect corn kernels and cobs and keep corn fresh so that it is easier for livestock to consume. Therefore, corn in its complete form, including the husk and cobs, is preferable to just corn kernels. Corn cobs can be used as feed for ruminants, although the quality of this feed is relatively low.

Data from Table 1 shows that the harvested area of corn in Toari District varies. Anawua Village and Wonua Raya Village have the largest harvested areas, 128 ha and 116 ha, respectively. In comparison, the total harvested area in Toari District reaches 864 ha, producing corn straw, which can be used as animal feed, especially when grass is difficult to find, such as in the dry season. Corn straw preserved by sun drying produces various by-products beneficial to livestock.

Table 1. Harvested area and production corn in Toari district.

Village	Harvest Area (Ha)	Production (Tons)
Toari	62	465.00
Lakito	55	401.50
Ranomentaa	103	733.36
Wowoli	113	803.43
Anawua	128	921.60
Rano Jaya	60	432.00
Harongkuli	53	386.90
Wonua Raya	116	835.20
Rahabite	72	518.40
Rano Sangia	102	714.00
Total	864	6,211.39

Source: Agricultural census results 2023

3.2 *Nutritional content of fermented and non-fermented corn straw*

One of the reasons why corn plants have not developed as animal feed in Indonesia is because farmers and breeders do not understand how to use corn waste. Therefore, more intensive economic studies and development of corn farming are needed, as well as efforts to educate farmers and livestock breeders about how to grow corn and use it as a source of animal feed. Corn cobs are used as feed for ruminants. This crude fiber mainly consists of cellulose, lignin, and hemicellulose, which reduces the level of digestibility when consumed by livestock (Amna *et al.* 2021).

Fermented corn straw usually has higher nutritional value than in its native state. This is caused by the ability of microbes to break down complex components into simpler substances, making them easier to digest. The nutritional composition of corn straw before and after fermentation in this study can be seen in Table 2.

Table 2. Chemical composition of corn straw before and after fermentation.

	Content (%)	
Nutrients	Corn Straw	Corn Straw Fermentation
Water content	6.28	8.59
Dry Ingredients	93.72	91.41
Ash	7.26	12.48
Organic Ingredients	86.46	78.93
Crude protein	9.64	7.12
Crude Fiber	30.99	23.45

Source: Nutrition Science and Feed Technology Laboratory, Universitas Halu Oleo (2023)

Utilizing fermented corn straw has several benefits, namely reducing feed costs, especially for goats, by replacing forage as the main feed. This can also increase agricultural land productivity because goat farms no longer need to prepare special land for planting forage. The use of corn straw can also provide added value for farmers, who may see it as a business opportunity, making it not a waste that interferes with production but a product that can generate income.

Table 2 describes changes in chemical components in corn straw before and after processing. The research results showed that processing using EM-4 decreased crude fiber content from 30.99% to 23.45% or decreased it. This decrease in crude fiber content can be caused by the microorganisms in EM-4, which produce fiber-digesting enzymes, such as cellulase and mannose, and because the bacteria in EM-4 do not produce crude fiber in their activities. This research also paid attention to the physical characteristics of fermented corn straw, such as color, odor, and texture, presented in Table 3.

Table 3. Physical characteristics of corn straw fermentation results.

Physical Observation	Observation Result
Color	Brown in color and almost resembles the original
Smell	Fragrant and sour
Texture	A bit soft

Source: Researcher's direct observation, 2023

Table 3 describes the physical characteristics of corn straw after fermentation with EM-4, including changes in color, aroma, and texture. Regarding color, fermented corn straw resembles the original plant before it was ensiled. Silage color can describe the fermentation process results, with the dominance of acetic acid, which tends to produce a yellowish color.

3.3 *In vitro digestibility of feed*

Ruminant feed digestibility is influenced by feed concentration and chemical composition. Traditional in vivo and sacco methods for assessing digestibility have drawbacks, such as high costs and the need for livestock with fistulas and large feed quantities. In response, in vitro digestibility methods have emerged, offering simplicity, efficiency, and cost-effectiveness by simulating ruminant digestive processes in the laboratory. This method allows for simultaneous evaluation of multiple feed ingredients and measures dry matter and organic matter loss after incubation, as presented in Table 4.

Table 4. Average digestibility of dry matter and organic matter of research feed.

	Treatment			
Digestibility	P0	P1	P2	P3
DM^{ns}	60.96	52.30	55.81	56.18
OM*	50.56^{ab}	45.54^{c}	49.09^{a}	51.99^{b}

Information: NS= Non-Significant, ^{a,b,c}different superscripts in the column there show significant differences (*P<0.05*), DM/OM = Dry matter/organic matter

Basically, *in vitro* techniques attempt to imitate the conditions in the rumen of livestock animals. Various conditions are modified in this method, such as buffer solution, fermentation container, stirring, gas phase, fermentation temperature, optimal pH, inoculum source, anaerobic conditions, fermentation period, and the end of the fermentation process.

3.3.1 *Dry matter digestibility*

The digestibility of dry and organic matter is a crucial factor in evaluating feed quality, as it determines the nutrients available for livestock. Analysis from Table 4 indicates higher dry matter digestibility in treatment P1, utilizing Gamal leaves without additional fermented corn straw with EM-4, compared to treatments P2 and P3. Despite incorporating fermented corn straw up to 30%, statistical analysis reveals no significant difference. This suggests that the low nutrient content in corn straw may hinder digestibility in ruminants' rumen, even after fermentation with EM-4, as observed in this study.

3.3.2 *Digestibility of organic materials*

The study observed varying organic matter digestibility values, ranging from 45.54% in treatment P1 to 51.99% in treatment P3. Statistical analysis indicated that the level of fermented corn straw substitution significantly influenced organic matter digestibility (P<0.01). Further Duncan tests revealed significant differences between treatments: P0 differed from P1, while P1 differed from P2 and P3. The increase in digestibility is attributed to EM-4 inoculation in corn straw fermentation, reducing crude fiber content through fiber-digesting enzymes production. However, no increase in crude protein levels in fermented corn straw was observed.

3.4 *Production performance*

Production performance is the results that can be achieved regarding milk, meat production, body weight gain, and reproduction related to livestock in a certain rearing system or environment. The performance parameters of *Peranakan etawa* goats measured in this study were feed consumption, body weight gain, and feed conversion. The results of research on the use of Gamal leaf feed with fermented corn straw on the performance of *Peranakan etawa* goats can be presented in Table 5.

Table 5. Average performance of *peranakan etawa* feeding gamal leaves and fermented corn straw.

	Treatment			
Digestibility	P0	P1	P2	P3
Feed Consumption (kg/head/month)*	124.63^{a}	126.40^{ab}	136.14^{b}	129.21^{ab}
Body Weight Gain (kg/head/month)*	3.37^{a}	4.07^{a}	4.40^{a}	6.37^{b}
Feed Conversion *	41.16^{a}	31.70^{ab}	31.24^{ab}	20.39^{b}

Information: a,b,c different superscripts in the same column show significant differences (*P<0.05*)

3.4.1 *Feed consumption*

Feed consumption, crucial for assessing livestock intake, was calculated by deducting uneaten and dried feed from the total. Peranakan Etawa goats, fed Gamal leaves with fermented corn straw, consumed an average of 123.63 to 129.21 kg/head/month, averaging 4.30 kg/head/day. Consumption tended to rise during the study, notably in treatment P2 (up by 136.14%), with a slight decrease at 30% corn straw addition in P3. Statistical analysis revealed significant differences (P<0.05) in feed consumption with fermented corn straw substitution. Taste, texture, and nutritional value likely influenced consumption levels, along with potential effects of EM-4 on corn straw. Crude fiber degradation by EM-4 could affect feed consumption levels in Peranakan Etawa goats.

3.4.2 *Increase in body weight*

Feed quality's impact on livestock is evident in weight gain measurements. Peranakan Etawa goats fed Gamal leaves and a mixture with fermented corn straw exhibited weight gains ranging from 3.37 to 6.37 kg/head/month. Higher corn straw additions correlated with increased weight gains, with treatment P3 showing the highest gain. Conversely, the control group (P0) achieved the lowest weight gain, indicating the importance of feed composition. Statistical analysis revealed significant differences (P<0.05) in weight gain between feeding regimes, emphasizing the influence of feed quality on livestock growth. Factors such as protein intake, livestock type, age, genetics, environment, and management practices contribute to variations in weight gain.

3.4.3 *Feed conversion*

Feed conversion, the ratio between feed consumption and livestock production, is vital for measuring production efficiency, with lower values indicating higher feed use efficiency. In this study, feed conversion values ranged from 20.39 to 41.16, with significant differences (P<0.05) observed between feeding regimes. Treatment P0, the control group fed only Gamal leaves, exhibited the highest conversion value, decreasing with the inclusion of fermented corn straw. These findings underscore the importance of feed quality, body weight gain, and digestibility in influencing feed conversion, particularly in ruminant livestock.

4 CONCLUSION

The utilization of corn straw waste, with the potential to reach 864 with a production of 6,211.39 tons through fermentation using EM-4 inoculum, has been proven to improve the chemical and physical quality and digestibility of corn straw in vitro. The use of corn straw that has been fermented and mixed with Gamal leaves to reach a level of 30% in the feed of *Peranakan etawa* goats has also succeeded in increasing feed consumption, body weight gain, and feed conversion efficiency in *Peranakan etawa* goats.

ACKNOWLEDGMENTS

We thank the Rector and Dean of the Faculty of Animal Science, Halu Oleo University, for their support in completing this research because, in general, this research can solve the problem of scarcity of animal feed in Southeast Sulawesi.

REFERENCES

Amna, L., Sariubang, M., & Nurhayu, A. (2021a). Increasing production of integration system of corn and beef cattle in Gowa, South Sulawesi. *E3S Web of Conferences*, 306, 05005. https://doi.org/10.1051/e3sconf/202130605005

Amna, L., Sariubang, M., & Nurhayu, A. (2021b). Increasing production of integration system of corn and beef cattle in Gowa, South Sulawesi. In Rubiyo & C. Indrawanto (Eds.), *E3S Web of Conferences* (Vol. 306, p. 05005). https://doi.org/10.1051/e3sconf/202130605005.

Elly, F. H., Lomboan, A., Kaunang, C. L., Rundengan, M., Poli, Z., & Syarifuddin, S. (2020). Development potential of integrated farming system (Local Cattle—Food Crops). *Animal Production*, 21(3), Article 3. https://doi.org/10.20884/1.jap.2019.21.3.739

Gong, X., Zou, H., Qian, C., Yu, Y., Hao, Y., Li, L., Wang, Q., Jiang, Y., & Ma, J. (2020). Construction of in situ degradation bacteria of corn straw and analysis of its degradation efficiency. *Annals of Microbiology*, 70(1), 62. https://doi.org/10.1186/s13213-020-01601-9

Hatmi, R. U., Purwaningsih, Nurhikmat, A., Wirasti, C. A., & Gunawan. (2023). Resource potential in agricultural areas is based on farmer corporations in Nglanggeran Village, Patuk, Gunungkidul, and Yogyakarta. *AIP Conference Proceedings*, 2583, 060011. https://doi.org/10.1063/5.0117008.

Miller, B. A., & Lu, C. D. (2019). Current status of global dairy goat production: An overview. *Asian-Australasian Journal of Animal Sciences*, 32(8 Suppl), 1219–1232. https://doi.org/10.5713/ajas.19.0253

Mogiye, S. L., Nafiu, L. O., & Pagala, M. A. (2020). Reproductive characteristics of *Peranakan etawa* and kacang goats in different maintenance systems in the Toari District, Kolaka Regency. *International Journal of Scientific Research in Science, Engineering and Technology*, 7(2), 442–446. https://doi.org/10.32628/IJSRSET207291

Mudawamah, M., Ciptadi, G., & Retnaningtyas, I. D. (2021). The prolific variation, body morphometrics, and breeding value of indonesian local etawah goat based in east java. *Animal Production*, 23(1), Article 1. https://doi.org/10.20884/1.jap.2021.23.1.85

Trisnadewi, S. A. A. A., Cakra, I. G. L. O., & Suarna, I. W. (2017). Kandungan nutrisi silase jerami jagung melalui fermentasi pollard dan molases. *Majalah Ilmiah Peternakan*, 20(2), 55–59. https://doi.org/10.24843/MIP.2017.v20.i02.p03.

Technological Innovations in Tropical Livestock Development for Environmental Sustainability and Food Security – P. Dhian Isnaeni et al. (eds)

Optimizing the utilization of plantation waste for carrying capacity of beef cattle feed in Southeast Sulawesi, Indonesia

L.O.M. Munadi*
Faculty of Animal Science, Universitas Halu Oleo, Kendari, Southeast Sulawesi, Indonesia

B. Purwanti & F. Sasmita
Faculty of Agriculture, Universitas Sulawesi Tenggara, Kendari, Southeast Sulawesi, Indonesia

R.D. Haloho
Faculty of Animal Science and Fisheries, Universitas Sulawesi Barat, Majene, West Sulawesi, Indonesia

F.M.S. Telupere
Faculty of Animal Science, Universitas Nusa Cendana, Kupang, Nusa Tenggara Timur, Indonesia

Y. Mekiuw, M. Rizal & A. Adrianus
Faculty of Agriculture, Universitas Musamus, Merauke, South Papua, Indonesia

S. Rosmalah
Faculty of Agriculture, Universitas Muhammadiyah, Kendari, Southeast Sulawesi, Indonesia

M.O. Kasmin
Faculty of Agriculture, Universitas Sembilanbelas November, Kolaka, Southeast Sulawesi, Indonesia

ABSTRACT: The availability of feed, especially forages, in terms of quality, quantity, and sustainability, plays a crucial role in determining the success of ruminant livestock farming. Continuous efforts are needed to provide food that meets the nutritional needs of livestock to ensure an adequate supply of feed. The main constraint in meeting the demand for forage is the limited availability of suitable land for its production. Currently, the land used for producing livestock forage tends to be located in regions with low soil fertility. This study specifically reveals the phenomenon of alternative feed from plantation waste, including oil palm, coconut, coffee, cocoa, cashew, and sago plants, using a carrying capacity formula to assess the potential of plantation waste as livestock feed. The analysis utilizes data from various supporting documents. The findings indicate that the potential for developing beef cattle in Southeast Sulawesi is quite promising when utilizing plantation waste as a source of livestock feed. This is evident from the carrying capacity analysis, which shows that plantation waste can provide year-round feed with variable carrying capacities depending on the extent of plantation areas.

Keywords: Optimization, Plantation Waste, Carrying Capacity, Beef Cattle

1 INTRODUCTION

Indonesia, as one of the countries with the largest population in the world, has a crucial task in ensuring an adequate food supply to meet the needs of its people. In this context, the livestock industry plays a key role in providing essential animal protein sources for the nutritional needs of

*Corresponding Author: lmmunadi@uho.ac.id

DOI: 10.1201/9781003468943-26

the population (Asrika *et al.* 2023; Aku *et al.* 2022). One crucial commodity in the livestock industry is animal feed. The demand for animal feed continues to rise in tandem with the growth of the human population and the increased demand for livestock products such as meat, milk, and eggs. This puts great pressure on the supply of adequate and quality animal feed (Astuty *et al.* 2023). In recent years, there has been a trend of increasing demand for quality livestock products, which requires the livestock industry to ensure high-quality feed for livestock.

In addition, the livestock sector also has a significant environmental impact, and efficient use of animal feed can help reduce this impact. Within this framework, it is important to look for sustainable and environmentally friendly feed sources (Munadi *et al.* 2023). Due to Indonesia's diverse climates and geographical conditions, the required animal feed also varies. This includes forages, concentrates, and other alternative feed sources that can provide suitable nutrition for various types of livestock. This diversity supports food security, environmental sustainability, and the growth of a sustainable livestock industry. It helps meet the increasing demand for animal feed and ensures that natural resources utilized for feed production are used efficiently.

Plantation waste in Southeast Sulawesi, arising as by-products from various plantation activities, holds significant potential as an alternative animal feed. Waste from crops such as oil palm, coconut, coffee, cocoa, cashew, and sago, when properly managed, can serve as a nutritious feed source for beef cattle. Although some previous research has identified the potential of plantation residues as animal feed, there is still a need for further investigation into maximizing nutritional value, efficient processing techniques, and the economic and environmental impacts of using plantation residues as feed for beef cattle. Moreover, the limited access to relevant literature on optimization techniques suitable for the local conditions of Southeast Sulawesi has not shown positive trends, indicating the necessity for more specific and in-depth research on this issue.

2 RESEARCH METHODS

This research, specifically focused on the intentionally chosen region of Southeast Sulawesi, examines the province's active development of a beef cattle husbandry program in extensive plantation areas, including oil palm, coconut, coffee, cocoa, cashew, and sago plantations, all of which have the potential to serve as a source of ruminant animal feed, particularly for beef cattle. Employing a literature review method, the research retrieves secondary data from relevant previous studies, official documents, and important records from various government agencies and related institutions up to the year 2023. The initial phase involves identifying regions with the potential to develop beef cattle farming based on oil palm, coconut, coffee, cocoa, cashew, and sago plantations, followed by an analysis to determine the number of beef cattle and the extent of oil palm plantations in each respective area.

This analysis focuses on evaluating the viability of using waste from oil palm, coconut, coffee, cocoa, cashew, and sago plantations as feed for beef cattle in Southeast Sulawesi. It involves identifying the relevant districts or cities with these plantations, assessing their extent, both community and privately managed, and measuring the potential of their waste for animal feed based on available land area. To assess the potential of oil palm, coconut, coffee, cocoa, cashew, and sago plantation waste that can be used as animal feed in Southeast Sulawesi, the following calculations were conducted:

Palm oil:
Production of fresh fronds and leaves (ha) = land area (ha) × 21450, Note: Average production of fronds and leaves = 21450 kg/ha.
Production of fresh palm mud material = land area (ha) × 1050 kg, Note: Average production of fresh palm mud = 1050 kg/ha.
Fresh palm oil meal production = land area (ha) × 567 kg, Note: Average palm oil sludge production = 567 kg/ha.
Production of fresh material from empty palm fruit bunches = land area (ha) × 1500 kg, Note: Average production of fresh material from empty palm fruit bunches = 1500 kg/ha.

Coconut Plantation:
Coconut cake = Amount of coconut production (tons) × 3.293%, Note: The composition of the coconut fruit components is 35% fiber, 28% flesh, 25% water, and 12% shell. On average, 1000 coconut seeds produce 180 kg (18%) of copra, 110 kg (11%) of oil, and 55 kg (5.5%) of coconut cake.

Coffee Plantation:
Potential coffee skin by-products = Coffee production (tons/year) × 51%, Note: Coffee beans range between 49.25 kg (49%), and coffee skin by-products range from 50.75 kg (51%).

Cocoa Plantation:
PKBK = (PBK × (100/24)). Cocoa fruit comprises 74% CBC, 2% placenta, and 24% seeds.

Cashew Plantation:
Pseudo Fruit Production (Tons) = (Number of Cashew Seed Production × (100/10)) × 90%, Note: Potential production of cashew nuts at the age of 5 years ranges from 6–8 kg/tree or 900–1,250 kg/ha with a population of 156 trees/ha and guava production consists of 90% false fruit and 10% seeds.

Sago Plantation:
Weight of wet sago dregs (tons) = Land area (ha) × 12,012 (tons/ha), Note: Average production of sago dregs per hectare = 12,012 tons with the assumption that in one hectare, 20 sago trees can be harvested.

3 RESULTS AND DISCUSSION

3.1 *Palm oil plantation waste*

Waste from oil palm plantations is generated in the cultivation process of oil palm. As one of the primary plantation commodities in many tropical countries, such as Indonesia and Malaysia, oil palm plantations produce various types of waste that can be processed or utilized as feed for beef cattle, as outlined in Table 1.

Table 1. Carrying capacity of palm oil plantation waste.

Regency	Palm Oil (Ha)	Calf Cattle Total LU	Young Cattle Total LU	Adult Cattle Total LU
Muna	135.50	57.42	26.35	12.65
Konawe	2,062.00	870.62	399.53	191.74
Kolaka	4,926.44	2,080.29	954.65	458.15
Konawe Selatan	3,839.00	1,620.91	743.84	356.98
Bombana	205.00	86.56	39.72	19.06
Konawe Utara	741.00	312.87	143.58	68.90
Kolaka Timur	806.60	340.73	156.36	75.04
Muna Barat	349.50	147.78	67.82	32.55

Source: Data Analysis, 2023, Information: LU (Livestock Unit)

The results of the analysis presented in Table 1 indicate that the utilization of plantation waste as a source of animal feed has high potential. This is reflected in the carrying capacity analysis, where each district has varied values depending on the extent of oil palm plantation areas it possesses. For example, Kolaka Regency, with an oil palm plantation area of 4,926.44 thousand hectares, can provide year-round feed for cattle, including 2,080.29 units of calf, 954.65 units of young cattle, and 458.15 units of adult cattle. Ensuring the increase in the population and meat production of ruminant livestock requires serious attention to the quantity, quality, and sustainability of feed supplies. Moreover, utilizing other natural resources, such as plantation waste, can play a crucial role in enhancing feed availability (Amalina *et al.* 2021).

3.2 *Coconut plantation waste*

The results of the analysis of the potential of coconut waste as a source of feed for beef cattle in Southeast Sulawesi are presented in Table 2. The utilization of coconut plantation waste holds tremendous potential when optimized, as illustrated in Table 2, where the carrying capacity values for coconut plantation waste vary significantly depending on the land area. To date, its potential utilization has not been optimal due to several factors, including low livestock resources and the use of traditional technologies. However, with the application of bioprocess technology using mannanolytic Eupenicillium javanicum or Aspergillus niger on coconut kernel cake, it is possible to enhance the protein content in vitro. Biotechnological approaches to feed play a crucial role in improving the nutritional quality of coconut kernel cake, especially through fermentation methods (Ho & Ofomaja 2006).

Table 2. Carrying capacity of coconut plantation waste.

Regency	Coconut (Ha)	Calf Cattle Total LU	Young Cattle Total LU	Adult Cattle Total LU
Buton	2,970.00	18.86	8.66	4.15
Muna	4,855.85	30.84	14.15	6.79
Konawe	2,410.50	15.31	7.03	3.37
Kolaka	4,026.12	25.58	11.74	5.63
Konawe Selatan	7,173.00	45.56	20.91	10.03
Bombana	15,197.80	96.53	44.30	21.26
Wakatobi	1,570.40	9.98	4.58	2.20
Kolaka Utara	3,715.75	23.60	10.83	5.20
Buton Utara	5,350.00	33.98	15.59	7.48
Konawe Utara	2,313.00	14.69	6.74	3.24
Kolaka Timur	2,806.50	17.83	8.18	3.93
Konawe Kepulauan	4,585.50	29.13	13.37	6.42
Muna Barat	3,406.30	21.64	9.93	4.77
Buton Tengah	1,586.00	10.07	4.62	2.22
Buton Selatan	750.00	4.76	2.19	1.05
Kota Kendari	293.29	1.87	0.86	0.41
Kota Baubau	185.15	1.18	0.54	0.26

Source: Data Analysis, 2023, Information: LU (Livestock Unit)

3.3 *Coffee plantation waste*

Coffee husks can serve as an alternative food option for ruminant animals such as cows, goats, buffaloes, and sheep to fulfill their basic production and reproductive needs. Therefore, livestock needs to receive food that aligns with their requirements, both in terms of the quantity consumed and the nutritional content provided. The potential of coffee husks as an alternative feed source to enhance beef cattle production in Southeast Sulawesi is presented in Table 3.

Table 3. Carrying capacity of coffee plantation waste.

Regency	Coffee (Ha)	Calf Cattle Total LU	Young Cattle Total LU	Adult Cattle Total LU
Buton	703.00	4.47	2.05	0.98
Muna	372.50	2.37	1.09	0.52
Konawe	1,065.50	6.77	3.11	1.49
Kolaka	520.04	3.31	1.52	0.73
Konawe Selatan	1,340.00	8.51	3.91	1.87
Bombana	1,725.70	10.96	5.03	2.41
Wakatobi	32.30	0.21	0.1	0.05

(continued)

Table 3. Continued

Regency	Coffee (Ha)	Calf Cattle Total LU	Young Cattle Total LU	Adult Cattle Total LU
Kolaka Utara	477.60	3.04	1.39	0.67
Buton Utara	48.00	0.30	0.14	0.07
Konawe Utara	479.00	3.04	1.40	0.67
Kolaka Timur	1,937.30	12.31	5.65	2.71
Konawe Kepulauan	45.25	0.29	0.13	0.06
Muna Barat	188.10	1.20	0.55	0.26
Buton Tengah	51.00	0.32	0.15	0.07
Buton Selatan	95.00	0.60	0.28	0.13
Kota Kendari	54.50	0.35	0.16	0.08
Kota Baubau	50.70	0.32	0.15	0.07

Source: Data Analysis, 2023, Information: LU (Livestock Unit)

Coffee husks are not widely utilized for animal feed and are mostly discarded as fertilizer. The direct utilization of coffee husks as animal feed has some drawbacks, including the presence of tannin compounds that can disrupt digestion when given in high amounts in their fresh form. Coffee husks are a byproduct of coffee fruit processing. If not managed properly, this waste can lead to environmental pollution (Hoseini *et al.* 2021).

3.4 *Cocoa plantation waste*

Cocoa pod husks are often discarded without clear utilization. Currently, cocoa pod husk waste is typically used as direct feed for cattle and goats without prior fermentation processes. However, in terms of its potential, cocoa pod husks can become a highly nutritious alternative feed for livestock if properly fermented, suitable for both ruminant animals and poultry. Many farmers dispose of cocoa pod husk waste around their plantations, which in turn has the potential to become a breeding ground for the "cocoa pod borer," a pest that harms farmers (Carta *et al.* 2020). The potential of cocoa pod husks as an alternative feed source to enhance beef cattle production in Southeast Sulawesi is presented in Table 4.

Table 4. Carrying capacity of cocoa plantation waste.

Regency	Cocoa (Ha)	Calf Cattle Total LU	Young Cattle Total LU	Adult Cattle Total LU
Buton	1,726.00	31.42	14.42	6.92
Muna	8,316.50	51.38	23.58	11.32
Konawe	12,911.00	25.51	11.71	5.62
Kolaka	25,591.08	42.61	19.55	9.38
Konawe Selatan	18,411.00	75.89	34.83	16.71
Bombana	9,620.00	160.8	73.79	35.41
Wakatobi	15.00	16.62	7.63	3.66
Kolaka Utara	78,970.90	39.32	18.04	8.66
Buton Utara	1,623.00	56.61	25.98	12.47
Konawe Utara	3,916.00	24.47	11.23	5.39
Kolaka Timur	56,859.43	29.7	13.63	6.54
Konawe Kepulauan	3,338.82	48.52	22.27	10.69
Muna Barat	5,409.97	36.05	16.54	7.94
Buton Tengah	57.00	16.78	7.70	3.70
Buton Selatan	34.00	7.94	3.64	1.75
Kota Kendari	94.31	3.11	1.43	0.69
Kota Baubau	134.69	1.97	0.9	0.43

Source: Data Analysis, 2023, Information: LU (Livestock Unit)

To create a suitable integrated farming model, it is necessary to consider livestock commodities that can utilize cocoa shell waste and ensure that farmers can apply this technology easily. Cocoa pod husks have promising potential in creating a cocoa-beef cattle integration model.

3.5 *Cashew plantation waste*

Various fruits can be transformed into high-quality animal feed through a fermentation process. This process is crucial to enhance the nutritional value of initially low-nutrient fruits. Through fermentation, the protein and calorie content of the fruits can be increased while the level of crude fiber can be reduced.

Processing fermented fruits into powder extends their viability for up to six months, offering practical benefits in storage and transportation for animal feed. This method ensures a consistent supply of feed throughout the year. Cashew processing generates waste in the form of cashew apples, often discarded but can be utilized as feed material, particularly when combined with legumes. However, cashew apples contain anacardic acid, which may cause throat irritation and coughing in livestock.

3.6 *Sago plantation waste*

During sago processing, bark and dregs are generated, comprising about 14% (Zulkarnain *et al.* 2016) of the sago stem's wet weight. Sadly, these dregs are typically discarded, leading to environmental pollution. Despite their high carbohydrate content and organic materials, they remain underutilized, accumulating in sago flour processing areas. However, their potential as an alternative feed source for beef cattle in Southeast Sulawesi is highlighted in Table 6.

The potential of local raw materials derived from agricultural, plantation, and agro-industrial waste is vast, but only a small fraction of these resources is utilized as feed. One method employed to enhance the utilization of such waste is the complete feed technology. This technology involves processing through physical treatment and supplementation to produce complete feed for poultry. Waste generated from the sago processing falls into the category of wet by-products since it still retains a moisture level of around 70–80%. Therefore, it is necessary to develop alternative technologies to utilize these sago waste products more efficiently.

Table 5. Carrying apacity of cashew plantation waste.

Regency	Cashew (Ha)	Calf Cattle Total LU	Young Cattle Total LU	Adult Cattle Total LU
Buton	6,024.00	12.09	5.55	2.66
Muna	25,799.80	51.77	23.76	11.4
Konawe	4,437.00	8.90	4.09	1.96
Kolaka	1,247.83	2.50	1.15	0.55
Konawe Selatan	13,479.00	27.05	12.41	5.96
Bombana	17,324.00	34.76	15.95	7.66
Wakatobi	547.50	1.10	0.50	0.24
Kolaka Utara	70.90	0.14	0.07	0.03
Buton Utara	6,033.00	12.11	5.56	2.67
Konawe Utara	4,465.00	8.96	4.11	1.97
Kolaka Timur	667.00	1.34	0.61	0.29
Konawe Kepulauan	5,591.33	11.22	5.15	2.47
Muna Barat	9,352.10	18.77	8.61	4.13
Buton Tengah	12,836.00	25.76	11.82	5.67

(*continued*)

Table 5. Continued

Regency	Cashew (Ha)	Calf Cattle Total LU	Young Cattle Total LU	Adult Cattle Total LU
Buton Selatan	3,539.50	7.10	3.26	1.56
Kota Kendari	235.19	0.47	0.22	0.10
Kota Baubau	764.40	1.54	0.70	0.34

Source: Data Analysis, 2023, Information: LU (Livestock Unit)

Table 6. Carrying capacity of sago plantation waste.

Regency	Sago (Ha)	Calf Cattle Total LU	Young Cattle Total LU	Adult Cattle Total LU
Konawe	1,562.00	181.97	83.51	40.08
Kolaka	106.49	12.47	5.72	2.75
Konawe Selatan	1,287.00	149.94	68.81	33.02
Bombana	6.90	0.82	0.37	0.18
Wakatobi	6.00	0.70	0.32	0.15
Kolaka Utara	104.28	12.23	5.61	2.69
Konawe Utara	254.00	29.59	13.58	6.52
Kolaka Timur	688.90	80.27	36.84	17.68
Konawe Kepulauan	207.35	24.23	11.12	5.34
Kota Kendari	72.00	8.39	3.85	1.85

Source: Data Analysis, 2023, Information: LU (Livestock Unit)

4 CONCLUSION

The study found that the potential utilization of industrial plantation waste in Southeast Sulawesi is quite promising, as reflected in various by-products generated to meet the feed requirements of beef cattle. However, a significant challenge is the insufficient knowledge among farmers about utilizing plantation waste as a feed source, which is attributed to inadequate human resources and the need for advanced technologies in feed processing. Specifically, to enhance the potential of waste as a feed source, support is needed from various stakeholders, including the government, agricultural extension officers, and the farmers themselves.

REFERENCES

Aku, A. S., Yaddi, Y., Saili, T., Hafid, H., Munadi, L. O. M., Dewi, F., & Kete, S. C. R. (2022). Mapping of reproduction disorders caused by infectious diseases in Bali cattle (Bos sundaicus) in muna regency, Indonesia. *Indian Journal of Animal Research*, *57*(2), 241–244. https://doi.org/10.18805/IJAR.BF-1424

Amalina Ishak, F., Haziq Jamil, M., Syukor Abd Razak, A., Huwaida Anuar Zamani, N., & Rashid Ab Hamid, M. (2019). Development of animal feed from waste to wealth using Napier grass and palm acid oil (PAO) from palm oil mill effluent (POME). *Materials Today: Proceedings*, *19*, 1618–1627. https://doi.org/10.1016/j.matpr.2019.11.190

Asrika, R., Tawai, A., Sani, L. O. A., Pagala, M. A., Zulkarnain, D., Munadi, L. O. M., Aku, A. S., Abadi, M., & Jabuddin, L. O. (2023). Extension performance and satisfaction level of bali cattle farmers in South Konawe Regency, Indonesia. *Revista de Gestão Social e Ambiental*, *17*(8), Article 8. https://doi.org/10.24857/rgsa.v17n8-004

Astuty Auza, F., Purwanti, S., A. Syamsu, J., Natsir, A., Badaruddin, R., Zulkarnain, D., & Ode Muh. Munadi, L. (2023). Effects of using black soldier fly larvae meal (Hermetia illucens L) as a source of protein on boosting performance, carcass quality, and nutrient digestibility of village chicken. *Journal of Animal Health and Production*, *11*(2), 193–198. https://doi.org/10.17582/journal.jahp/2023/11.2.193.198

Carta, S., Nudda, A., Cappai, M. G., Lunesu, M. F., Atzori, A. S., Battacone, G., & Pulina, G. (2020). Short communication: Cocoa husks can effectively replace soybean hulls in dairy sheep diets—Effects on milk production traits and hematological parameters. *Journal of Dairy Science*, *103*(2), 1553–1558. https://doi.org/10.3168/jds.2019-17550

Daru, T. P., Sunaryo, W., Pagoray, H., Suhardi, S., Mayulu, H., Ibrahim, I., & Safitri, A. (2023). Diversity, nutrient contents and production of forage plants in an integrated cattle livestock-oil palm plantation in East Kalimantan, Indonesia. *Biodiversitas Journal of Biological Diversity*, *24*(4), Article 4. https://doi.org/10.13057/biodiv/d240406

Ho, Y. S., & Ofomaja, A. E. (2006). Biosorption thermodynamics of cadmium on coconut copra meal as biosorbent. *Biochemical Engineering Journal*, *30*(2), 117–123. https://doi.org/10.1016/j.bej.2006.02.012

Hoseini, M., Cocco, S., Casucci, C., Cardelli, V., & Corti, G. (2021). Coffee by-products derived resources. A review. *Biomass and Bioenergy*, *148*, 106009. https://doi.org/10.1016/j.biombioe.2021.106009

Munadi, L. O. M., Pagala, M. A., Nafiu, L. O., & Zulkarnain, D. (2023). Oil Palm Plantation and Plant Species Diversity in Kolaka District, Indonesia. *WSEAS Transactions on Systems*, *22*, 249–254. https://doi.org/10.37394/23202.2023.22.26

Van Selm, B., Hijbeek, R., van Ittersum, M. K., van Hal, O., van Middelaar, C. E., & de Boer, I. J. M. (2023). Recoupling livestock and feed production in the Netherlands to reduce environmental impacts. *Science of The Total Environment*, *899*, 165540. https://doi.org/10.1016/j.scitotenv.2023.165540

Yafetto, L., Odamtten, G. T., & Wiafe-Kwagyan, M. (2023). Valorization of agro-industrial wastes into animal feed through microbial fermentation: A review of the global and Ghanaian case. *Heliyon*, *9*(4), e14814. https://doi.org/10.1016/j.heliyon.2023.e14814

Zulkarnain, D., Zuprizal, Wihandoyo, & Supadmo. (2016). Effect of cellulase supplementation on in vitro digestibility and energy, crude fiber and cellulose content of sago palm (Metroxylon sp.) waste as broiler chicken feed. *Pakistan Journal of Nutrition*, *15*(11), 997–1002. https://doi.org/10.3923/pjn.2016.997.10023

Technological Innovations in Tropical Livestock Development for Environmental Sustainability and Food Security – P. Dhian Isnaeni et al. (eds)
© 2025 The Author(s), ISBN 978-1-032-74373-8

Potential of cocoa by-products (*Theobroma cocoa*) for livestock feed in Southeast Sulawesi

Syamsuddin
Postgraduate Student of Agricultural Science Study Program, Universitas Oleo, Kendari, Southeast Sulawesi, Indonesia

A. Bain, N.S. Asminaya & T. Saili*
Department of Animal Science, Faculty of Animal Science, Universitas Oleo, Kendari, Southeast Sulawesi, Indonesia

ABSTRACT: This research endeavors to evaluate the viability of utilizing cocoa by-products for livestock feed in Southeast Sulawesi. The primary focus includes assessing the carrying capacity and potential availability of livestock feed derived from cocoa by-products across various districts/cities in the region. The analytical methods encompass the examination of cocoa plantation areas, livestock populations, and other factors influencing the carrying capacity of livestock feed. The research findings highlight Kolaka Utara Regency as the primary producer of cocoa by-products, supported by a substantial plantation area of 78,971 hectares. The biomass production of cocoa husks in this region amounts to 79,115 tons/ha/year in dry matter. This production can potentially provide livestock feeds for approximately 131.2 heads of calves, 60.21 heads of heifers, and 28.9 units of adult cattle. Carrying capacity analysis indicates that this region exhibits a high potential for providing significant livestock feed. Furthermore, the study identifies influential factors affecting carrying capacity, such as livestock population and cocoa plantation area. The overall analysis presents a positive outlook on the potential development of livestock activities in Southeast Sulawesi based on cocoa by-products. Additionally, the research contributes to a deeper understanding of the optimal utilization of cocoa by-products as a source of livestock feed, laying the groundwork for policy development and the promotion of sustainable livestock practices in Southeast Sulawesi.

Keywords: Cocoa, by-products, feed, livestock, regency

1 INTRODUCTION

Indonesia, as the country with the world's largest population, has a significant responsibility to ensure an adequate food supply to meet the needs of its people. In this context, the livestock industry plays a central role in providing essential animal protein for the nutritional needs of the population.

Improving livestock productivity requires efforts to provide feed that is not only of high quality but also sufficient in quantity and sustainable. In Southeast Sulawesi, the availability of forage is highly influenced by climate fluctuations and diverse geographical conditions throughout the year.

An essential component in livestock production is animal feed (Bain *et al.* 2020). The increasing demand for animal feed aligns with the expanding human population and a growing desire for livestock products, including meat, milk, and eggs. This surge in demand

*Corresponding Author: takdir69@uho.ac.id

places considerable strain on the availability of sufficient and top-quality animal feed (Bain *et al.* 2017; Kurinawan *et al.* 2019).

Southeast Sulawesi, as one of the regions in Indonesia, plays a strategic role in the agricultural sector, particularly in cocoa production. By-products of cocoa consist of leaves, stems, and fruit skins, which are often left unused or discarded without being optimally utilized.

The exploration of cocoa by-products as livestock feed presents itself as a compelling alternative, addressing the demand for high-quality feed to promote livestock growth in Southeast Sulawesi. Establishing a livestock feed system centered on cocoa by-products has the potential to be a sustainable solution, offering the prospect of increased income for farmers (Torres 2021; Velasquez *et al.* 2023), and concurrently mitigating the adverse environmental consequences linked to the disposal of cocoa by-products.

Although the potential of cocoa by-products as livestock feed has been identified, further research is still needed to optimize the utilization of cocoa by-products as livestock feed. Therefore, this research aimed to provide detailed information on the potential of cocoa by-products as feed for livestock in Southeast Sulawesi through a comprehensive scientific approach.

2 RESEARCH METHODS

This research utilized a survey method involving the collection of primary and secondary data as well as literature studies. The initial phase involves identifying regions with the potential to develop cattle farming.

The feed requirements for livestock were calculated based on animal unit (AU) standards. The feed requirements based on standard animal units for each type of livestock are as follows: calves (1.65kg dry matter/head/day equivalent to 602.25kg/head/year; young livestock (3.6kg dry matter/head/day equivalent to 1,314 kg per head per year, and adult livestock (7.5kg dry matter/head/day equivalent to 2,737.5kg/head/year (Nell and Rollinson 1974).

The analysis of the potential of cocoa by-products involved the available production throughout the year with the assumption that everything was well-spent. The percentage of cocoa by-products consists of four components: pod husk (73.7%), pulp (10.1%), placenta (2.0%), and seeds (4.2%) (Chandrasekaran 2012). Therefore, the formula to obtain cocoa pod husk production (PKBK) is PKBK (tons/year) = (73.7/14.2) × PBK (Watson *et al.* 2012).

3 RESULTS AND DISCUSSION

3.1 *Text and indenting*

The analysis listed in Table 1 showed that the Kolaka Utara Regency is the region with the highest biomass production of cocoa by-products. This factor can be distributed over the plantation area, which reaches 78,971 hectares with the production of by-product biomass in the form of cocoa shells of 79,115 tons/ha/year in dry matter and can meet the livestock needs of 131.2 AU for calves, 60.21 AU for heifers, and 28.9 AU for adult cattle. On the other hand, Kolaka Regency also attracted attention to the analysis of carrying capacity. The results of research on the production potential of cocoa plants and their use for cattle feed in Southeast Sulawesi were presented in Table 1.

The examination of cocoa plantation areas revealed that Kolaka Utara Regency, encompassing a vast plantation area of 78,971 hectares, has the capacity to produce 79,115 tons of dry matter (DM) from cocoa by-products. This production is sufficient to provide feed for 131 calves, 60 heifers, or 29 adult cattle. In summary, the analysis paints a positive picture of the potential growth of livestock in Southeast Sulawesi. The carrying capacity analysis underscores the promising prospects for the development of livestock activities in this region.

The carrying capacity values outlined in Table 1 for each district/city are shaped by two primary factors: the cocoa plantation area and the livestock population. Notably, areas characterized by a comparatively modest livestock population yet substantial cocoa plantation area inherently yield high carrying capacity. Conversely, regions featuring a significant livestock population but a limited cocoa plantation area experience a detrimental effect on carrying capacity, particularly concerning the provision of feed derived from cocoa by-products.

The carrying capacity of cocoa by-products (Table 1) as livestock feed can vary depending on cocoa biomass production. For example, Kolaka Timur Regency, with an area of 57,916 hectares could produce wet Cocoa Pod Husk Biomass as much as 94,409 ton/year which is equal to 26,236 ton/year dry matter. These results have a positive impact on providing livestock support, capable of supporting approximately 44 heads of calf or 20 heads of heifer livestock, or 10 heads of adult cattle.

The utilization of cocoa husks as livestock feed is not only economically beneficial for farmers but also supports sustainable farming practices by reducing by-product waste, preserving the environment, and minimizing negative impacts. The management of cocoa husks as livestock feed still needs to improve due to time constraints, human resource limitations, and storage facility constraints.

Table 1. Carrying capacity of cocoa by-products as livestock feed in Southeast Sulawesi.

			Cocoa Husk Biomass Production (Ton/Year)			Feed Fulfillments (head/Year)		
Regency/City	Cocoa Plantation Area (Ha)	Cocoa Production (Ton/year)	Wet	Dry matter (%)	Dry matter production (ton/year Ingredients)	Calf	Heifer	Adult
Buton	2,412	174	903	27.79	251	0.42	0.19	0.09
Muna	8,317	2.581	13.396	27.79	3.723	6.17	2.83	1.36
Konawe	14,894	9.218	47.843	27.79	13.295	22.05	10.12	4.86
Kolaka	29,507	10.338	53.656	27.79	14.911	24.73	11.35	5.45
Konawe Selatan	20,152	8.391	43.55	27.79	12.103	20.07	9.21	4.42
Bombana	9,954	4.363	22.645	27.79	6.293	10.44	4.79	2.3
Wakatobi	16	2	10	27.79	3	0	0	0
Kolaka Utara	78,971	54.852	284.69	27.79	79.115	131.2	60.21	28.9
Buton Utara	2,304	69	358	27.79	100	0.17	0.08	0.04
Konawe Utara	3,974	586	3.041	27.79	845	1.4	0.64	0.31
Kolaka Timur	57,916	18.19	94.409	27.79	26.236	43.51	19.97	9.58
Konawe Kepulauan	3,341	1	5	27.79	1	0	0	0
Muna Barat	5,877	1.921	9.97	27.79	2.771	4.59	2.11	1.01
Buton Tengah	59	4	21	27.79	6	0.01	0	0
Buton Selatan	36	0	0	27.79	0	0	0	0
Kota Kendari	128	21	109	27.79	30	0.05	0.02	0.01
Kota Baubau	154	59	306	27.79	85	0.14	0.06	0.03

Beyond the mainland areas, the island regions of Southeast Sulawesi also exhibit potential availability of livestock feed derived from cocoa by-products, as indicated in Table 1. As an example, Muna Barat Regency, with 5,877 hectares of cocoa plantation, has the potential to produce approximately 9.97 tons per year of wet Cocoa Pod Husk Biomass, equivalent to 2,771 tons per year of dry matter. This potential in Muna Barat Regency can play a pivotal role in supplying feed for livestock, supporting approximately 5 calves, 2 heifers, or 1 adult cattle.

The disposal of cocoa husks around the plantation area has the potential to cause pest problems, harming farmers. An integrated farming approach between cocoa and beef cattle has proven to be an effective solution to address this issue. This system not only creates efficiency in the management of plantations and livestock but also enhances the income of farmers in rural areas.

The carrying capacity of livestock feed is notably influenced by factors such as livestock population and the cocoa plantation area. Kolaka Utara Regency stands out as an exemplary case, characterized by an appropriate livestock population and an extensive cocoa plantation area, creating favorable conditions for maximizing the utilization of cocoa by-products. In summary, this research provides valuable insights into the potential of utilizing cocoa by-products for ruminant livestock feed in Southeast Sulawesi. The practical recommendations derived from this study can be instrumental in shaping policies and strategies for sustainable livestock development, leveraging local resources to optimize the growth of the livestock sector in Southeast Sulawesi.

In this scenario, there are promising opportunities for the development of livestock business programs that can capitalize on the utilization of cocoa husk by-products as a valuable source of livestock feed. To establish an effective integrated farming model, careful consideration should be given to the selection of livestock commodities that can efficiently utilize cocoa husks, ensuring that farmers can readily implement this technology. Cocoa fruit husks show potential as an integral material in a cocoa-beef cattle model, alleviating the need for grass typically required by farmers, especially in intensive patterns or full-stall maintenance. The capacity of cocoa husks as a livestock feed source hinges on cocoa production per unit of land and its distribution throughout the year.

4 CONCLUSION

This study underscores the substantial potential of cocoa plant by-products as a valuable source of ruminant livestock feed in Southeast Sulawesi. North Kolaka Regency, in particular, stands out as a key producer, boasting a vast plantation area of 78,971 hectares and a significant biomass production of cocoa pod husks amounting to 79,115 tons/ha/year in dry matter. This production can effectively meet the livestock requirements for 131.2 units of calves, 60.21 units of heifers, and 28.9 units of adult cattle. The carrying capacity analysis reveals that this region possesses a high capacity to provide feed for ruminant livestock, presenting noteworthy opportunities for the advancement of the livestock sector.

ACKNOWLEDGMENTS

Thank you to the promoter and co-promoter for their assistance and dedication in helping the author complete this research. Hopefully, it will be a spur in the next stages.

REFERENCES

Bain A, Wiryawan I K G, Astuti D A, Arman C and Suharti S. 2017 Fermentability and nutrient digestibility of ration supplemented with Soybean oil Calcium soap and Cashew fruit flour *Pak. J. Nutr.* **16** 945–53.

Bain A, Wiryawan K G, Astuti D, Suharti S, Arman C and Nasiu F. 2020 Characteristics of in vitro fermentation and nutrient digestibility of ration supplemented with different level of Soybean oil calcium soap. *IOP Conference Series: Earth and Environmental Science* vol 465 (IOP Publishing) p 012020

Chandrasekaran M. 2012. *Valorization of food processing by-products.* New West: CRC Press, Taylor and Prancis Group.

Kurniawan W, Bain A, Syamsuddin, Abadi M and Sandy Y N. 2019 Quality and fermentation characteristic of corn stover – rubber cassava (Manihot glaziovii M.A) combination silage *IOP Conference Series: Earth and Environmental Science* vol 287 p 012022

Nell A J dan Rollinson D H L. 1974 *Kebutuhan dan Ketersediaan Pakan Ternak di Indonesia.* UNDP/FAO, Washington DC.

Torres Castillo N E, Ochoa Sierra J S, Oyervides-Muñoz M A, Sosa-Hernández J E, Iqbal H M N, Parra-Saldívar R and Melchor-Martínez E M 2021 Exploring the potential of coffee husk as caffeine bio-adsorbent – A mini-review *Case Stud. Chem. Environ. Eng.* **3** 100070

Velásquez-Jiménez D, Luzardo-Ocampo I, Gaytán-Martínez M and Campos-Vega R 2023 Design and characterization of a solid-state fermented cacao pods and husk-based functional ingredient to potentially modulate circadian rhythm-associated proteins *Food Biosci.* **56** 103199

Watson R R, Preedy V R, Zibadi S. 2012 *Chocolate in Health and Nutrition.* New York: Humana Press brand of Springer.

Technological Innovations in Tropical Livestock Development for Environmental Sustainability and Food Security – P. Dhian Isnaeni et al. (eds)

Optimizing the use of revenue sharing funds from palm oil to enhance governance and environmental quality of sustainable palm oil plantations

V.S. Arhian
Student in Environmental Science Doctoral Program at Gadjah Mada University, Indonesia

S.H. Murti*
Faculty of Geography, Gadjah Mada University, Indonesia

E. Baliarti
Graduate School Gadjah Mada University, Indonesia

ABSTRACT: Plantation expansion impacts socio-ecology in Indonesian palm oil plantations. The environmental issues stem from alterations in land use and landscape. Realizing the Indonesian Sustainable Palm Oil (ISPO) certification is a crucial step towards establishing sustainable and trustworthy practices in the country's palm oil industry. The Government of the Republic of Indonesia offers revenue-sharing funds to palm oil plantations, which incentivizes the development of regional infrastructure and boosts economic growth. These measures aim to promote sustainable and responsible palm oil production from the upstream to downstream sectors, and mitigate any concerns about unsustainable processes. The oil palm plantations in Sintang Regency cover an area of 195,779.74 hectares, and the revenue generated from 46 oil palm companies in 2023 DBH Sawit was Rp. 20,492,470.000. The majority of this revenue (80%) is allocated for road and bridge infrastructure development. Out of all the current oil palm companies, only 6 have implemented sustainable waste management practices, and 10 have adopted sustainable land management practices.

Keywords: Socio Ecology, ISPO, Sustainable Palm Oil

1 INTRODUCTION

The Government of the Republic of Indonesia issued Regulation of the Minister of Agriculture No. 11/Permentan/OT.140/3/2015 to establish ISPO. The Indonesian Sustainable Palm Oil Certification System (ISPO) is a business system in the oil palm plantation industry that adheres to applicable laws and regulations. It is economically, socially, and environmentally responsible. ISPO implementation aims to minimize the detrimental effects of environmental damage, greenhouse gas emissions, and deforestation. This implementation should be conducted with proper adherence to ethical and fair practices (Arifandy 2018).

The ISPO refers to Law No. 40 of 2007, which mandates that companies involved in natural resource-related business activities must shoulder social and environmental responsibilities. Based on ISPO standards, social responsibility is demonstrated through programs aimed at enhancing the well-being of indigenous communities and preserving local

*Corresponding Author: sigit.heru.m@ugm.ac.id

DOI: 10.1201/9781003468943-28

knowledge. This concept reflects a dedication to sustainable development, as well as the effective management of social, economic, and environmental performance.

Revenue sharing funds (DBH) are funds sourced from APBN revenues allocated to regions based on their potential for production. These funds are used to meet regional needs in the context of implementing decentralization. DBH functions as a fiscal balance between the center and the regions from taxes and natural resources (SDA) that are shared, including as a correction factor for the exploitation of natural resources (Alvaro 2022). Currently, DBH is primarily utilized in the mining, oil, and gas sectors. This issue remains unresolved. However, there is widespread dissatisfaction among local Indonesian governments regarding the unequal distribution of DBH between the central and local governments (Hadna 2016).

In Sintang District, the oil palm plantation area covers 195,779.74 hectares, with only twelve companies currently holding ISPO certification. In 2023, Sintang Regency for the first time received revenue sharing funds from the oil palm plantation sector. Revenue Sharing Funds are part of the balancing funds, in accordance with Law No. 33 of 2004 on Central and Regional Financial Balance, which brings fundamental changes to the system and mechanism of regional government management, confirms that for the implementation of the authority of regional government, the central government will transfer balancing funds to the regional government. With the transfer of funds from the center, it is expected that local governments will be able to better allocate the local revenues they receive to finance local expenditures in their regions (Mulyati 2017).

2 MATERIAL AND METHODS

2.1 *Material*

This study was conducted in Sintang Regency, located in West Kalimantan Province. The area comprises 195,779.74 hectares of oil palm plantations, including those owned by 46 companies and smallholders. In 2021, the total production amounted to 319,464.99 tons, and this region has six palm oil processing plants, each with a production capacity of 30–60 tons per hour.

2.2 *Methods*

The research methodology implemented is qualitative, relying on data obtained from technical agencies within the Sintang district. The data is subsequently analyzed and compared to revenue sharing funds received by the district in 2023 (Agustina 2022).

3 RESULTS AND DISCUSSION

3.1 *Plantation crop area and production in Sintang Regency*

Based on the 2015–2035 spatial map of Sintang district, the land allocated for oil palm plantations is evenly dispersed among 14 sub-districts. This distribution could contribute to the expeditious growth of Sintang district. In particular, these oil palm plantations have a palpable positive impact on the community in terms of accessibility, allowing easier mobility between sub-districts and villages. With an area of 21,638 square kilometers, the process of developing infrastructure in Sintang District will be slow due to limited funds in the APBD that can only be allocated for infrastructure development. Sintang District also directly borders Malaysia in the Ketungau Hulu and Ketungau Tengah sub-districts with a border area of 4,320 square kilometers and a population of 53,056. There is also a 295,478-hectare oil palm plantation along the border.

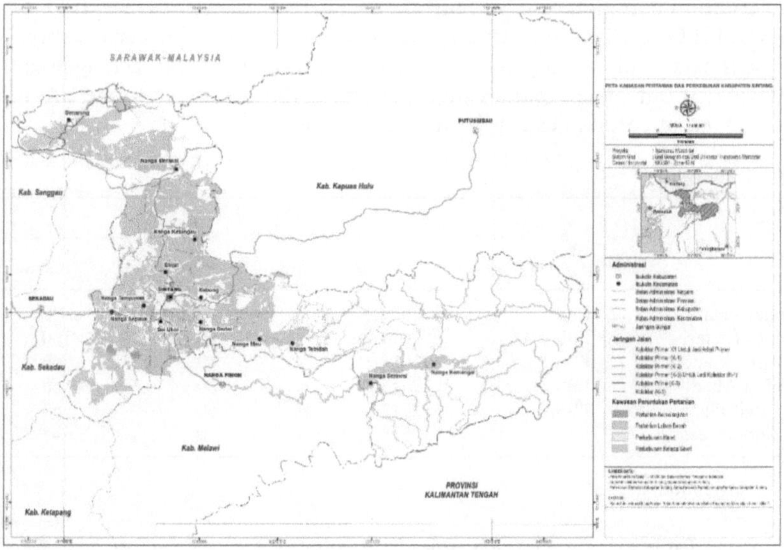

Figure 1. Map of agriculture and plantation areas of Sintang regency.

3.2 *Palm plantation development*

The palm oil is a significant commodity in Sintang district, dominating both in terms of area and total production, as Table 1 illustrates.

Table 1. Plantation commodities in Sintang regency.

Commodity Type	In hectares			In Tons		
Palm Oil	185,500	193,184.89	195,779.74	282,569	323,703.21	195,779.74
Hybrid Coconut	1,505	1,326.95	1,312.70	350	309.40	1,312.70
Rubber	96,397	98,587.00	102,320.00	39,264	39,267.00	102,320.00
Coffee	368	346.50	352.50	91	83.07	352.50
Cocoa	91	82.40	82.70	10	–	82.70

Source : DPMPTSP Sintang

Regarding the progress of plantation production, the number of oil palm plants has risen from 2017 to 2021 and is outlined in Table 2.

Table 2. Development of plantation crop production by type (tons) in 2017–2021.

Plant Type	2017	2018	2019	2020	2021
Palm Oil	206,291	280,771	280,771	323,703.89	319,464.99
Hybrid Coconut	205	211	211	208.50	207.50
Rubber	39,609	39.274	39.254	39,269.00	40,359.00
Coffee	99	95	99	83.07	82.00
Cocoa	10	10	10	8.00	8.00

Source : DPMPTSP Sintang

Not all of the 46 companies in Sintang District have processing plants as only one processing plant is allowed per group of companies. According to current data, there are six palm oil processing factories in Sintang District.

Twelve plantation companies in Sintang District are members of the RSPO, all of which already possess ISPO certification. Among the 12, eight possess ISPO certification, while two are RSPO members. This arrangement results in sustainable land management practices being solely carried out by companies that meet both ISPO standards and are members of the RSPO. The list of companies can be found in Table 4.

Table 3. Palm oil mill.

Company	Raw Materials	Year of Operation	Capacity		
			Permissions	Installed	Used
PT. Bontipermai Jayaraya	TBS	2009	60	30	30
PT. Agro Sukses Lestari	TBS	2014	80	100	60
PT. Sintang Agro Mandiri	TBS	2014	60	60	45
PT. Buana Hijau Abadi	TBS	2015	60	60	30
PT. Perdana Sawit Plantation	TBS	2017	60	60	60
PT. Permata Subur Lestari	TBS	2018	30	45	30

Source: DPMPTSP Sintang

Table 4. Data of companies that have ISPO.

No	Company Name	Land Area (Ha)
1	PT Grand Mandiri Utama	19,200
2	PT Palmindo Lestari	5,700
3	PT Duta Sejahtera Utama	17,000
4	PT Bukitprima Plantindo	19,500
5	PT Bukit hijau Lestari	7,000
6	PT Buana Hijau Abadi	24,500
7	PT Kiara Sawit Andalan	28,000
8	PT. Sintang Agro Mandiri	17,190
9	PT Mitra Nusa Sarana	19,000
10	PT Palma Agro Lestari Jaya	13,900
11	PT Mitra Nusa Sarana	19,000
12	PT Palma Agro Lestari Jaya	13,900
Total Area		203,890

Source : *Landscale* Kab. Sintang 2022

To achieve zero waste in plantations and adopt sustainable waste management practices, six companies implement the use of liquid waste from palm oil processing as fertilizer through land application. They do so in compliance with Minister of Environment Decree No. 29 of 2003, which outlines guidelines for requirements and procedures for licensing the utilization of palm oil industry wastewater in oil palm plantations. The utilization of wastewater as fertilizer and animal feed has potential benefits. Its use can prevent waste accumulation in the environment.

Table 5. Land application.

No	Company Name	Land Area (Ha)
1	PT. Agro Sukses Lestari	Kecamatan Kelam Permai
2	PT. Perdana Sawit Plantation	Kecamatan Ketungau Tengah
3	PT. Permata Subur Lestari	Kecamatan Sungai Tebelian
4	PT. Bintara Tani Nusantara	Kecamatan Kayan Hilir
5	PT. Cahaya Unggul Prima	Kecamatan Ketungau Hilir
6	PT Buana Hijau Abadi	Kecamatan Ketungau Hilir

Source: *Landscale* Kab. Sintang 2022

3.3 *Infrastructure in Sintang regency*

The district roads in Sintang Regency span 2,289,620 kilometers, mainly comprising of unpaved and damaged roads. The regency covers an area of 21,638 square kilometers, comprising of 14 sub-districts, 16 villages and 390 hamlets. The inadequate infrastructure adversely affects the development in the region, impeding trade and mobility. In remote areas outside the city center, the cost of goods rises, forcing border residents to choose between purchasing necessities at high prices or selling their own crops to Malaysia instead of traveling to the district city. Table 6 and Figure 2 provide an overview of the road conditions in Sintang Regency.

Table 6. District road condition.

Pavement Type (Km)	Good (Km)	Medium (Km)	Lightly Damaged (Km)	Severely Damaged (Km)
Hotmix	72.230	26.589	9.218	51.723
Macadam	0.034	3.755	9.377	29.655
Concrete	26.268	60.505	12.934	6.964
Gravel	0.000	1,311.374	184.100	90.490
Dirt	0.000	0.400	119.990	274.014
Total	98.532	1,402.623	335.619	452.846

Source: DPU Sintang 2023

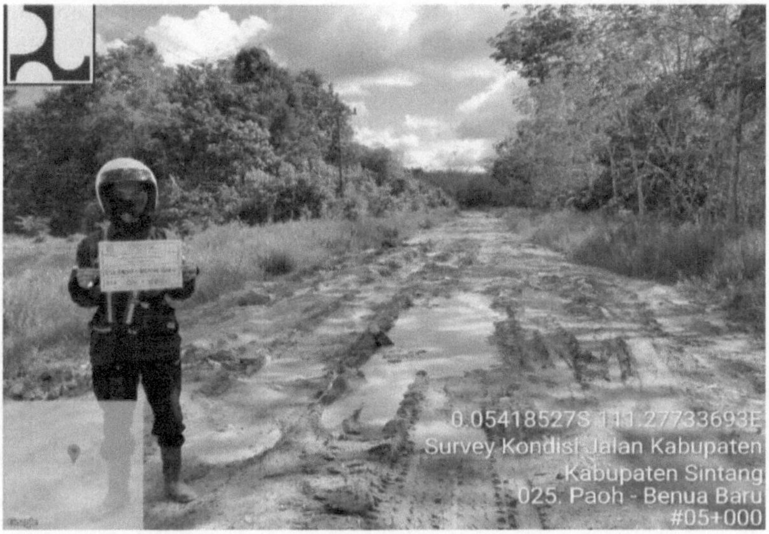

Figure 2. Road conditions in Sintang regency. Source: DPU Sintang 2023.

3.4 *Optimizing palm oil revenue sharing fund*

The determination of oil palm plantation DBH is based on Government Regulation Number 38 of 2020. The regulation stipulates that the source of oil palm DBH comes from export duties and export levies imposed on oil palm, with a DBH ceiling set at a minimum of 4%. The 4% DBH is then divided among the Provincial Government (20%), other bordering districts/cities (20%), and producing districts (60%). As a result, in 2023, Sintang Regency received oil palm DBH amounting to Rp. 20,492,470,000.

Sintang Regency received revenue sharing funds in 2023 and will be included in the regional revenue and expenditure budget in 2024, in accordance with the finance minister's regulation number 91 of 2023 concerning the management of revenue sharing funds for oil palm plantations. At least 80% of the revenue sharing funds must be allocated to activities related to road and bridge infrastructure. Oil palm plantations do not significantly contribute to regional revenue. They only provide local revenue through land and building tax payments and Income Tax on Land and Buildings.

Local governments that produce oil palm plantation products often face pressure from the community due to concerns about environmental damage caused by land exploitation. In Sintang district, the majority of people in the plantation area still have a low standard of living. This is in contrast to the potential of the existing natural resources, which is not being fully utilized to improve social welfare. According to data from the Central Bureau of Statistics, there is no positive correlation between natural resources in the plantation sector and the level of community welfare. In West Kalimantan, the number of people living in poverty is 367.89 thousand, with the highest concentration of poverty found in Sintang district, where 53.04 thousand people live below the poverty line. According to chrisendo (2022), oil palm cultivation is expected to have a positive impact on people's living standards, education, nutrition, living conditions, and asset ownership.

The data presented in Tables 1 and 2 show the area of oil palm plantations and the amount of CPO production in the Sintang district. However, it is important to note that the DBH of oil palm is very small per year for the district as a producing region. Establishing fiscal policy in producing regions can be challenging due to limited natural resources (Azhgaliyeva 2014). Therefore, it is crucial for policy makers to prioritize the effectiveness of revenue sharing funds to ensure optimal utilization of palm oil revenue sharing funds. The central and local governments have not prioritized revenue sharing funds for activities related to environmental management in land use activities used for plantations. It is important to consider the environmental impact of these activities and allocate funds accordingly. This statement does not align with the principles outlined in the ISPO regulations, which require environmentally sound and sustainable land use.

4 CONCLUSION

The government should study the revenue sharing amount for palm oil-producing regions since these regions receive direct benefits from palm oil plantation activities.

ACKNOWLEDGEMENT

The authors send their gratitude to Indonesia Endowment Fund for Education Agency for the funding of the research.

REFERENCES

Agustina D, Heryadi, and Saharuddin. 2014. Analisis lingkungan sosial ekonomi pengelolaan perkebunan kelapa sawit berkelanjutan berdasarkan kriteria ISPO PT. Tapian nadenggan. *Jurnal pengelolaan sumberdaya alam dan lingkungan*. Vol 4 No 1: 43–48.

Agustina, I. Kebijakan dana bagi hasil (DBH) berdasarkan perimbangan keunagn pusat dan daerah. *Jurnal ekonomi dan keuangan publik* vol.9. Juni 2022: 51–60.

Alvaro, R. The effect of local revenue, general allocation fund, revenue sharing fund, specific allocation fund, and regional expenditures on economic growth in district regions of undeveloped regions. *Jurnal Budget* Vol.7 Edisi 2, 2022.

Amalia R, dkk. Perubahan tutupan lahan akibat ekspansi perkebunan kelapa sawit: dampak sosial, ekonomi dan ekologi. *Jurnal ilmu lingkungan.*

Azhgaliyeva D. The effect of fiscal policy on oil revenue fund: The case of Kazakhstan. *Journal of Eurasian Studies* 5 (2014) 157–183.

Arifandy M, Hariyadi, and S. Adiwibowo. 2018. Analisis pengaruh adopsi ISPO terhadap perbaikan kinerja pengelolaan lingkungan dan perubahan sosial ekonomi masyarakat. *Jurnal pengelolaan sumberdaya alam dan lingkungan.* Vol 8(2): 199–206.

Badan Pusat Statistik. 2023. *Indikator kesejahteraan rakyat kabupaten Sintang.*

Chrisendo D *et al.* Oil palm cultivation improves living standards and human capital formation in smallholder farm households. *World Development* 159 (2022) 106034

Dharmawan, A. H., F. T. Nasdia, B. Barus, R. A. Kinseng, Y. Indaryanti, H. Indriana, D.I. Mardianingsih, F. Rahmadian, H. N. Hidayah, and A. M. Roslinawati.2019. Kesiapan petani kelapa sawit swadaya dalam implementasi ISPO: persoalan lingkungan hidup, legalitas dan keberlanjutan. *Jurnal ilmu lingkungan* Vol 17(2): 304–315.

Hadna, A. 2016. Formulating an oil and gas revenue sharing fund based on right based approach. *International journal of administrative science & organization*, volume 23 number 1.

Hovis M, F. Cubbage, J. C. Hollinger, T. Shear, B. Doll, J. J. Kurki-Fox, D. Line, M. Lovejoy, B Evans. T. Potter. 2022. Determining the costs, revenues, and cost-share payments for the "floodwise" program: Nature-based solutions to mitigate flooding in eastern, rural North Carolina. *Nature-Based Solutions* Vol 2 (2022) 100016.

Juniyanti L, L.B. Prasetyo, D.P. Aprianto, H. Purnomo, H. Kartodihardjo. 2020. Perubahan penggunaan dan tutupan lahan, serta faktor penyebabnya di pulau bengkalis, provinsi riau (periode 1990–2019). *Journal of natural resources and environmental management.* Vol 10 (3): 419–435

Matti S, J. Nassen, and J. Larsson. 2022. Are fee-and-dividend schemes the savior of environmental taxation? Analyses of how different revenue use alternatives affect public support for Sweden's air passenger tax. *Enviromental Science and Policy* Vol 132 (2022)181–189.

Mulyasari G, I. N. Djarot, N. A. Sasongko, and A. S. Putra. 2023. Social-life cycle assessment of oil palm plantation smallholders in Bengkulu province, Indonesia. *Heliyon* Vol 9 (8) e19123.

Mulyati, S, Yusriardi. 2017. Dana bagi hasil dan dana alokasi umum terhadap belanja daerah pada provinsi aceh. *agregat: Jurnal ekonomi dan bisnis.*

Oliphant, E., and Simon, A.C. 2022. The cost of sustainable palm oil: Should an Indonesian smallholder pursue RSPO-certification?. *World Development Perspectives* 26 (C).

Ordway, E.M., Rosamond, L.N., Raymond, N.N, and Eric, F. L. 2019. Oil palm expansion and deforestation in Southwest Cameroon associated with proliferation of informal mills. *Nature Communications* Vol 10: 1–11.

Paoli, G.P., Betsy, Y., Philip, L. W., and Aisyah. S. 2010. CSR, Oil palm and the rspo: translating boardroom philosophy into conservation action on the ground. *Tropical conservation science* Vol 3(4):438–446.

Papilo. P, Marimin, M., Erliza, H., Machfud, Yani, M., Asrol, M., Evanila, Hermawan, P., and Mahmud, J. 2022. Palm oil-based bioenergy sustainability and policy in Indonesia and Malaysia: A systematic review and future agendas. *Heliyon* 8 (2022) e10919.

Rosanne, E.de V, Suwarno, A., Slingerland, M., Peter, J. van der M., and Jennifer, M. L. 2023. Pre-certification conditions of independent oil palm smallholders in Indonesia. Assessing prospects for RSPO certification. *Land Use Policy.* 130 (2023) 106660

Rowland, D., Zanello, G., Aliyo, E., and Ickowitz, A. 2022. Oil palm and gendered time use: A mixed-methods case study from West Kalimantan, Indonesia. *Forest Policy and Economic* Vol 137 (2022) 102682

Suryadi, S., Dermawan, A. H., and Barus, B. 2020. Ekspansi perkebunan kelapa sawit: persoalan sosial, ekonomi dan lingkungan hidup (studi kasus kab. palalawan riau). *Jurnal ilmu lingkungan* Vol 18(2): 367–374.

Utami, R., Putri, E. I. K., and Ekayani., M. 2018. Biaya eksternal dan internalisasi limbah pabrik kelapa sawit. *Jurnal pengelolaan sumberdaya alam dan lingkungan* Vol 8(2): 143–150

Technological Innovations in Tropical Livestock Development for Environmental Sustainability and Food Security – P. Dhian Isnaeni et al. (eds)
© 2025 The Author(s), ISBN 978-1-032-74373-8
Open Access: www.taylorfrancis.com, CC BY-NC-ND 4.0 license

The abundance of flies associated with cow dung collected in Besut, Terengganu, Malaysia

N.A. Md Yusof*, M.A. Rosdi & F. Lananan
Netherlands School of Animal Science, Aquatic Science and Environment, Faculty of Bioresources, Universiti Sultan Zainal Abidin (UniSZA), Besut Campus, Besut, Terengganu, Malaysia

ABSTRACT: Flies are important vectors for many pathogens that transmit diseases to humans and animals. They breed on decayed, fermenting or rotting organic materials. Elements such as humidity, temperature and rainfall can highly influence the condition of breeding sites and the survival of eggs and larvae. Livestock animals are usually raised in open ranges in areas close to people. Therefore, animal dung such as cow dung may attract flies to the areas. Considering these factors, this study aimed to identify flies associated with cow dung in Besut, Terengganu and their population abundance. The cow dung samples were collected from three different locations around Universiti Sultan Zainal Abidin (UniSZA) Besut Campus, Besut, Terengganu. Samples were collected once a week for three consecutive weeks in January 2022 for the rainy season and in April 2022 for the hot season. A total of 1078 individuals from six families were identified: Calliphoridae, Muscidae, Psychodidae, Scatophagidae, Sepsidae, and Sphaeroceridae. The hot season recorded more Diptera families than in the rainy season. The most abundant family obtained was Sepsidae and the least abundant was Scathophagidae for both seasons. Analysis showed that there was no significant difference ($p>0.05$) in the abundance of the Diptera population in the rainy and hot seasons. This study serves as an initial step towards advancing ecological research for developing public health objectives aimed at reducing the spread of pathogenic microorganisms, particularly flies as potential vectors.

Keywords: Ectoparasite, Diptera, vector, livestock, seasonal abundance

1 INTRODUCTION

The members of the order Diptera (Class: Insecta) are commonly known as true flies. They are easily distinguished from other insect groups by halteres, which are their modified hind wings (Marsyal 2017). Some species are important vectors for pathogens such as bacteria, protozoa, nematodes and viruses (Preze *et al.* 2020). The transmission of pathogens by flies can cause many diseases in humans and livestock and subsequently cause public health issues (Short *et al.* 2017).

Flies breed on decayed, fermenting or rotting organic materials including cow dung. Cattle manure contains organic matter and bacteria, rendering it an optimal substrate for fly larvae that consume the microorganisms found during the decomposition of the manure (Naupane *et al.* 2021). Elements such as humidity, temperature and rainfall can highly influence the condition of breeding sites and the survival of eggs and larvae of many insect vectors (Short *et al.* 2017). A study conducted by (Sontigun *et al.* 2018) on the temporal density of the oriental latrine fly (*Chrysomya megacephala*) showed a high number of this species during summer and the number of flies declined at the end of the season. The abundance of *C. megacephala* rose again in the early rainy season and eventually declined through the rainy season.

*Corresponding Author: athiqahmdyusof@unisza.edu.my

 DOI: 10.1201/9781003468943-29

Universiti Sultan Zainal Abidin (UniSZA) Besut Campus is situated on the East Coast of Peninsular Malaysia. The rains are a lot heavier in this area from November to January, while the weather is usually sunny from March to October every year. This study was predominantly motivated by recent outbreaks of flies during the rainy season in the Besut Campus area in November 2021. The surrounding Besut Campus, UniSZA has many free grazing livestock and the campus is also near to many small farms. Assumptions were made that this factor may contribute to the increasing number of flies on the campus during that season due to the cattle manures that provide good breeding sites for the flies.

Some studies have explored the relationship between weather conditions and fly abundance in Malaysia (Sahahar *et al.* 2011; Tahir *et al.* 2007), however lack of research investigating the relationship between fly abundance and cattle manure during the summer and rainy seasons. Therefore, this study aimed to investigate the type and abundance of flies associated with cattle dung in UniSZA Besut Campus, Terengganu, Malaysia.

2 METHODOLOGY

2.1 *Study site*

This study was conducted around Universiti Sultan Zainal Abidin (UniSZa), Besut Campus, Terengganu, Malaysia (5.754144129155157, 102.62753295164114). Samples of cow dung were collected from three different locations around UnisZA Besut Campus: a) Near the mosque, b) Near the hostel and c) Near the cow shed.

2.2 *Sampling period*

Sample collections were conducted in three consecutive weeks for both rainy and hot seasons. For the rainy season, the samples were collected starting 17th January 2022 until 31st February 2022. For the hot season, the samples were collected from 29th March until 12th April 2022. The dung samples were collected at the same time, between 11 am to 4 pm, where most of the flies are biologically active.

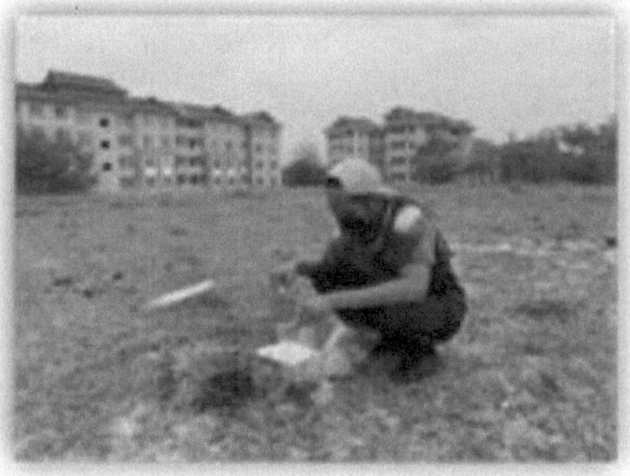

Figure 1. Cow dung collection near the hostel, UniSZA Besut Campus.

2.3 *Cow dung sampling*

The freshly collected cow dung was placed in airtight zip-lock bags and each bag was labelled with the collection date and location. At each location, three pats of dung samples were collected. Then, the samples were brought to the Entomology laboratory, Faculty of Bioresources and Food Industry, UniSZA for a rearing process to observe the emergence of adult flies.

In the laboratory, the dung samples from each location were placed in a separate container for the rearing process. Several tiny holes were made on the coverlid of the container to allow airflow and respiration. A small amount of water was added ad libitum into the rearing container to maintain dung moisture (Khofar *et al.* 2019). Samples were observed every day for the emergence of adult flies. The emerging adult flies were collected and killed in the killing jar containing ethyl acetate. Flies are immediately stored in 70% ethanol for preservation and further identification. The steps were repeated until the adult flies finished emerging.

2.4 *Identification of flies*

The emerged adult flies were identified at the family level based on the characteristics described by (Mashall 2012). The family present and their frequency for each family were recorded based on the week for each season

2.5 *Statistical analysis*

The differences in the population abundance of Diptera families between sampling locations were analysed with One-way ANOVA. The analysis was performed using Minitab Software version 17.

3 RESULTS AND DISCUSSIONS

In this study, an assessment was carried out of Diptera specimens from samples of cow manure during two different seasons: the rainy season and the hot season. A total of 1078 individuals from six families were identified: Calliphoridae, Muscidae, Psychodidae, Scatophagidae, Sepsidae, and Sphaeroceridae. Our findings revealed a significant difference in the number of flies collected between the two seasons. A significantly higher count of 777 individuals was observed during the hot season, whereas a comparatively lower count of 301 individuals was recorded during the rainy season, as depicted in Table 1. However, there was no significant difference ($p>0.05$) between the number of flies for both seasons. The results are comparable to a study conducted by (Heo *et al.* 2010). Sixteen dipteran families, including the Muscidae, Sepsidae, Calliphoridae, Sphaeroceridae, and Psychodidae were found in the samples of cow dung collected.

Table 1. Number of flies collected from cow dung in rainy and hot seasons.

Season	Family	No. of individual	Total
Rainy	Calliphoridae	36	301
	Muscidae	120	
	Psychodidae	26	
	Sepsidae	67	
	Sphaeroceridae	52	
Hot	Calliphoridae	54	777
	Muscidae	170	
	Psychodidae	127	
	Scatophagidae	11	
	Sepsidae	340	
	Sphaeroceridae	75	
		Total	1,078

Muscidae, with 120 individuals during the rainy season, was the leading family among the six families that were recorded. The family Muscidae is the most serious coprophagous pests, which include house flies, stable flies, and horn flies (Grzywacz *et al.* 2016). The success of fly larvae development is largely dependent on the quality of the larval substrate. The increased prevalence of muscid flies during the rainy season in this study could be attributed to favourable environmental conditions, including adequate moisture levels and suitable temperatures within the manure, which create an optimal habitat for larval development (Hogsette 1996).

On the other hand, the family Sepsidae was the most abundant with 340 individuals were emerged in the hot season. Sepsid are often superabundant around fresh cow or horse dung, and also on other decomposing materials such as carrion and compost (Marshall 2012). A study by Rohner *et al.* (2019) on the seasonal occurrence of sepsid showed that some sepsid species are abundant throughout the year with a peak in summer, hence these species are classified as worm-loving. Although Sepsidae plays an important role in the decomposition of cattle dung, however, they may be considered potentially harmful to humans because they regularly carry pathogens due to their high degree of synanthropy (Pont & Meier 2002).

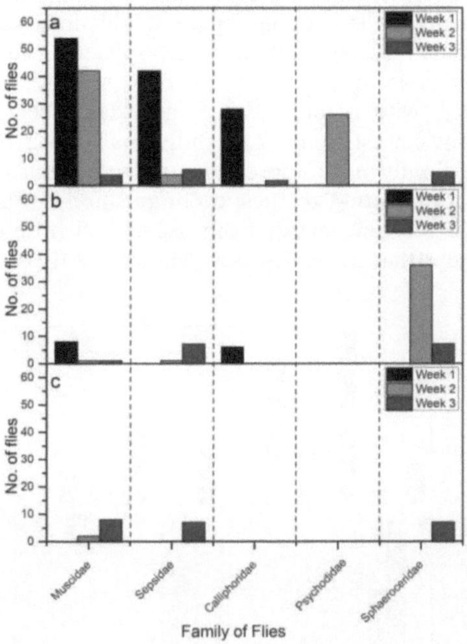

Figure 2. Distribution of abundance by family of flies collected in rainy season according to the location of cattle manure collected.

According to the data presented in Figure 2, the area close to the mosque (a) exhibited the greatest abundance of flies throughout the three-week sampling period, with a total of 213 specimens collected. For the first two weeks of the sampling, the family Muscidae had the highest number among the five families. The Sepsidae also showed a high abundance throughout the three weeks of sampling with 52 individuals sampled. The other three families: Calliphoridae, Pshycodidae and Sphaeroceridae also occurred in this location, however, their numbers were low.

The flies that were gathered near the hostel (b) exhibited the second highest level of abundance, totalling 67 individuals. It was observed that the families Muscidae and Calliphoridae displayed significant levels of abundance during the first week. The family Sphaeroceridae exhibited the highest number of individuals that were collected during the second week. Sphaeroceridae was the most numerous with 36 individuals collected in the second week of sampling. Sphaeroceridae, or lesser dung flies are a common fly in any humid terrestrial environment. Larval sphaerocerids fulfil the role of microbial grazers in a variety of habitats that are abundant in bacteria and exhibit high levels of humidity, such as dung and carrion. Based on their symbiotic relationship with microbes, sphaerocerids have the potential to harbour numerous pathogenic microorganisms. While their solitary lifestyles prohibit them from playing a significant part in the spread of disease, occasionally they may pose a risk to public health or serve as indicators of one. A study by Bertolini *et al.* (2022) revealed that sphaerocerids carry one pathogen, *Staphylococcus sciuri*, that is contagious and related to bovine mastitis in Brazil.

During the first week of sampling, no Diptera was detected in the vicinity of the cow shed (c). The presence of the Muscidae family was observed during the second week. During the last week of sampling, a low number of three families, namely Muscidae, Sepsidae, and Sphaeroceridae, were identified. In general, the results from the third week of sampling indicated the lowest fly population across all three sampling locations.

Similar to the rainy season, the sampling conducted near the mosque (a) yielded the highest number of flies that emerged from cow dung, totalling 431 individuals over three weeks during the hot season, as depicted in Figure 3. This location documented the most diverse Diptera family, encompassing Calliphoridae, Sphaeroceridae, Muscidae, Sepsidae, Pshycodidae, and Scatophagidae. In contrast to the rainy season, the Sepsidae exhibited the highest level of abundance, with a total of 236 individuals being collected. The family Scatophagidae recorded the fewest number of individuals, with only 11. Certain species within the Scatophagidae family have coprophagous larvae that consume the manure of large mammals, thereby contributing to their decomposition. Adults, in general, are predators of other insects and get their energy from nectar and fresh dung, so they are not a potential vector of pathogens that cause diseases (Marshall 2012).

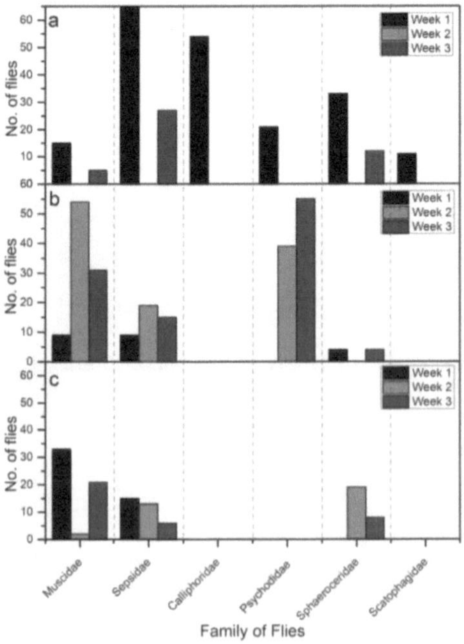

Figure 3. Distribution of abundance by family of flies collected in the hot season according to the location of cattle manure collected.

The number of flies collected at the location near the hostel (b) was notably low in week one, totalling only 22 individuals. However, in week two, the fly population increased substantially, increasing to 112 individuals. Muscidae exhibited the highest count, comprising 55 specimens were collected. An abundance of Muscidae was anticipated at this sampling site, which was near the hostel. This is due to the group's established association with human beings, where they proliferate in effluvia, garbage dumps, and human and domestic animal waste that is rich in bacteria (Geden *et al.* 2021). Continuously moving between unsanitary environments and food sources, the adults carry a collection of pathogens and the enteric diseases linked to them (Nayduch *et al.* 2017). Hence, it is imperative to consider the substantial prevalence of this particular family as a proactive measure to mitigate the transmission of diseases in a region.

During the third week of sampling, a broader range of fly families was observed at the hostel location, including Sphaeroceridae, Muscidae, Sepsidae, and Psychodidae. The family Psychodidae exhibited the highest abundance of flies, with a total of 55 individuals collected. The majority of members within the family Psychodidae are non-biting species. However, a subfamily known as Phlebotominae, which are biting flies that are responsible for transmitting various disease-causing agents such as viruses, bacteria, and protists to both humans and domestic animals (Marshall 2012). A study by Sahahar *et al.* (2011) documented the seasonal abundance of the Phlebotomus genus in Gunung Senyum, Pahang. The results align with our research, indicating that the prevalence of biting flies was minimal by the end of March, but experienced an increase in early April.

The location near the cow shed (c) had the fewest flies collected, with only 117 flies collected over three weeks of sampling. The overall abundance of flies was high in the first week of sampling, with Muscidae dominating, and decreased slightly towards the end of sampling events.

4 CONCLUSION

In summary, research on the distribution and abundance of flies associated with cow dung is crucial for developing public health objectives aimed at reducing the spread of pathogenic microorganisms, particularly flies as potential vectors. Even though the data in this study are only preliminary, they serve as an initial step towards advancing ecological research and enhancing pest management practices in the future. Future research should take into account an extended sampling period and should also prioritize the identification of the flies to the species level to clarify and provide a deeper understanding of the environmental factors of the flies associated with cow dung.

AUTHORS' CONTRIBUTIONS

Nur Athiqah Md Yusof designed the study and drafted the manuscript, Muhammad Alhafiz Rosdi conducted the study and Fathurrahman Lananan performed the statistical analysis.

ACKNOWLEDGMENTS

We would like to thank the Universiti Sultan Zainal Abidin (UniSZA) for the facilities provided for this study.

REFERENCES

Bertolini, A. B., Prado, A. M., Thyssen, P. J., De Souza Ribeiro Mioni, M., De Gouvea, F. L. R., Da Silva Leite, D., Langoni, H., De Figueiredo Pantoja, J. C., Rall, V. M., Guimarães, F. F., Joaquim, S. F., Guerra, S. T., Hernandes, R. T., Lucheis, S. B., & Ribeiro, M. G. (2022). Prevalence of bovine mastitis-related pathogens, identified by mass spectrometry in flies (Insecta, Diptera) captured in the milking environment. *Letters in Applied Microbiology*, 75(5), 1232–1245. https://doi.org/10.1111/lam.13791

Geden, C. J., Nayduch, D., Scott, J. G., Burgess, E. R., Gerry, A. C., Kaufman, P. E., Thomson, J. L., Pickens, & Machtinger, E. T. (2021). House fly (Diptera: Muscidae): biology, pest status, current management prospects, and research needs. *Journal of Integrated Pest Management*, 12(1). https://doi.org/10.1093/jipm/pmaa021

Grzywacz, A., Hall, M. J. R., Pape, T., & Szpila, K. (2016). Muscidae (Diptera) of forensic importance—an identification key to third instar larvae of the western Palaearctic region and a catalogue of the muscid carrion community. *International Journal of Legal Medicine*, 131(3), 855–866. https://doi.org/10.1007/s00414-016-1495-0

Heo, C. C., Ahmad, N. W., Kian, C. W., Kurahashi, H., Jeffery, J., Kiang, H. S., Omar, B., Pahang, J., & Lumpur, K. (2010). A study of cow dung diptera in Sentul Timur, Kuala Lumpur, Malaysia. *The Journal of Tropical Medicine and Parasitology*, 33(2), 53–61. https://www.researchgate.net/profile/Chong_Chin_Heo/publication/214689944_A_Study_of_Cow_Dung_Diptera_in_Sentul_Timur_Kuala_Lumpur_Malaysia/links/08430947661d4b1ad3e4a531.pdf

Hogsette, J. A. 1996. Development of house flies (Diptera: Muscidae) in sand containing varying amounts of manure solids and moisture. *Journal of Economic Entomology*, 89(4), 940–945.

Khofar, P. N., Kurahashi, H., Zainal, N. S., Isa, M. S., & Heo, C. C. (2019). Diversity of Coprophilic Diptera associated with buffalo dung in Selangor, Malaysia. *Journal of Wildlife and Parks*, 34, 63–80. Retrieved from https://jwp.wildlife.gov.my/index.php/jwp/article/view/8

Marshall, S. A. (2012). Flies: The natural history and diversity of Diptera. *Ontario*, Canada: Firefly Books Ltd.

Marshall, S. A. (2017). Insects: Their natural history and diversity: with a photographic guide to insects of Eastern North America (2nd ed.). *Ontario*, Canada: Firefly Books Ltd.

Nayduch, D., & Burrus, R. G. (2017). Flourishing in filth: house fly–microbe interactions across life history. *Annals of the Entomological Society of America*, 110(1), 6–18. https://doi.org/10.1093/aesa/saw083

Neupane, S., Saski, C., & Nayduch, D. (2021). House fly larval grazing alters dairy cattle manure microbial communities. *BMC Microbiology*, 21(1). https://doi.org/10.1186/s12866-021-02418-5

Pérez de León, A. A., Mitchell, R. D., & Watson, D. W. (2020). Ectoparasites of cattle. *Veterinary Clinics: Food Animal Practice*, 36(1), 173–185.

Pont, A C & Meier, R 2002 The Sepsidae (Diptera) of Europe — Fauna Entomologica Scandinavica 37 1–221.

Rohner, P. T., Haenni, J., Giesen, A., Busso, J. P., Schäfer, M. A., Püchel-Wieling, F., & Blanckenhorn, W. U. (2019). Temporal niche partitioning of Swiss black scavenger flies in relation to season and substrate age (Diptera, Sepsidae). *Alpine Entomology*, 3, 1–10. https://doi.org/10.3897/alpento.3.28366

Shahar, M. K., Hassan, A., Lee, H. L., & Soua, M. (2011). Studies of phlebotomine sand fly (Diptera: Psychodidae) populations in limestone areas and caves of western Malaysia. *PubMed*, 42(1), 83–93. https://pubmed.ncbi.nlm.nih.gov/21323169

Short, E. E., Caminade, C., & Thomas, B. N. (2017). Climate change contribution to the emergence or re-emergence of parasitic diseases. *Infectious Diseases*, 10, 117863361773229. https://doi.org/10.1177/1178633617732296

Sontigun, N., Sukontason, K. L., Klong-Klaew, T., Sanit, S., Samerjai, C., Somboon, P., Thanapornpoonpong, S., Amendt, J., & Sukontason, K. (2018). Bionomics of the oriental latrine fly Chrysomya megacephala (Fabricius) (Diptera: Calliphoridae): temporal fluctuation and reproductive potential. *Parasites & Vectors*, 11(1). https://doi.org/10.1186/s13071-018-2986-2

Tahir, N. A., Ahmad, A. H., Hashim, N. A., & Basari, N. (2007b). The seasonal abundance of synanthropic fly populations in two selected food outlets in Pulau Pinang, *Malaysia. Jurnal Biosains*, 18(1), 81–91.

Technological Innovations in Tropical Livestock Development for Environmental Sustainability and Food Security – P. Dhian Isnaeni et al. (eds)

Correlation between vegetation biomass and soil carbon on various types of drylands use in Aceh Besar district

U.H. Abdullah* & R. Salima
Department of Plantation Management, Politeknik Indonesia Venezuela, Aceh Besar, Indonesia

S. Sufardi
Department of Soil Science, Faculty of Agriculture, Universitas Syiah Kuala, Darussalam, Banda Aceh, Indonesia

ABSTRACT: Soil carbon or more accurately referred to as soil organic carbon (SOC), because most of the soil carbon is in the form of organic matter, is very important as the main indicator of soil fertility or productivity and sustainability of terrestrial ecosystems but is also an important component in the global c cycle. Its existence will have an impact on the global climate in the future. As a c storehouse with the largest capacity to store and release organic c on land, soil interacts strongly with changes in atmospheric composition, climate, and land cover. Changes in the amount of soc on land can have a significant global effect and can reduce or increase climate change. Therefore, it is necessary to study the correlation between vegetation biomass and soil carbon in various types of dry land use in aceh besar district. Study this implemented on one unity land in the area dry in regency aceh big with wide area studies 239,439.63 ha. The laboratory of soil and plant sciences and the laboratory of physics faculty land university agriculture Shia Kuala conducted analyses of soil samples and biomass samples. Writing instruments, other supporting tools, and a set of PCs running Microsoft Windows 10 with analysis software was among the tools used in this study. Soil samples, tree diameter measurement data, and land use maps containing information on topography, geology, climate, slope class, and soil were the primary resources used in this study. A value of 0.6076 was revealed by the correlation analysis test results. This shows that the relationship between vegetation biomass and soil c potential at a soil depth of 30 cm is a strong correlation. The relationship between soil carbon and carbon biomass in various types of dry land use is very close. The more plant stands and the diameter of the stem, the more carbon biomass will increase in a type of land use.

Keywords: Aceh Besar district, correlation, dry land, soil carbon, vegetation biomass

1 INTRODUCTION

Land, water, and biodiversity make up the majority of soil, which serves as the foundation for sustainable livelihoods, social development, and economic cohesiveness through the products and services provided by ecosystems. This resource has been used for hundreds of thousands of years and is quite necessary. However, they are versatile and perennial in the exploitation of many resource yields, such: as unsuitable agricultural techniques, overgrazing of grasslands, and excessive deforestation of barren soils, which are more prone to the derivation of various types of soil or soil degradation. Soil degradation is the ongoing

*Corresponding Author: umarah_1977@yahoo.co.id

DOI: 10.1201/9781003468943-30

damage to environmental soils due to natural and anthropogenic activities, or as defined by the UNCCD (United Nations Convention to Combat Desertification) a "reduction or loss of biological or economic productivity and complexity of rainfed, irrigated agricultural land, or ranges, grasslands, forests, and woodlands resulting from land use or a process or combination of processes arising from human activity" (Chidozie *et al.* 2021).

Variations in land characteristics in the form of topography, climate, geology, soil, and vegetation covering the soil in watersheds will affect the physical properties of the soil. In addition, vegetation can make soil conditions looser and refine aggregates. Finer soils will result in reduced bulk density and high porosity. This will produce a lot of macropores and micropores, which will allow faster penetration and increase soil moisture. Soil physical properties determine the penetration of plant roots, water retention, drainage, aeration, and plant nutrition. The physical properties of the soil on the use of paddy fields, dry land, mixed garden land, and land experiencing disturbances such as forest fires with each different slope, have varying physical properties, the soil texture is dominated by the dust and sand fractions with a dusty loam texture class, has a moderate organic matter, moderate permeability, poor porosity, field capacity and low to high saturated moisture content (Naharuddin *et al.* 2020).

Dryland forest ecosystems in Indonesia have a very strategic role in fulfilling the functions of protection, conservation, and social culture of the community, in addition to economic functions. The existence and maintenance of these forest ecosystems have been proven to contribute and have a positive impact on improving the quality of the environment and the quality of life of the people. The implementation of a forest management system that considers the ecosystem's carrying capacity, flexibility, and recovery capacity is crucial to the sustainable fulfillment of these functions. Tropical rainforests have heterogeneous species composition with varying tree age structures at each site. Stand structure describes the distribution of stand dimensions for various tree diameter sizes. Density, basal area, frequency distribution, and diameter class (Raden Mas Sukarna *et al.* 2022).

Species coexisting with contrasting ecological differences can increase overall resource utilization, or by chance, high plant diversity can include trees that have a significant impact on the dynamics of forest biomass (i.e., large diameter trees), which can also promote biomass production. One of the most important markers of the general resilience, habitat quality, and ecosystem function of natural forests is the structural diversity of a stand. High tree stand uniformity is helpful in forecasting the growth and dynamics of tree stands in forests and is linked to a higher rate of uptake of forest stand biomass (Yuan *et al.* 2021).

Soil is one of the three carbon pools on land. Other storage is in live plant biomass and dead plants or necro mass and litter (Muller and Munroe 2014). Based on research by Usmadi *et al.*, in 2015 it was explained that in the Balikpapan Botanical Garden, it was known the average carbon stock was 141.6 tons/ha. The largest component contributing to carbon stocks from the five components of the carbon pool was found in the living vegetation component at 48.50% and soil contributing 28.15% or 39.84 tons/ha and the rest in necro mass and other components. The value of soil carbon stock in the Balikpapan Botanical Gardens is almost the same as the secondary forest after the fire at PT. Inhutani I Batu Ampar, Province of East Kalimantan at a soil layer depth of 0 – 30 cm. Based on a report by Sahid *et al.* (2018) it has been explained that the average carbon stock in scrubland is 9.54 tons/ha. Then Edwin (2016) also found low carbon stocks of organic soil carbon at soil depths of up to 30 cm in the Bukit Pelangi Botanical Gardens, which is an average of 6.90 tons/ha.

Soil plays a very important role in the dynamics of carbon (C) in the biosphere and has great potential to be a source or store of atmospheric C because soil stores about 81% of C in terrestrial ecosystems. Soil carbon or more accurately referred to as soil organic carbon (SOC), because most of the soil carbon is in the form of organic matter, is very important as the main indicator of soil fertility or productivity and sustainability of terrestrial and but is also an important component in the global C cycle. Its existence will have an impact on the global climate in the future. As a C storehouse with the largest capacity to store and release organic C on land, soil interacts strongly with changes in atmospheric composition, climate, and land cover. Changes in the amount of SOC on land can have a significant global effect and can reduce or increase climate change. (Siringoringo 2014). Therefore, it is necessary to study the correlation between vegetation biomass and soil carbon in various types of dry land use in Aceh Besar District.

2 MATERIALS AND METHODS

The study area of 239,439.63 ha was a unit of land in the dry area of Aceh Besar District that was used for this research. At the Faculty of Agriculture, Soil and Plant Science Laboratory and Soil Physics Laboratory of Syiah Kuala University, biomass samples and soil samples were analyzed. Sampling was carried out on one land use, three sample points were taken with five replications and the average data was taken.

Biomass measurement and sampling techniques use methods developed by the Indonesian National Standards Agency (BSN) in 2011 with the number: SNI 7724:2011. For biomass sampling, rectangular or square sample plots with a size of 20 m $\times$ 20 m or 400 m^2 were made. Furthermore, each plot was divided into four subplots according to the level of vegetation, namely: subplot A (size 2 m $\times$ 2 m or 4 m^2). This subplot is also called the "seedling" subplot which is used to calculate the weight of litter and small plants with a diameter of $\leq$ 2.0 cm, subplot B (size 5 m $\times$ 5 m or 25 m^2). This subplot is also called the "sapling" subplot which is used to count the number and biomass weight of plants with a stem diameter of 2 – 10 cm, subplot C (size 10 m $\times$ 10 m or 100 m^2). This subplot is also called the "pole" subplot which is used to count the number and biomass weight of plants with a diameter of 10 – 20 cm, and subplot D (size 20 m x 20 m or 400 m^2). This subplot is also called the "tree" subplot which is used to count the number and weight of plant biomass with a diameter of > 20 cm.

To collect soil samples in plot A (under-storey), the plants were pruned. Estimation of tree root biomass can be done using default values, which are based on the ratio of crown to root. Estimating the general ratio between crown and root biomass for wet tropical forests in drylands is 4:1. For wetlands it is 10:1 and for trees on poor soils it is 1:1. All living organic matter, including wood or branches that are in or on top of the soil, living plants, and litter, is referred to as biomass in this study. By measuring the moisture content and examining the carbon content of the biomass in the lab, the C content of the biomass in plot A was determined. Understory biomass is biomass whose stem diameter is < 2 cm. Measured using the destructive method in a 2 m $\times$ 2 m plot.

By drilling the soil, soil samples were taken from the top layer at a depth of 30 cm. Analyzing soil chemical properties, such as the organic C content, was done using samples of disturbed soil. The Walkley and Black method was used to analyze the carbon content of the soil.

The percentage value of carbon content, which is 0.47, or the percent value of carbon produced in the laboratory are multiplied by the depth of the soil sample, which is expressed in centimeters (cm), the bulk density of the soil, which is expressed in grams/cm^3, and the amount of soil. Next, the obtained soil carbon is multiplied by 100 and converted from grams per centimeter to tons per hectare.

A set of PCs running Microsoft Windows 10 with analysis software, writing instruments, and additional tools like a GPS, sewing tape, compass, earth ring, and drill were among the instruments used in this study. soil, a machete, a knife, plastic bags, brown envelopes, tally sheets, scales, and label paper. Microsoft Office Excel 2010 was one of the programs used for tabulations and calculations. b. The Statistical Package for the Social Sciences 25 (SPSS 25) for examining the relationship between the carbon stored in the soil and the characteristics under study. Soil samples, tree diameter measurement data, and land use maps containing information on topography, geology, climate, slope class, and soil were the primary resources used in this study.

Plots are calculated and consist of five 20 m × 20 m plots. Plants like stakes, poles, trees, and soil samples were measured using the plots. Meanwhile, ten 1 m × 1 m sub-plots were created for the sampling of seedlings and undergrowth. A general assessment of the plots' vegetation or a census of the trees, poles, and saplings was conducted. Three dimensions were measured: total height, branch-free height, and diameter at breast height (DBH = 1.3 m from the ground). A selection of litter and undergrowth. To calculate the wet weight, all of the litter and undergrowth above the soil surface in the 2 m × 2 m sub-plots were removed and weighed. Subsequently, the undergrowth and litter were placed inside a brown envelope and baked to ascertain the moisture content and dry weight.

Two techniques were used to collect soil samples: 1. Composite (or disturbed) soil samples, and 2. Undisturbed (or intact) soil samples. baker. To determine the dry weight and moisture content of the litter and undergrowth, baking was done for 48 hours at 80°C. The sample to be baked in the oven is considered to be the weight if its wet weight is less than 200 grams. In the meantime, the wet weight taken is up to 200 grams if the wet weight is greater than 200 grams. In addition to under-storeys and litter, the oven also contained undisturbed soil samples. The bulk density, soil porosity, and dry weight of this undisturbed soil sample were measured. For a full day, the soil samples were kept undisturbed in the oven at 105°C. Following that, the samples' dry weight and ring weight were determined. Bulk density and soil porosity will be determined using this data. Calculating the Standing Carbon and Biomass. A non-destructive method was used to estimate standing biomass using allometric equations that were tested based on earlier research (Rusdiana 2012). The criteria analysis test correlation could be seen in Table 1 (Manurung and Dewanto 2021).

Table 1. Criteria analysis test correlation.

No.	Correlation value	Information
1	0	There is no correlation between the two variables
2	> 0 – 0.25	The correlation is very weak
3	> 0.25 – 0.5	Correlation enough
4	> 0.50 – 0.75	Strong correlation
5	> 0.75 – 0.99	The correlation is very strong
6	. = 1	The perfect correlation is positive
7	. = −1	Negative perfect correlation

3 RESULTS AND DISCUSSION

Tables 2 and 3 show that the results of the correlation analysis test show a value of 0.6076. This shows that the relationship between vegetation biomass and soil C potential at a soil depth of 30 cm is a strong correlation. The relationship between soil carbon and carbon biomass in various types of dry land use is very close. The more plant stands and the diameter of the stems, the more biomass carbon will increase in a type of land use. Litter and necro mass produced from plant biomass will be able to increase soil carbon in a type of land use, especially in the topsoil layer of 0 – 30 cm. Soil carbon provides input for soil quality index criteria in determining soil quality index parameters.

The distribution of SOC is typically concentrated on the land layer and decreases with soil depth, according to research by (Sufardi *et al.* 2020) on different soil orders in Aceh Large's dry land. Similar findings are also reported by (McLeod *et al.* 2021), who reports that the majority of soil organic matter in Acehnese agricultural systems on dry land is found on the ground. The type of vegetation, land use patterns, and agricultural systems all have a significant influence on the amount of carbon that is added to the atmosphere from outside the soil. When it comes to biomass production, the forest has the highest biomass when compared to other vegetation types. Every land has content ingredient organic which is different in soil characteristics and land use. Changes in the land's vegetation, land use, or management style affect the organic land's content (McLeod *et al.* 2021; Natalia *et al.* 2017; Priyadarshini *et al.* 2021; Sufardi *et al.* 2020; Yasin and Gusnidar 2019).

Potency absorption carbon could be determined by backup SOC on vegetation experience before conversion to type use land other and influence land use to carbon loss. Use and management of lands that reduce carbon inputs or increase losses are compared with vegetation experience producing subtraction SOC from time to time, creating a soil carbon deficit relative to pre-existing carbon levels in the ground. This deficit is an opportunity to save carbon from conversion use and management of land when changing the product enhancement input or dropping loose carbon (Harden *et al.* 2018).

Table 2. Analysis correlation among potency C land with plant biomass.

No.	Land Use Type	Potential C Biomass	Potential C 0 – 30 cm
1	Forest primary	290.17	207.798
		221.93	204.452
		213.04	201.106
2	Forest secondary	243.17	73.268
		107.22	74.294
		105.77	70.856
3	Forest pine	249.29	614.295
		128.61	57.741
		143.18	64.506
4	Forest eucalyptus	186.70	70.414
		158.12	69,236
		105.25	71.592
5	Forest teak	204.13	553.875
		66.62	57.148
		52.68	53.246
6	Forest bush	228.12	42.800
		55.34	43.524
		33.54	44.248
7	Shrubs	29.66	44,862
		22.13	45,396
		21.71	44,328
8	Grasslands	17.85	728.145
		15.17	739.805
		12.43	716.485
9	Mixed garden	204.02	65.720
		143.72	68.152
		67.32	67.912
10	Moor	62.35	40.811
		57.06	41.632
		27.95	42.453
11	Rainfed fields	5.12	31.882
		4.97	32.833
		4.79	30.931
12	Bare land	0.59	40.963
		0.55	40.119
		0.53	41.807

Table 3. Mark correlation among potency C land with plant biomass.

Correlation Relationship	Potency C Biomass	Potency C 0 – 30 cm
Potency C Biomass	1	
Potency C 0 – 30 cm	0.607 6	1

Biomass in tree stands affects the carbon potential stored. All parameters which influence biomass in a manner no live will also affect carbon storage in biomass and ecosystems namely individual density, stem diameter, tree species diversity, and soil. Density trees which there are in some regions will influence to increase in carbon stocks through increased biomass. The growth of forest stands plays an important role in forest structure, biomass, and the content of a hard ground (Goebes *et al.* 2019).

4 CONCLUSIONS

A value of 0.6076 was revealed by the correlation analysis test results. This shows that the relationship between vegetation biomass and soil C potential at a soil depth of 30 cm is a strong correlation. The relationship between soil carbon and carbon biomass in various types of dry land use is very close. The more plant stands and the diameter of the stem, the more carbon biomass will increase in a type of land use. Litter and necromass produced from plant biomass will be able to increase soil carbon in a type of land use, especially in the topsoil layer of 0 – 30 cm. Soil carbon provides input for soil quality index criteria in determining soil quality index parameters. Various soil order in the dry land of Aceh Large also shows that the distribution of SOC is generally concentrated on the land layer and more reduce with soil depth. The type of vegetation, land use patterns, and agricultural systems all have a significant influence on the amount of carbon that is added to the atmosphere from outside the soil. When it comes to biomass production, the forest has the highest biomass when compared to other vegetation types. Every land has content ingredient organic which is different by soil characteristics and land use. Variations in the land's vegetation, land use, and management practices result in variations in the organic land's constituent elements. The growth of forest stands plays an important role in forest structure, biomass, and the content of hard land.

ACKNOWLEDGMENTS

We extend our gratitude to everyone who has received this article and our best wishes to the entire conference committee.

REFERENCES

Chidozie E. Ongechi O., Chukwurah M., Raza T., Qadir M.F., Chibuikem U., Onyechere A., Winifred I. Estimating land degradation neutrality (LDN) using carbon sequestration pedotransfer function on dissimilar land use and land cover in humid tropics', *Soil and Environment*, vol. 40, no. 2, pp. 102–109. 2021 doi: 10.25252/SE/2021/202535.

Edwin M. Assessment of organic soil Carbon stocks in several land use types in East Kutai, East Kalimantan. *Jurnal Agrifor*, vol. 15, no. 2, pp. 279–288. 2016.

Goebes P., Schmidth K., Seitz S., Both S., Bruelheide H., Erfmeier A., Scholten T., Kuhn P. 'The strength of soil-plant interactions under forest is related to a Critical Soil Depth', *Sci Rep*, vol. 9, no. 1, pp. 1–12, 2019, doi: 10.1038/s41598-019-45156-5

Harden J. W., Hugelius G., Ahlstrom A., Blankinship J.C., Bond-Lamberty B., Lawrence C.R., Loisel J., Malhota A., Jackson R.B., Ogle S., Phillips C., Ryals R., Todd-Brown K., Vargas R., Vergara S.E., Cutrufo M.F., Keiluweit M., Heckman K.A., Crow S.E., Silver W.L., DeLonge M., Nave L.E. Networking our science to characterize the state, vulnerabilities, and management opportunities of soil organic matter, *Glob Chang Biol*, vol. 24, no. 2, pp. e705–e718, 2018, doi: 10.1111/gcb.13896.

Lubis S. and O. Rusdiana. Correlation estimation between soil characteristics and Carbon stock in secondary forests. *Jurnal Silvikultur Tropika*, vol. 03, no. 01, pp. 14–21. 2013.

Manurung P.L. and O. Dewanto. Calculation and correlation of Total Organic Carbon (TOC) values in the North East Java Basin area. *Journal of Geoscience, Engineering, Environment, and Technology*, vol. xx, no. xx, pp. 1–7. 2021.

McLeod M. K., S. Sufardi, and S. Harden, 'Soil fertility constraints and management to increase crop yields in the dryland farming systems of Aceh, Indonesia', *Soil Research*, vol. 59, no. 1, pp. 68–82, 2021, doi: 10.1071/SR19324.

Müller D. and D. K. Munroe. Current and future challenges in land-use science', *J Land Use Sci*, vol. 9, no. 2, pp. 133–142. 2014. doi: 10.1080/1747423X.2014 doi: 10.1080/1747423X.2014.883731.

Naharuddin N., I. Sari, H. Harijanto, and A. Wahid. Physical characteristics of soil in agroforestry land and secondary dryland forest in Wuno Sub-Das, Palu basin. *Jurnal Pertanian Terpadu*, vol. 8, no. 2, pp. 189–200. 2020. doi: 10.36084/jpt..v8i2.251.

Natalia D., E. Arisoesilaningsih, and K. Hairiah, 'Are high carbon stocks in agroforests and forest associated with high plant species diversity?', *Agrivita*, vol. 39, no. 1, pp. 74–82, 2017, doi: 10.17503/agrivita.v39i1.676

Priyadarshini R., K. Hairiah, D. Suprayogo, and J. B. Baon. Diversity of pepper plants and their impact on ecosystem services. *Berk. Penel. Hayati Edisi Khusus*, vol. 7, no. F, pp. 81–85. 2021.

Sahid, D. Rohmat, Y. Malik, and L. Wahyuni, 'An investigation of oxygen need based on green open space in Indonesia university of education (UPI) campus bandung', *IOP Conf Ser Mater Sci Eng*, vol. 434, no. 1, 2018, doi: 10.1088/1757-899X/434/1/012234.

Sufardi, T. Arabia, Khairullah, Karnilawati, and Z. Fuadi, 'Distribution of carbon and soil quality in drylands of Aceh Besar, Indonesia', *IOP Conf Ser Earth Environ Sci*, vol. 458, no. 1, 2020, doi: 10.1088/1755-1315/458/1/012040.

Sukarna R.M., N. Hidayat, and M.S. Tambunan. Dryland tropical forest conditions based on structure and composition of stand types (Case Study at PT. Sindo Lumber, Central Kalimantan Province, Indonesia). *Journal of Environment and Management*, vol. 3, no. 1, pp. 80–88, 2022, doi: 10.37304/jem.v3i1.4294.

Syafrimen D. I. Yasin, *Gusnidar. Land Degradation in Mixed and Moor Gardens in Dharmasraya District*. vol. IV, no. 1, pp. 5–9. 2019.

Usmadi D., D., Hidayat, S., Yuzammi., dan Asikin. Biomass potential and carbon reserves of balikpapan botanical garden, East Kalimantan. *Buletin Kebun Raya*, vol. 18, no. 1, pp. 1–14, 2015.

Yuan Z., Ali A., Sanaei A., Ruiz-Benito P., Jucker T., Fang L., Bai E., Ye J., Lin F., Feng S., Hao Z., Wang X. Few large trees, rather than plant diversity and composition, drive the above-ground biomass stock and dynamics of temperate forests in northeast China', *For Ecol Manage*, vol. 481, no. October 2020, 2021, doi: 10.1016/j.foreco.2020.118698.

Technological Innovations in Tropical Livestock Development for Environmental Sustainability and Food Security – P. Dhian Isnaeni et al. (eds)
© 2025 The Author(s), ISBN 978-1-032-74373-8

Recommendations for rice fertilizing based on soil nutrient status

Harwindah, F. Rosbarnawan & R. Wati
Development Planning Agency at Sub-National Level Province of Bengkulu, Indonesia

Yahumri, T. Hidayat*, A. Ishak, E. Fauzi, T. Rahman, S. Rosmanah, Alfayanti & Afrizon
National Research and Innovation Agency of Indonesia, Indonesia

S. Rohiat
University of Bengkulu, Indonesia

ABSTRACT: The average productivity of lowland rice in Seluma Regency has only reached 3.5 t/ha, which is still low compared to the average rice productivity at the Bengkulu Province level, which has reached 4.5 t/ha. The low productivity of rice is caused by farming management that is not optimal; the type and dose of fertilizer given are not balanced, is still general and is not based on soil nutrient status. To overcome this problem, efforts need to be made to improve technical cultivation through the application of location-specific types and doses of fertilizers based on the nutrient status of field soil. This research aims to develop recommendations for fertilizing lowland rice based on nutrient status in the South Seluma District. The nutrient status of paddy field soil was obtained from 7 land units obtained from previous research. Nutrient status is categorized into three classes, namely low, medium, and high; nutrient status P and K refer to Minister of Agriculture Regulation No. 13 in 2022. Furthermore, the preparation of recommended dosages refers to the reference for determining recommendations for N, P and K fertilizers based on Minister of Agriculture Regulation No. 13 of 2022 and Paddy Soil Test Kit Version 1.2. Fertilization recommendations based on soil nutrient status were analyzed descriptively to describe recommendations based on 7 land units. The research results showed that the pH status on the 7 land units was slightly acidic to acidic, the N nutrient status was predominantly moderate, the P nutrient status was all low, and the K status was very low-high. Recommendations for N fertilizer doses for target yields of 5–6 t/ha at medium-very high nutrient status in the form of Urea (200–250 kg ha^{-1}), P fertilizer doses in the form of SP-36 (100 kg ha^{-1}), and fertilizer doses K in the form of KCl for very low nutrient status (100–150 kg ha^{-1}), medium-high nutrient status (50 kg ha^{-1}).

Keywords: Rice Fertilizing, Soil, Nutrien

1 INTRODUCTION

Lowland rice farming is the primary sector in the Indonesian economy (Kusumaningrum 2019), especially in rural areas such as South Seluma District, Seluma Regency, Bengkulu Province. However, agricultural productivity is often hampered by the problem of low soil quality (Widjajanto *et al.* 2020; Wihardjaka & Harsanti 2021) and inappropriate fertilization practices. This condition affects farmers' potential yields and welfare, so it is essential to develop fertilizer recommendations appropriate to the soil nutrient status in the area.

*Corresponding Author: taufikhidayatveydo@gmail.com

DOI: 10.1201/9781003468943-31

Rice is the world's most important staple food crop, being the main source of calories for more than half of the world's population (Tripathi *et al.* 2018); in West Africa, consumption levels have multiplied over time in line with population growth, urbanization and increasing purchasing power (Fofana *et al.* 2014). Almost all countries that use rice as a staple food are experiencing a food crisis that forces countries like Senegal to import rice to meet domestic needs (Abdoulaye & Fambaye 2020). In Indonesia, rice is one of the strategically important food crop commodities and the level of rice consumption is increasing daily along with the increase in Indonesia's population (Ichwan & Tope 2020). To meet the need for these basic commodities, the government strives to maintain national rice production.

National rice production in 2020 reached 31.36 million tons but tend to fall to 31.33 million tons in 2021(Kemeterian Pertanian 2021). The national average rice production in 2020 was 5.4 tons per ha, higher than the rice productivity of Bengkulu Province, which was 4.5 tons per ha, while the rice productivity in Seluma Regency was 3.5 tons per ha, lower than the productivity of rice in Bengkulu Province (BPS 2021).

South Seluma District, Seluma Regency, Bengkulu Province, has various soil characteristics, ranging from sandy loam to clay. Environmental factors such as uneven rainfall and improper land management also affect the balance of soil nutrients. Apart from that, continuous planting patterns without paying attention to the nutritional needs of plants have also resulted in a gradual decline in soil quality.

In this context, it is vital to conduct more in-depth research on soil nutrient status in the South Seluma District to provide fertilizer recommendations that suit the needs of rice plants. Information obtained from analyzing soil nutrient status, such as nitrogen, phosphorus, and potassium content, will be the basis for developing optimal and sustainable fertilization strategies.

The decline in lowland rice production is caused by many factors, including: the ever-changing climate, water availability, soil fertility, varieties, plant management systems, and the development of pests and diseases. Apart from that, lowland rice production, which is cultivated intensively, has experienced a slowdown, where the increase in additional input units is not followed by an economic increase in production (Hilalullaily *et al.* 2021). The decline in production is mainly caused by a decrease in soil organic matter levels, reduced addition of N_2 in the air, a decrease in the rate of supply of N, P, and K nutrients in the soil, organic acids, nutrient imbalance, deficiency of Cu and Zn nutrients, soil that is too reductive, irregularities climate and biotic pressures and varieties (Suarjana *et al.* 2015).

Based on the problems above, the low production results achieved are closely related to the level of soil fertility, fertilization that is not in accordance with specific locations, or there are no specific location recommendations (Wang *et al.* 2021) and also considering the unique soil and environmental conditions in South Seluma District, research on recommendations for fertilizing lowland rice based on soil nutrient status in this area is expected to provide appropriate guidance for local farmers. It is also hoped that these recommendations can increase agricultural productivity, reduce dependence on chemical fertilizers, and support environmental sustainability and farmer welfare in the long term. The research aims to develop specific fertilizer recommendations for the South Seluma District based on the nutrient status of paddy fields.

2 MATERIALS AND METHODS

This research was carried out in South Seluma District, Seluma Regency in seven units of rice fields. Map of research locations and land map units of South Seluma District (Figure 1). The research was carried out from August to October 2023.

Data on the nutrient status of paddy fields were obtained from seven land units that had been carried out in a previous research process with land unit codes, namely Af.1.2.1, Au.1.1.1, Bfq.1.2, Hab.1.1.1, Pf.8.2, Tf.2.1, and Tf.3.2. Nutrient status assessment was

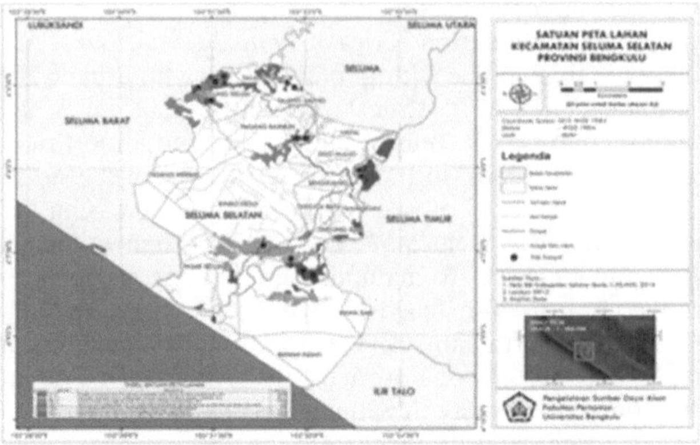

Figure 1. Research location and land map units of South Seluma district.
Source: Afrisa *et al.* (2023)

carried out by referring to the research results of the P and K nutrient status map of paddy fields Afrisa *et al.* (2023), regarding the nutrient status of rice fields in South Seluma District. Preparation of nutrient status with 3 classes of nutrient status P and K based on Minister of Agriculture Regulation No. 13 in 2022, namely low, medium, and high (Table 1).

Furthermore, the preparation of recommended dosages refers to the Reference for Determining Recommendations for N, P and K Fertilizers on Location-Specific Rice Fields as an Attachment to Minister of Agriculture Regulation No. 13 of 2022 and recommendations based on target results refer to (Setyorini *et al.* 2019). Nutrient requirements based on Minister of Agriculture Regulation No. 13 of 2022 are the type and amount of nutrients plants need for optimal production. The types of nutrients are nitrogen (N), phosphorus (P), and potassium (K).

This fertilizer recommendation is made based on variations between 3 soil P nutrient statuses (low, medium, and high) and 3 K nutrient statuses (Table 2). Fertilization recommendations based on soil nutrient status were analyzed descriptively to describe recommendations based on 7 land units previously obtained.

Table 1. Results of assessing the status of P and K nutrients in rice fields.

	Nutrient	
Nutrient tatus	P_2O_5	K_2O
Low	< 20 mg 100 g^{-1} soil	< 10 mg 100 g^{-1} soil
Medium	20–40 mg 100 g^{-1} soil	10–20 mg 100 g^{-1} soil
High	> 40 mg 100 g^{-1} soil	> 20 mg 100 g^{-1} soil

Source: Minister of Agriculture Regulation No. 13 year 2022.

Table 2. Recommendations for fertilizer doses are based on nutrient status.

	Recommendation (kg ha^{-1})		
Nutrient Status	Urea	SP-36	KCl
Low	Based on target results	100	100
Medium		75	50
High		50	50

Source: Minister of Agriculture Regulation No. 13 year 2022.

3 RESULTS AND DISCUSSION

3.1 *Characteristics of nutrient status of rice field soil in research locations*

The characteristics of the soil nutrient status of the research location are quite diverse (Table 3). There are seven land units in South Seluma District, namely Af.1.2.1, Au.1.1.1, Bfq.1.2, Hab.1.1.1, Pf.8.2, Tf.2.1, and Tf.3.2. Land units Af.1.2.1, Au.1.1.1, and Pf.8.2 are inseptisol soil types with flat to slightly steep slopes. Land unit Bfq.1.2 is an entisol soil type with a flat slope. Furthermore, land units Hab.1.1.1, Tf.2.1, and Tf.3.2 are ultisol soil types with flat to gentle slopes.

The soil's acidity status (pH) in all land units is acidic to slightly acidic. Nitrogen status is classified as moderate to very high, phosphorus status as low, and potassium status as very low to high. The status of the soil nitrogen element in each land unit at the research location is classified as moderate to very high. In contrast, the status of the P_2O_5 element is low in all land units, and the status of the soil K_2O element in each land unit at the research location is classified as a value criterion from very low to tall (Afrisa *et al.* 2023).

Table 3. Land characteristics in each land unit.

		Chemical Properties and Status of Soil Nutrients			
No.	Land Units	pH	Nitrogen (%)	P_2O_5 (Mg 100 gr^{-1})	K_2O (Mg 100 gr^{-1})
1	Af.1.2.1	5.433	0.30	11.27	33.93
2	Au.1.1.1	5.529	0.33	15.37	37.14
3	Bfq.1.2	4.909	0.24	13.84	24.70
4	Hab.1.1.1	5.054	0.45	14.09	9.88
5	Pf.8.2	4.990	0.33	11.76	45.36
6	Tf.2.1	5.430	2.07	16.50	23.79
7	Tf.3.2	4.892	0.53	14.23	11.99

Source: (Afrisa *et al.* 2023).

3.2 *Fertilization recommendations*

Based on the P and K status of rice field soil, recommendations for fertilizer doses for each land unit in South Seluma District were obtained. The nitrogen element is given in the form of Urea fertilizer at a dose of 250 kg ha^{-1}, and the P_2O_5 element in the form of SP-36 fertilizer at 100 kg ha^{-1}, while the fulfilment of the K_2O element is given in the form of KCl fertilizer at varying doses between 50 kg ha^{-1} to 100 kg ha^{-1}. Apart from single fertilizer recommendations, recommendations for compound fertilizers in the form of NPK fertilizer (15-10-12) and additional urea fertilizer have also been prepared. Recommended NPK fertilizer dosage of 300 kg ha^{-1} to 375 kg ha^{-1} and additional Urea fertilizer of 125 kg ha^{-1} to 150 kg ha^{-1} (Table 4).

Table 4. Recommended single and compound fertilizer (kg ha^{-1}).

	Recommended Single and Compound Fertilizer (kg ha^{-1})				
Land Units	Urea	SP-36	KCl	NPK 15-10-12	Urea
Af.1.2.1	250	100	50	300	150
Au.1.1.1	250	100	50	300	150
Bfq.1.2	250	100	50	300	150
Hab.1.1.1	250	100	100	375	125
Pf.8.2	250	100	50	300	150
Tf.2.1	250	100	50	300	150
Tf.3.2	250	100	100	375	125

Source: Data is processed 2023.

The change in the type of subsidized fertilizer from NPK 15-15-15 fertilizer to NPK 15-10-12 fertilizer causes an increase in the dose of NPK fertilizer given, but still requires a single fertilizer to meet the N, P or K nutrient deficiency (Hartono *et al.* 2022).

Based on Table 1, the doses of Urea and SP-36 fertilizer are the same for each unit of land. The same dose of SP-36 fertilizer for each unit of land shows that the status of the P_2O_5 element in rice fields in South Seluma District is all low. The low P_2O_5 status in all paddy field units requires efforts to fulfil phosphorus reserves. The nutrient element phosphorus is an essential macro nutrient that is very useful for the growth of rice plants, which functions to stimulate root growth, especially at the beginning of plant growth, flower, and fruit formation (Muzaki 2019; Tito 2022). Therefore, efforts need to be made to fulfill and provide P in paddy fields through the provision of organic material in the form of organic fertilizer. Organic materials can form complex compounds that can cheat Al and Fe metals so that P nutrients can be available in the soil (Murnita & Taher 2021).

Another essential macro nutrient is potassium. Potassium nutrients are needed by plants to stimulate the process of opening and closing stomata through increasing cell turgor activity, translocating assimilates, and strengthening plant stems (Apriliani 2022), and is one of the limiting factors for rice plant growth (Darma 2022; Sareh & Rayes 2019).

Fertilization recommendations are also prepared based on a yield target of 5–7 tons/ha using single and compound fertilizers. Single and compound fertilizer doses were arranged into three groups, namely without organic matter, straw compost, and return of organic matter (Table 5 and 6).

Table 5. Recommendations for Single NPK fertilizer for paddy rice plants target yield 5–6 t ha^{-1} GKP.

		Recommendations for Single NPK fertilizer for paddy rice plants								
		Without Organic Matter			Straw Compost			With Organic Matter		
No.	Land Unit	Urea	SP-36	KCl	Urea	SP-36	KCl	Urea	SP-36	KCl
1.	Af.1.2.1	250	100	50	230	100	0	225	50	30
2.	Au.1.1.1	250	100	50	230	100	0	225	50	30
3.	Bfq.1.2	250	100	50	230	100	0	225	50	30
4.	Hab.1.1.1	250	100	100	230	100	50	225	50	80
5.	Pf.8.2	250	100	50	230	100	0	225	50	30
6.	Tf.2.1	250	100	50	230	100	0	225	50	30
7.	Tf.3.2	250	100	100	230	100	50	225	50	80

Source: Data is processed 2023.
Note: Straw Compost = 2 t ha^{-1}; Minimum fresh straw = 5 t ha^{-1}.

Furthermore, fertilizer recommendations are also prepared based on a yield target of 7 t ha^{-1} using single and compound fertilizers. Single and compound fertilizer doses were arranged into three groups, namely without organic matter, straw compost, and return of organic matter (Table 7 and 8).

Recommendations for a single fertilizer dose in South Seluma District with a target yield of 7 t/ha on seven land units without organic material are 300 kg ha^{-1} Urea, 100 kg ha^{-1} SP-36, and 50–100 kg ha^{-1} KCl. Fertilizer dosage by applying 2 t ha^{-1} straw compost was 280 kg ha^{-1} Urea, 100 kg ha^{-1} SP-36, without applying KCl fertilizer on five land units, namely Af.1.2.1, Au.1.1.1, Bfq.1.2, Pf.8.2, and Tf.2.1, the need for potassium elements is met because the nutrient status is moderate, while the two land units Hab.1.1.1 and Tf.3.2 require additional KCl fertilizer of 50 kg ha^{-1} because the nutrient status on these two land units is

Table 6. Recommended NPK 15-15-15 (kg/ha) fertilizer for lowland rice plants target yield 5-7 t GKP/ha.

		Recommended NPK 15-15-15 (kg/ha) fertilizer for lowland rice plants					
		Without Organic Matter		Straw Compost		With Organic Matter	
No.	Land Units	NPK 15-15-15	Urea	NPK 15-15-15	Urea	NPK 15-15-15	Urea
1.	Af.1.2.1	250	175	225	150	125	200
2.	Au.1.1.1	250	175	225	150	125	200
3.	Bfq.1.2	250	175	225	150	125	200
4.	Hab.1.1.1	350	150	225	150	250	150
5.	Pf.8.2	250	175	225	150	125	200
6.	Tf.2.1	250	175	225	150	125	200
7.	Tf.3.2	350	150	225	150	250	150

Source: Data is processed 2023.
Note: Straw Compost = 2 t ha^{-1}; Minimum fresh straw = 5 t ha^{-1}.

low. Next, a single fertilizer dose by applying fresh organic straw material is at least 5 t ha^{-1}, a dose of 275 kg ha^{-1} Urea, 50 kg ha^{-1} SP-36, and 30–80 kg ha^{-1} KCl (Table 7). Recommended compound fertilizer dosage is 225–350 kg ha^{-1} NPK 15-15-15 and plus 175–225 kg ha^{-1} Urea, 350 kg ha^{-1} NPK 15-10-12 and plus 175 kg ha^{-1} Urea (Table 8).

Fertilization recommendations based on the nutrient status of rice fields are prepared using the principle of balanced fertilization using either single fertilizer or compound fertilizer, each of which has advantages and disadvantages. Using compound fertilizers that are not in the correct dosage can cause excesses and deficiencies of certain elements (N, P, or K). Therefore, the application of compound fertilizer still requires additional single fertilizer, especially N fertilizer (Setyorini *et al.* 2019).

Applying location-specific fertilizer doses in accordance with recommendations is also able to save the use of NPK fertilizer by around 36.5%, does not reduce the yield of inbred rice, increases the efficiency of fertilizer use and profits from rice farming (Erythrina *et al.* 2023; Suyamto & Saeri 2018).

Table 7. Recommendations for single NPK fertilizer for paddy rice plants target yield 7 t ha^{-1} GKP.

		Recommendations for single NPK fertilizer for paddy rice plants								
		Without Organic Matter			Straw Compost			With Organic Matter		
No.	Land Unit	Urea	SP-36	KCl	Urea	SP-36	KCl	Urea	SP-36	KCl
1.	Af.1.2.1	300	100	50	280	100	0	275	50	30
2.	Au.1.1.1	300	100	50	280	100	0	275	50	30
3.	Bfq.1.2	300	100	50	280	100	0	275	50	30
4.	Hab.1.1.1	300	100	100	280	100	50	275	50	80
5.	Pf.8.2	300	100	50	280	100	0	275	50	30
6.	Tf.2.1	300	100	50	280	100	0	275	50	30
7.	Tf.3.2	300	100	100	280	100	50	275	50	80

Source: Data is processed 2023.
Note: Straw Compost = 2 t ha^{-1}; Minimum fresh straw = 5 t ha^{-1}.

Table 8. Compound fertilizer recommendations target yield 7 t ha^{-1} GKP.

No.	Land Units	Compound fertilizer recommendations (kg ha^{-1})			
		NPK 15-15-15	Urea	NPK 15-10-12	Urea
1.	Af.1.2.1	225	225	350	175
2.	Au.1.1.1	225	225	350	175
3.	Bfq.1.2	225	225	350	175
4.	Hab.1.1.1	350	175	350	175
5.	Pf.8.2	225	225	350	175
6.	Tf.2.1	225	225	350	175
7.	Tf.3.2	350	175	350	175

3.3 *Recommended fertilization method and time*

Effective and efficient fertilization of rice plants requires the proper method, time, and amount of fertilizer to suit the plant's needs at each stage of plant growth. Providing balanced fertilizers and fertilizer combinations can also prevent greenhouse gas (GHG) emissions comprehensively and objectively (Wu *et al.* 2021). Recommended methods and times of single and compound fertilization are shown in Table 9.

Table 9. Methods and times of fertilizing single and compound fertilizers.

Fertilizer Type	Basic Fertilizer (1-2 WAP)	Supplementary Fertilizer I (3-5 WAP)	Supplementary Fertilizer II (6-7 WAP)
Single:			
– Urea	– 1/3 doses of Urea	– 1/3 dose of Urea	– 1/3 dose of Urea
– SP-36	– All doses of SP-36	– 0	
– KCl	– ½ dose of KCl	– ½ dose of KCl	
Compound:			
– NPK 15-10-12	– All doses of NPK	– ½ dose of Urea – All dose of KCl	– Additional urea Urea

Source: (Setyorini *et al.* 2019).
Note: WAP = Week After Planting.

4 CONCLUSIONS

Recommended N fertilizer doses for target yields of 5–6 t ha^{-1} at medium-very high nutrient status in the form of Urea 200–250 kg ha^{-1}, P fertilizer doses in the form of SP-36 100 kg ha^{-1}, and K fertilizer doses in the form of KCl for very low nutrient status 100–150 kg ha^{-1}, medium-high nutrient status 50 kg ha^{-1}.

Recommendations for a single fertilizer dose in South Seluma District with a target yield of 7 t ha^{-1} on seven land units without organic material are 300 kg ha^{-1} Urea, 100 kg ha^{-1} SP-36, and 50–100 kg ha^{-1} KCl. Recommended compound fertilizer dosage is 225–350 kg ha^{-1} NPK 15-15-15 and 175–225 kg ha^{-1} Urea, 350 kg ha^{-1} NPK 15-10-12 and 175 kg ha^{-1} Urea.

Fertilization recommendations based on the nutrient status of rice fields are prepared using the principle of balanced fertilization using either single fertilizer or compound fertilizer, each of which has advantages and disadvantages. Using compound fertilizers that are not in the correct dosage can cause excesses and deficiencies of certain elements (N, P, or K). Effective and efficient fertilization of rice plants requires the proper method, time, and amount of fertilizer to suit the plant's needs at each stage of plant growth.

ACKNOWLEDGEMENT

Thanks to the Head and Head of the Division Development Planning Agency at Sub-National Level Province of Bengkulu for research facilitation.

REFERENCES

Abdoulaye, F. A., & Fambaye, B. N. (2020). Impact of marketing contracts on the rice yield of Senegal River Valley producers. *Agri Res & Tech: Open Access Journal*, *23*(4), 16–22. https://doi.org/10.19080/ARTOAJ.2020.23.556240

Afrisa, H., Barchia, M. F., & Ganefianti, D. W. (2023). Evaluasi kesesuaian lahan sawah berdasarkan status hara di Kecamatan Seluma Selatan Kabupaten Seluma. *NATURALIS: Jurnal Penelitian Pengelolaan Sumberdaya Alam Dan Lingkungan*, *12*(1), 66–77. https://doi.org/DOI: https://doi.org/10.31186/naturalis.12.1.26715

Apriliani, I. N. (2022). Pengaruh Kalium pada pertumbuhan dan hasil dua varietas tanaman ubi jalar (Ipomea batatas (L.) Lamb). *JIMTANI*, *2*, 148–157. http://jurnalmahasiswa.umsu.ac.id/index.php/jimtani

BPS. (2021). *Provinsi Bengkulu Dalam Angka.*

Darma, S. (2022). Land suitability of rice fields in Bumi Rapak Village and Selangkau Village East Kutai Regency. *Jurnal Ilmu Tanah Dan Lingkungan*, *24*(1), 32–38. https://doi.org/10.29244/jitl.24.1.32-38

Erythrina, E., Pratiwi, G. R., Agustiani, N., & Nurrahma, A. H. I. (2023). Nitrogen fertilizers and plant spacing in organic rice cultivation: a review. *Journal of Applied Agricultural Science and Technology*, *7*(3), 314–328. https://doi.org/10.55043/jaast.v7i3.143

Fofana, I., Goundan, A., Vicky, L., & Domgho, M. (2014). Impact Simulation of ECOWAS Rice Self-Sufficiency Policy. In *International Food Policy Research Institute* (1st ed., Vol. 1, pp. 1–26). www.ifri.go.id.

Hartono, A., Firdaus, M., Purwono, P., Barus, B., Aminah, M., & Simanihuruk, D. M. P. (2022). Evaluation of fertilization dose recommendation of Ministry of Agriculture for rice). *Jurnal Ilmu Pertanian Indonesia*, *27*(2), 153–164. https://doi.org/10.18343/jipi.27.2.153

Hilalullaily, R., Kusnadi, N., & Rachmina, D. (2021). Analisis efisiensi usahatani padi di jawa dan luar jawa: Kajian prospek peningkatan produksi adi nasional. *Jurnal Agribisnis Indonesia*, *9*(2), 143–153. https://doi.org/10.29244/jai.2021.9.2.143-153

Ichwan, M., & Tope, P. (2020). Essential commodity consumption: a study on food consumption expenditure of rural society. *AGROLAND: The Agricultural Sciences Journal*, *7*(2), 116–125. http://103.245.72.23/index.php/agroland/article/download/628/1227

Kemeterian Pertanian. (2021). Buletin Konsumsi Pangan Tahun 2021. *Pusat Data Dan Sistem Informasi Pertanian*, *12*, 1–100.

Kusumaningrum, S. I. (2019). Pemanfaatan sektor pertanian sebagai penunjang pertumbuhan perekonomian Indonesia. *Jurnal Transaksi*, *11*(1). http://ejournal.atmajaya.ac.id/index.php/transaksi/article/download/477/283

Murnita, & Taher, Y. A. (2021). Effect of organic and inorganic fertilizers on soil chemical properties and rice plant production (Oriza sativa L.). *Menara Ilmu*, *15*(2), 67–76.

Muzaki, A. (2019). *Study of nutrient status and recommendations for phosphorus fertilization on land used for lowland rice cultivation (Oryza sativa l.) in Sokaraja District, Banyumas Regency*. Universitas Jenderal Soedirman.

Sareh, A. F. F., & Rayes, M. L. (2019). Land suitability evaluation of rice on irrigated rice field at Junrejo District of Batu City. *Jurnal Tanah Dan Sumberdaya Lahan*, *06*(01), 1193–1200. https://doi.org/10.21776/ub.jtsl.2019.006.1.18

Setyorini, D., Widowati, L. R., & Kasno, A. (2019). *Petunjuk Penggunaan Perangkat Uji Tanah Sawah versi 1.2* (Vol. 1). KPRI Puspita, Balai Penelitian Tanah.

Suarjana, I. W., Supadma, A. A. N., & Arthagama, I. D. M. (2015). Study status of fertility paddy soil to determine instigation balanced fertilization specific location rice plants in Manggis District. *E-Jurnal Agroekoteknologi Tropika*, *4*(4), 314–323. http://ojs.unud.ac.id/index.php/JAT

Suyamto, S., & Saeri, M. (2018). Evaluation of site-specific nutrient management recommendation for low-land rice in East Java. *Jurnal Penelitian Pertanian Tanaman Pangan*, *2*(1), 1. https://doi.org/10.21082/jpptp.v2n1.2018.p1-8

Tito, J. (2022). *Pengaruh Fosfor terhadap Pertumbuhan dan Produksi Galur Mutan M5 Pare Ambo.*

Tripathi, A. D., Mishra, R., Maurya, K. K., Singh, R. B., & Wilson, D. W. (2018). Estimates for world population and global food availability for global health. In *The Role of Functional Food Security in Global Health* (pp. 3–24). Elsevier. https://doi.org/10.1016/B978-0-12-813148-0.00001-3

Wang, J. L., Liu, K. Lou, Zhao, X. Q., Zhang, H. Q., Li, D., Li, J. J., & Shen, R. F. (2021). Balanced fertilization over four decades has sustained soil microbial communities and improved soil fertility and rice productivity in red paddy soil. *Science of the Total Environment*, *793*. https://doi.org/10.1016/j.scitotenv.2021.148664

Widjajanto, D., Hasanah, U., Sukmawati, S., Sari, N., & Mufida Handayani, S. R. (2020). Application of organic fertilizer enriched on paddy soils in village of Bolapapu District of Kulawi Regency of Sigi. *Mosintuvu: Jurnal Pengabdian Kepada Masyarakat*, *1*(1), 23–31. http://jurnal.faperta.untad.ac.id/index.php/MOSINTUVU/article/download/454/506

Wihardjaka, A., & Harsanti, E. S. (2021). Management of environmentally friendly rice fields by means of organic fertilizer utilization to improve soil quality. *Jurnal Pangan*, *30*(1), 53–64.

Wu, H., MacDonald, G. K., Galloway, J. N., Zhang, L., Gao, L., Yang, L., Yang, J., Li, X., Li, H., & Yang, T. (2021). The influence of crop and chemical fertilizer combinations on greenhouse gas emissions: A partial life-cycle assessment of fertilizer production and use in China. *Resources, Conservation and Recycling*, *168*. https://doi.org/10.1016/j.resconrec.2020.105303

Technological Innovations in Tropical Livestock Development for Environmental Sustainability and Food Security – P. Dhian Isnaeni et al. (eds)

Availability of animal waste resources as an alternative energy source in Muna Regency

A.S. Aku*, H. Hafid, N. Sandiah, L.O. Sahaba, Y. Yaddi, Surahmanto, R. Aka, H. Has, R. Libriani, Fitrianingsih, H.A. Hadini & P.N.K. Pransanjaya
Faculty of Animal Science, Halu Oleo University, Indonesia

M. Taufik & Gusnawati
Faculty of Agriculture, Halu Oleo University, Indonesia

Kahirun
Faculty of Forestry and Environmental Science, Halu Oleo University, Indonesia

W.O. Hinarti
Research and Development Agency of Muna Regency, Indonesia

L. Sinaini
National Research and Innovation Agency, Indonesia

ABSTRACT: The study aimed to investigate the feasibility of using livestock waste as an alternative energy source in Muna Regency. The research was carried out through a survey conducted in 112 villages across 22 sub-districts, involving 1207 respondents over a period of six months. The research results revealed that the raw materials available in Muna Regency can be used in building biogas installations at a household level. A total of 17,921 units can be built, but only 549 units can be constructed due to the availability of supporting facilities such as livestock pens. The study also found that farmers in Muna Regency have not been utilizing livestock waste and waste for alternative energy or fertilizer production. In conclusion, the research shows that there is a significant potential for using livestock waste as an alternative energy source in Muna Regency.

Keywords: resources, livestock waste, alternative energy

1 INTRODUCTION

To reduce reliance on fuel oil, the government has issued Presidential Regulation of the Republic of Indonesia number 5 of 2006 concerning national energy policy to develop alternative energy sources as a substitute for fuel oil. This policy emphasizes renewable resources as an alternative to fuel oil. One alternative energy source is biogas. This gas comes from various kinds of organic waste such as garbage, biomass, human waste, animal waste, and home industry waste (such as tofu and tempeh production waste), and can be used as energy through an anaerobic digestion process.

Biogas is a process of producing biogas from organic material with the help of bacteria. This process of degradation of organic material without involving oxygen is called anaerobic digestion. The gas produced is mostly (more than 50%) in the form of methane (Darwis *et al.* 2018; Oktavia & Firmansyah 2017).

*Corresponding Author: achmad.s.aku@uho.ac.id

DOI: 10.1201/9781003468943-32

The organic material collected in the digester (reactor) will be broken down into two stages with the help of two types of bacteria. In the first stage, organic material will be degraded into weak acids with the help of acid-forming bacteria. These bacteria will decompose waste at the hydrolysis and acidification levels. Hydrolysis is the breakdown of complex compounds or long-chain compounds such as fats, proteins, and carbohydrates into simple compounds. Meanwhile, acidification is the formation of acids from simple compounds.

Efforts to utilize various residual (waste) products as alternative energy sources are not only easy to adopt but also do not require large costs in their application (Padang *et al.* 2020; Romadhona *et al.* 2020). However, the availability of raw materials, especially the potential and distribution of waste and/or residual products from home industry production, is not well recorded, so alternative energy development programs are less focused. Based on such thinking, research was carried out to prepare a database and model for the use of livestock and home industry waste as an alternative energy source in Muna Regency.

2 RESEARCH METHODS AND MATERIALS

The research was carried out through a survey conducted in 112 villages across 22 sub-districts, involving 1207 respondents.

3 RESULTS AND DISCUSSION

The research data suggests that the raw materials identified in this study could be converted into alternative energy sources to replace oil fuels. Table 1 demonstrates the potential of alternative energy as a substitute for various types of fuel oil.

Table 1. Potential substitute for oil fuel: Biogas energy.

	Methane Gas Production (M3/Kg)						Conversion to Other Fuels (Per day)		
District	Dairy Cows	Cow	Buffalo	Goat	Pig	Total	LPG (Kg)	Kerosene (Litre)	Gas (Litre)
Tongkuno	0	48.02	0.00	92.25	–	140.27	64.52	86.97	112.22
Tongkuno Selatan	0	17.63	0.00	76.95	1.53	96.11	44.21	59.59	76.89
Parigi	0	42.15	0.13	89.10	0.80	132.18	60.80	81.95	105.75
Bone	0	16.16	0.18	93.60	–	109.94	50.57	68.16	87.95
Marobo	0	5.59	0.04	74.70	–	80.34	36.96	49.81	64.27
Kabawo	0	23.78	0.04	216.45	–	240.27	110.52	148.97	192.22
Kabangka	0.21	30.71	0.03	194.70	–	225.65	103.80	139.90	180.52
Kontukowuna	0	10.82	0.00	108.60	–	119.72	54.93	74.04	95.54
Kontunaga	0	6.37	0.00	193.35	–	199.72	91.87	123.83	159.78
Watopute	0	24.95	0.00	102.45	–	127.40	58.60	78.99	101.92
Katobu	0	1.21	0.00	58.80	–	60.01	27.60	37.20	48.01
Lohia	0	12.88	0.00	169.05	–	181.93	83.69	112.79	145.54
Duruka	0	4.40	0.00	153.15	–	157.55	72.47	97.68	126.04
Batalaiworu	0	6.81	0.00	49.20	–	56.01	25.67	34.72	44.81
Napabalano	0	31.49	0.23	76.65	–	108.37	49.85	67.19	86.70
Lasalepa	0	30.85	0.00	55.95	–	86.80	39.93	53.82	69.44
Towea	0	3.09	0.00	34.95	–	38.04	17.50	23.59	30.44
Wakorumba Selatan	0	6.47	0.03	84.60	–	91.09	41.90	56.48	72.88
Pasir Putih	0	6.23	0.00	69.75	–	75.98	34.95	47.11	60.79
Pasi Kolaga	0	8.61	0.00	64.80	–	73.41	33.77	45.52	58.73
Maligano	0	13.96	0.26	66.15	–	80.38	36.97	49.83	64.30
Bataukara	0	2.79	0.03	46.65	–	49.93	22.97	30.96	39.95
Muna	0.21	355.00	0.96	2,172	2.79	2,530.78	1,164.16	1,569.08	2,024.62

Information: Research data, processed (2020).

According to the data, the livestock waste in Muna Regency has the potential to replace 1164.16 Kg of LPG daily. This amount is equal to 388.05 LPG cylinders or has a monetary value of Rp. 6,948,945. Additionally, the same raw material can replace 1569.02 litres of kerosene every day or 47,072 liters every month. If converted to kerosene, this raw material can replace 2,024.62 kerosene every day or 60,738.65 liters every month.

Based on field research conducted in 2020, it is known that only 549 units of biogas installations can be built for the housed livestock. If we consider the cheapest price of 15,000,000 (the lowest price), then the economic potential would be around 15,000,000. Therefore, the maximum amount that can be proposed for funding construction is only Rp. 8,235,000,000 (Eight Billion Two Hundred and Thirty-Five Million Rupiah).

Table 2 presents the distribution of potential alternative energy raw materials in Muna Regency based on the availability of caged livestock throughout the area.

Table 2. Potential alternative energy installations can be built in Muna Regency from livestock waste.

		Potential for Built Biogas Installations							
No	District	Dairy Cows	Cow	Buffalo	Goat	Pig	Total	real	Potential
1	Tongkuno		1912		154		2,075	22	2,053
2	Tongkuno Selatan		705		128	31	864	20	844
3	Parigi		1686	5	149	16	1,856	47	1,809
4	Bone		647	7	156	0	810	34	776
5	Marobo		224	2	125	0	350	12	338
6	Kabawo		951	2	361	0	1,314	44	1,270
7	Kabangka	8.33	1229	1	325	0	1,562	53	1,509
8	Kontukowuna		433	0	181	0	614	36	578
9	Kontunaga		255	0	322	0	577	36	541
10	Watopute		998	0	171	0	1,169	34	1,135
11	Katobu		48	0	98	0	146	9	137
12	Lohia		515	0	282	0	797	56	741
13	Duruka		176	0	255	0	431	41	390
14	Batalaiworu		272	0	82	0	354	12	342
15	Napabalano		1260	9	128	0	1,397	17	1,380
16	Lasalepa		1234	0	93	0	1,327	17	1,310
17	Towea		124	0	58	0	182	10	172
18	Wakorumba Selatan		259	1	141	0	401	13	388
19	Pasir Putih		249	0	116	0	366	12	354
20	Pasi Kolaga		345	0	108	0	453	2	451
21	Maligano		559	11	110	0	769	20	669
22	Bataukara		112	1	78	9	200	2	198
	Muna	8.33	14,199	38.5	3,620	55.75	17,921	549	17,372

Information: Research data, processed (2020).

Field data was collected on the availability of penned livestock that could be used for the construction of biogas installations. The data was obtained from several sub-district areas in Muna Regency. The study revealed that only Lohia (56 units) and Kabangka (53 units) sub-districts have the potential to build more than 50 biogas installations. Parigi District, Kabawo, and Duruka District can build more than 40 units each. On the other hand, Tongkuno, Parigi, Kabawo, Kabangka, Watopute, Nanapabalano, and Lasalepa sub-districts have sufficient raw materials but cannot support livestock. These sub-districts have the potential to build an average of more than 1,000 biogas installations.

The traditional extensive rearing systems (Aku *et al.* 2022; Hafid 2008) and or raising livestock only as a part-time business are the main reasons why the raw materials for alternative energy are not utilized. To utilize this great potential, the government, especially extension workers, needs to play a significant role in providing knowledge and skills (Sutrianto *et al.* 2016). Field data was collected on the availability of penned livestock that could be used for the construction of biogas installations. The data was obtained from several sub-district areas in Muna Regency. The study revealed that only the Lohia (56 units) and Kabangka (53 units) sub-districts have the potential to build more than 50 biogas installations. Parigi District, Kabawo, and Duruka District can build more than 40 units each. On the other hand, Tongkuno, Parigi, Kabawo, Kabangka, Watopute, Nanapabalano, and Lasalepa sub-districts have sufficient raw materials but cannot support livestock. These sub-districts have the potential to build an average of more than 1000 biogas installations.

According to Kholiq (2015) and Oktavia & Firmansyah (2017) breeders have limited knowledge about animal husbandry and need to increase their knowledge in this field. Biogas technology is a useful method for processing livestock waste. Its application can provide multiple benefits, including: 1) reducing environmental pollution caused by livestock manure accumulation; 2) serving as an alternative fuel; 3) saving household expenses on fuel purchases; and 4) producing organic fertilizer (in both liquid and solid forms) from biogas by-products (Darwis *et al.* 2018).

4 CONCLUSION

The research results revealed that the raw materials available in Muna Regency can be used in building biogas installations at a household level. A total of 17,921 units can be built, but only 549 units can be constructed due to the availability of supporting facilities such as livestock pens. The study also found that farmers in Muna Regency have not been utilizing livestock waste and waste for alternative energy or fertilizer production. In conclusion, the research shows that there is a significant potential for using livestock waste as an alternative energy source in Muna Regency.

ACKNOWLEDGEMENTS

The author is grateful to the Government of Muna Regency, Southeast Sulawesi Province for funding this research.

REFERENCES

Aku A.S, Hafid H., Saili T., Nafiu L.O., Pagala M.A., Bain A., Zulkarnain D., Tasse A.M., Rusdin M., Yaddi Y., Daoed D.M., Libriani R. 'Production System of Bali Cattle on Smallscale Farms in Muna Regency: Case Study on People's Livestock in Muna Regency', presented at the International Conference on Improving Tropical Animal Production for Food Security (ITAPS 2021), Kendari, Indonesia, 2022. doi: 10.2991/absr.k.220309.041.

Darwis, A. Zaeni, and M. A. Pagala, *Biogas Solusi Menuju Desa Mandiri energi Bahan Bakar, Pupuk dan Pakan Ternak*, vol. 1. Yayasan Cipta Anak Bangsa, 2018.

Hafid H., 'Strategi Pengembangan Peternakan Sapi Potong Di Sulawesi Tenggara Sebagai Upaya Mendukung Pencapaian Swasembada Daging Nasional', p. 25, 2008.

Kholiq I., 'Pemanfaatan Energi Alternatif Sebagai Energi Terbarukan Untuk Mendukung Subtitusi BBM', no. 2, 2015.

Oktavia I., & Firmansyah A. (2017). Pemanfaatan Teknologi Biogas sebagai Sumber Bahan Bakar Alternatif di Sekitar Wilayah Operasional PT. Pertamina Asset 2 Prabumulih Field. *Jurnal Resolusi Konflik*, CSR Dan Pemberdayaan (CARE), 1(1)

Padang Y.A, Mirmanto M. M., Syahrul S. S., Sinarep S. S., and Pandiatmi P. P., 'Pemanfaatan Energi Alternatif Dan Terbarukan', *JKP*, vol. 2, no. 2, pp. 77–84, Oct. 2020, doi: 10.29303/jkp.v2i2.58.

Romadhona G., Winarso W., and Mukholik A., 'Pemanfaatan Biogas Sebagai Sumber Alternatif Tenaga Listrik Di BBPTU HPT Baturraden', *Techno*, vol. 21, no. 1, p. 21, Apr. 2020, doi: 10.30595/techno.v21i1.6885.

Sutrianto S., Aku A. S., and Pagala M. A., 'Analisis Potensi Energi Terbarukan Limbah Kotoran Dari Ternak Sapi Di Kecamatan Kusambi Kabupaten Muna Barat Provinsi Sulawesi Tenggara, *jitro*, vol. 3, no. 2, p. 64, May 2016, doi: 10.33772/jitro.v3i2.1689.

Technological Innovations in Tropical Livestock Development for Environmental Sustainability and Food Security – P. Dhian Isnaeni et al. (eds)
© 2025 The Author(s), ISBN 978-1-032-74373-8

Mapping analysis of flood vulnerability level in the Muna Regency based on geographical information system

L.O. Alwi*
Department of Agribusiness, Halu Oleo University, Kendari, Sulawesi Tenggara, Indonesia

Harisma
Department of Geological Engineering, Halu Oleo University, Kendari, Sulawesi Tenggara, Indonesia

ABSTRACT: Flood disasters almost constantly occur in the Muna Regency, especially when the rainy season arrives, which is caused by several factors, such as high rainfall levels, slope, and topography. The objective of this research is to determine the vulnerability level of flood disasters in the Muna Regency using a geographic information system. The data used in this study covered primary and secondary data, such as slope data, soil type, rainfall level, and land use. The data analysis was used in overlaying of flood vulnerability map and then continued by scoring and weighting the values. The result shows that the Muna Regency is divided into five levels of flood vulnerability, consisting of Flood Area, covering 4,859 ha; Flood Prone Area, covering 64,218 ha; Slightly Flood Prone Area, covering 112,345 ha; Less Flood Prone Area, covering 19,466 ha; and Non-Flood Prone Area, covering 4,881 ha.

Keywords: Muna Regency, Flood Vulnerability Level, Geographical Information System

1 INTRODUCTION

Flooding is the flow and overflow of water that exceeds the normal water level, which causes water to overflow from the riverbed resulting in inundation on low land on the side of the river (BNPB 2011). A change in the condition of land in a certain period can be a potential flood disaster, this is because the river's capacity is getting smaller due to silting, fluctuations in water discharge between the rainy season and the dry or hot season are getting higher, land conservation is occurring, and exploitation of groundwater. which is excessive. This flood disaster was largely caused by high rainfall above normal which resulted in water flowing and the drainage system being less able to accommodate rainwater. The slope, altitude, and land cover factors greatly influence the occurrence of flood disasters.

Muna Regency is one of the areas in the administrative region of Southeast Sulawesi Province with a geographical location between 4°06' – 5°15' South Latitude and 122°08' – 123°15' East Longitude with an area of 2,057.69 km^2 (BPS of Muna Regency 2021). Geographically, Muna Regency is an archipelagic region located at the meeting point of four tectonic plates. This condition is very potential and prone to disasters such as; earthquakes, tsunamis, floods and landslides. Muna Regency has a tropical climate with two seasons, namely hot and rainy, characterized by quite extreme changes in weather, temperature and wind direction. These climatic conditions combined with relatively diverse surface topography and rock conditions, both physically and chemically, produce fertile soil conditions.

*Corresponding Author: alwiode76@gmail.com

DOI: 10.1201/9781003468943-33

On the other hand, this condition can cause several bad consequences for humans, such as hydrometeorological disasters such as floods (Ahiablame *et al.* 2016; Ajuun *et al.* 2022; Ariyani *et al.* 2020, 2021; Auliagisni *et al.* 2022).

Floods are disasters that cause enormous losses to society (Fernandos *et al.* 2020; Rinaldi *et al.* 2021), which are destructive and dangerous, can claim lives cause material losses and require time to recover. To overcome the problem of flooding, the basic thing that must be understood is the causes of flood disasters and areas that have the potential to flood which depend on the characteristics of climatology, hydrology and physical conditions of an area (Asdak *et al.* 2018; Basri *et al.* 2021; Breinl *et al.* 2021; Knufer *et al.* 2008).

One technology that can be used to process data is using a Geographic Information System (GIS) to identify the level of flood vulnerability (Purnawali *et al.* 2017. Flood vulnerability can be seen quickly and accurately through GIS based on flood disaster vulnerability parameters (Chukwuma *et al.* 2021; Deepak *et al.* 2020; Falguni & Singh 2020; Haryadi 2016).

Using GIS, existing data and information can be easily integrated, modelling can be done easily and which areas are prone to flooding can be identified by displaying information output in the form of a map of flood vulnerability levels (Chukwuma *et al.* 2021; Deepak *et al.* 2020). In this way, predictions of the possibility of flooding and the resulting losses can be identified and preventive planning can be carried out (Gift *et al.* 2020; Herry *et al.* 2017; Hussain *et al.* 2021; Komolafe *et al.* 2020; Liu *et al.* 2018; Putra 2017).

2 METHODOLOGY

2.1 *Study site*

This study was conducted in Muna Regency, Southeast Sulawesi. Muna Regency directly borders several surrounding districts. The northern part borders the South Konawe Regency and the Tiworo Strait, the eastern part borders the North Buton Regency, the southern part borders the Central Buton Regency and the western part borders the West Muna Regency.

2.2 *Instrument and material*

The instruments used in this study are a laptop and Arcgis 10.8 software. The materials used in this study cover administrative, rainfall, slope, soil type, and land use maps of the Muna Regency.

2.3 *Data analysis*

Data analysis was used to identify the level of flood vulnerability in the Muna Regency by using the overlay technique. This technique is a duplication technique for two or more maps that uses geographic information system technology to retrieve new information. The maps that are overlaid are maps of the parameters for determining the level of flood vulnerability, including slope map, soil type map, rainfall map, and land use map of the Muna Regency. Meanwhile, determining areas prone to flooding is carried out using the overlay method, where each variable is weighted and given a score based on sensitivity to flooding (Table 1).

Table 1. Weight parameters for flood vulnerability levels (Haryadi 2016).

No.	Parameter	Level
1.	Slope	3
2.	Soil Type	3
3.	Rainfall	2
4.	Land use	2

The division of areas susceptible to flooding is analyzed by looking at the overall results of the flood vulnerability classification parameters for each land. This is based on the total value resulting from the sum of the variable scores and the weight of each parameter. Determining the classification of flood vulnerability classes uses the formula from Haryadi (2016):

$$Ki = (Xt - Xr)/k$$

where Ki = interval level; Xt = highest data; Xr = lowest data; and k = number of expected level.

3 RESULTS AND DISCUSSION

3.1 *Parameters of flood susceptibility*

3.1.1 *The slope*

The slope is the part that influences the occurrence of flooding, where the steeper of the slope, the higher the speed of surface water produced. The weights and scores for the slope parameter levels for the Muna Regency are presented in Table 2.

Table 2. Scores and weights of slope parameters in Muna Regency.

No.	Classification	Slope	Area (Ha)	Percentage (%)	S	B	S x B
1.	Flat	0 – 8 %	83,972	40.81	5	3	15
2.	Slope	8 – 15 %	50,529	24.56	4	3	12
3.	Rather steep	15 – 25 %	70,589	34.30	3	3	9
4.	Steep	25 – 40 %	600	0.29	2	3	6
5.	Very steep	>40 %	80	0.04	1	3	3
	Total		205,769	100%			

Abbreviation: S = Score; B = Weight.

The slope conditions of the Muna Regency obtained from Aster DEM data processing, showing that based on the parameter classification, the slope level of the slopes is divided into 5 levels, namely, flat (0–8%); gentle (8–15%), slightly steep (15–25%), steep (25–40%), and very steep (>40%). Based on these results, it was found that Muna Regency is dominated by slopes which are in the flat class covering an area of 83,972 ha of the total area of Muna Regency, namely 205,769 ha. These results show that the low slope of the slope results in slow water flow, thereby allowing water to pool on this land unit. The distribution of slopes in the study area can be seen in Figure 1.

3.1.2 *Soil type*

One of the physical factors that influence the occurrence of flooding or inundation is the soil type because this type of soil can absorb water in the soil. The higher the absorption process, the faster the amount of water will decrease and minimize the occurrence of flooding. Infiltration or the ability of the soil to absorb water above its surface greatly influences the length of time water is stored above the soil surface. The longer the water soaks into the ground, the more it can cause puddles and if this puddle lasts long enough it will cause problems, namely flooding.

Based on processed soil type data, it was found that Muna Regency has 5 distributions of soil types. Lithosol and organosols soil types with large infiltration are spread over an area

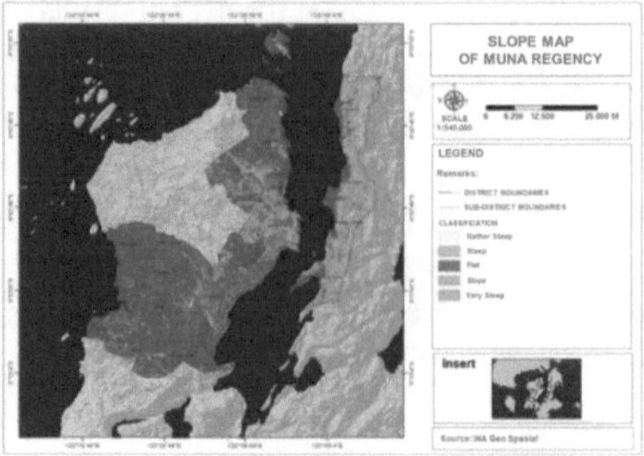

Figure 1. Slope map of Muna Regency.

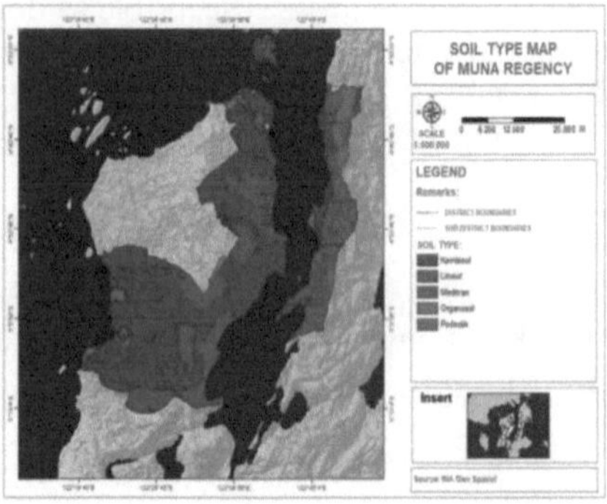

Figure 2. Soil type map of Muna Regency.

of 35,340 ha of the total area of Muna Regency, Mediterranean with moderate infiltration is 49,896 ha, and cambisols and podzolic soil types with rather large infiltration are 120,533 ha. The weights and scores for the Muna Regency soil type parameter classes are presented in Table 3, while the distribution of soil types is presented in Figure 2.

Table 3. Scour and weight parameters of soil type in Muna Regency.

Soil Type	Infiltration	Area (Ha)	Percentage (%)	S	B	S x B
Regosols, Lithosol, Organosols, Rendzina	Large	35,340	17	1	3	3
Andosol, Laterite, Grumusols, Podzol, Podzolic	Rather Large	120,533	59	2	3	6
Brown Forest Soil, Non-Calcic Brown, Mediterranean	Moderate	49,896	24	3	3	9
Latosol	Rather Small	0	0	0	3	0
Alluvial, planosol, Hydromorphic Kelanu	Small	0	0	0	3	0
Total		205,769	100%			

3.1.3 *Rainfall*

Muna Regency is an area with a tropical climate where there is a rainy season and a dry season. The intensity of rainfall in an area is one of the factors determining the level of flood vulnerability. Rainfall assessment is necessary because the soil is saturated resulting in a series of continuous heavy rains. The ability of high rainfall causes the soil to absorb water permanently. If the soil becomes saturated it will cause flooding. The rainfall needed for flood control planning is the average rainfall throughout the area concerned, not rainfall at a certain point which is usually called regional/regional rainfall. If a place has high rainfall, there is the potential for flooding, and conversely (Table 4).

Muna Regency's rainfall ranges between <25000 mm/year and 2500–3500 mm/year, meaning that based on class parameters the rainfall is at score 1 (very low) and score 2 (low). The results of this study show that Muna Regency is dominated by very low rainfall, so the potential for flooding in this area is very low (Figure 3).

Table 4. Weight and score of rainfall level in Muna Regency.

No.	Rainfall Level (mm/year)	Classification	Area (Ha)	Percentage (%)	S	B	S X B
1.	<2500	Very low	136,966	67	1	2	2
2.	2500–3500	Low	68,803	33	2	2	4
3.	3500–4500	Medium	0	0	0	2	0
4.	4500–5500	High	0	0	0	2	0
5.	>5500	Very high	0	0	0	2	0
	Total		205,769	100%			

Abbreviations: S = Score; B = Weight.

3.1.4 *Land use*

Land use in Muna Regency is classified into ten land cover classes, they are (1) forest; (2) mixed gardens; (3) open land; (4) Field; (5) residential; (6) rice field; (7) bush; (8) pond; (9) moor/field; and (10) water body. Land cover planted with plants is an area with a low potential for flooding. Most of Muna Regency's area is dominated by mixed gardens covering an area of 75,299 ha, forest covering an area of 44,425 ha, shrubs covering an area of 28,438 ha and moorland covering an area of 25,903 ha. This explains that Muna Regency is classified as an open area. The weights and scores for the Muna Regency rainfall class are presented in Table 5.

Table 5. Weight and score of the land use in the Muna Regency.

No.	Land Use	Remark	Area (ha)	Percentage (%)	S	B	S X B
1.	Forest	very good	44,425	21.59	1	2	2
2.	Mixed gardens	good	75,299	36.59	2	2	4
3.	Open land	not good	13,812	6.71	4	2	8
4.	Field	not good	9,930	4.83	4	2	8
5.	Residential	very not good	4,175	2.03	5	2	10
6.	Rice field	very not good	722	0.35	5	2	10
7.	Bush	moderate	28,438	13.82	3	2	6
8.	Pond	not good	1,930	0.94	4	2	8
9.	Moor/field	not good	25,903	12.59	4	2	8
10.	Waterbody	not good	1,126	0.55	4	2	8
	Total		205,769	100%			

Abbreviation: S = Score; and B = Weight.

The Muna Regency area is dominated by mixed plantations covering an area of 75,299 ha and most of the area has vegetation that is quite good for controlling floods. Areas that have high vegetation will influence the flow of falling rainwater which will be retained by vegetation before it falls to the ground. Land use was analyzed using Landsat 8 imagery which was then processed to obtain a land use map to calculate the area and influence of land use on the level of flood vulnerability in the Muna Regency.

3.2 *Flood vulnerability level*

Based on the results of the analysis of four parameters for classifying the level of flood vulnerability, namely: slope, soil type, rainfall, and land use in the Muna Regency, five classes of flood vulnerability were obtained (Table 6), namely: (1) flood area; (2) flood-prone area; (3) slightly flood-prone area; (4) less flood-prone area; and (5) not-flood prone area.

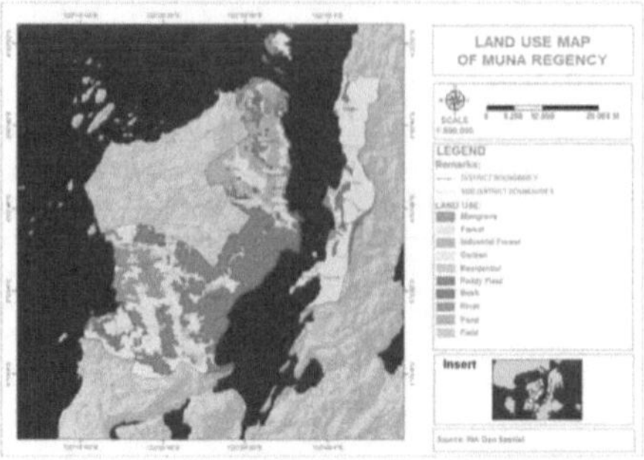

Figure 3. Land use map of the Muna Regency.

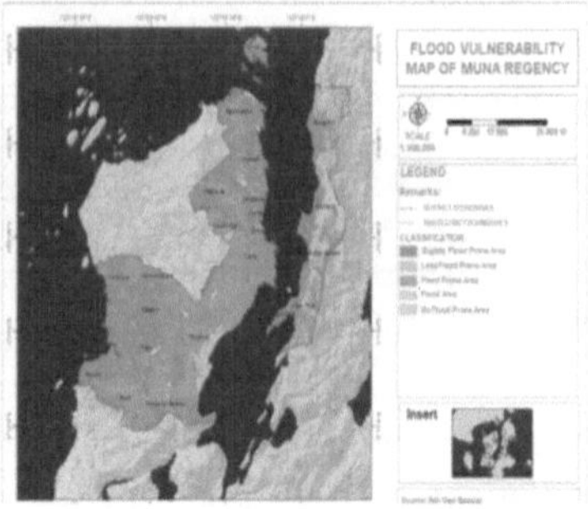

Figure 4. Flood vulnerability level map of the Muna Regency.

Table 6. Flood vulnerability level in the Muna Regency.

No.	Flood Vulnerability Level	Class Interval	Area (Ha)
1.	Flood area	34–39	4,859
2.	Flood prone area	28–33	64,218
3.	Slightly flood-prone area	22–27	112,345
4.	Less flood-prone area	16–21	19,466
5.	Not flood-prone area	10–15	4,881
	Total		205,769

Based on the results of the analysis of the level of flood vulnerability in the Muna Regency, it was found that the area is in the slightly flood-prone class covering an area of 112,345 ha, meaning that land units in this class are flood-prone areas with interval of 22 – 27. The largest area in this class is Kabawo District covering an area of 92,662 ha, and the lowest is located in South Tongkuno District covering an area of 84 ha. Based on four flood vulnerability parameters that most influence the slightly flood-prone area are areas located on flat slopes and polyciliate soil types which cause the possibility of stagnant water being very high.

The area in the flood class in Muna Regency is classified as not very large, only 4,859 ha of the total area of Muna Regency. The widest distribution is in Pasikolaga District covering an area of 2,915 ha. The most influencing parameter is that the land units in this class are on a flat slope. Agricultural plants and shrubs generally have roots that are less able to absorb water quickly and slow the absorption of water into the soil. The condition of the soil cover layer is related to the activities of residents in cultivating and processing land according to its function and potential.

4 CONCLUSION

The conclusions of this study are Muna Regency is divided into five flood vulnerability classes, they are (1) Flood area; (2) prone area; (3) Slightly flood-prone area; (4) Less flood-prone area; (5) and Not flood-prone area. The dominant flood vulnerability class is a slightly flood-prone area with an area of 112,345 ha. Based on four flood vulnerability classification parameters, the one that has the most influence on this class is the slope factor, where most of the Muna Regency area is on a flat slope which makes the land unit flood-prone area and also the podzolic soil type factor which mostly covers the Muna Regency.

REFERENCES

Ahiablame, L., & Shakya, R. (2016). Modelling flood reduction effects of low impact development at a watershed scale. *Journal of Environmental Management*, 171, 81–91. https://doi.org/http://dx.doi.org/10.1016/j.jenvman.2016.01.036

Ajun Purwanto, Rustam, Eviliyanto and Dony Andrasmoro, 2022. Flood risk mapping using GIS and multi-criteria analysis at Nanga Pinoh West Kalimantan area. *Indonesian Journal of Geography* Vol 54, No 3 (2022): 463–470. DOI: 10.22146/ijg.69879 website: htps://jurnal.ugm.ac.id/ijg

Ariyani D, Aprilia V, Tri Juniati A, Dewi A, Kurnia F. 2020. Curve number method to determine the runoff height in the upper Cimanuk watershed. *IOP Conf. Ser. Mater. Sci. Eng.* 852:12020.doi:10.1088/1757-899X/852/1/012020

Ariyani D, Wulandari A, Juniati A, Nur Arini R. 2021. Rainwater harvesting for water security in campus (case study Engineering Faculty in the University of Pancasila). *J. Phys. Conf. Ser.* 1858(1):1–9.doi:10.1088/1742-6596/1858/1/012020.

Asdak, C., Supian, S., & Subiyanto. (2018). Watershed management strategies for flood mitigation: A case study of Jakarta's flooding. *Weather and Climate Extremes*, 21, 117–122. https://doi.org/https://doi.org/10.1016/j.wace.2018.08.002

Basri, H., & Chandra, S. Y. (2021). Assessment of infiltration rate in the Lawe Menggamat Sub-Watershed, Aceh Province, Indonesia. *IOP Conference Series: Earth and Environmental Science*, 667(1), 12069.

Chukwuma, E. C., Okonkwo, C. C., Ojediran, J. O., Anizoba, D. C., Ubah, J. I., & Nwachukwu, C. P. (2021). A GIS-Based Flood Vulnerability Modelling of Anambra State Using An Integrated IVFRN-DEMATEL-ANP model. *Heliyon*, 7, e08048. https://doi.org/10.1016/j.heliyon.2021.e08048

Deepak, S., & Rajan, G., & Jairaj, P. G. (2020). Geospatial approach for assessment of vulnerability to flood in local Self-Governments. *Geoenvironmental disasters*, 7, Article No. 35. https://doi.org/10.1186/s40677-020-00172-w.

Fernandos, Tambunan M.P and Marko. (2020). Loss levels regarding flood affected areas in the upper citarum watershed. *IOP Conference Series: Earth and Environmental Science*

Haryadi, Yudi. (2016). Analisis Tingkat Kerawanan Kawasan Bencana Banjir Berbasis GIS di Kecamatan Payung Sakaki Kota Pekanbaru (Tugas Akhir). *Program Studi Perencanaan Wilayah dan Kota.* Universitas Islam Riau.

Knufer L.K. Peter & Burrel E Montz. (2008). Flooding and watershed management. *Journal of Contemporary Water research & education. Issue* 139, pp: 45–51

Komolafe, A. A., Awe, B. S., Olorunfemi, I. E., & Oguntunde, P. G. (2020). Modelling flood-prone areas and vulnerability using the integration of multi-criteria analysis and HAND model in the Ogun River Basin, Nigeria. *Hydrological Sciences Journal*, 65(10), 1766–1783.

Liu, J., Gao, G., Wang, S., Jiao, L., Wu, X., & Fu, B. (2018). The effects of vegetation on runoff and soil loss: Multidimensional structure analysis and scale characteristics. *Journal of Geographical Sciences*, 28(1), 59–78.

Mukhsan Putra Hatta, Sugiarto Badaruddin, Zulvyah Faisal and Devi Ayu Puspita, 2020. Flood hazard mapping using geographic information systems (GIS) in the Walanae river basin Wajo Regency of South Sulawesi province. *Journal of Engineering and Applied Science*, 15 (14): 2802–2810, 2020

Rinaldi Aulia and Heldi. (2021). Analysis of flood events in the Batang Kuranji Watershed environment based on Weather radar. *Science and Environmental Journals for Postgraduate*. Vol. 4(1). Pp 17–21. http://senjop.ppj.unp.ac.id/index.php/senjop

Sarkar, D., & Mondal, P. (2020). Flood vulnerability mapping using frequency ratio (FR) model: A case study on Kulik River basin, Indo-Bangladesh Barind region. *Applied Water Science*, 10, 1–13. https://doi.org/10.1007/s13201-019-1102-x

Sitorus, Santun R.P. (2016). Perencanaan Penggunaan Lahan. *Bogor*. IPB Press.

Tamiru, H., & Dinka, M. O. (2021). Artificial intelligence in Geospatial analysis for flood vulnerability assessment: A case of dire dawa watershed, Awash Basin, Ethiopia. *Scientific World Journal*, 2021, Article ID: 6128609. https://doi.org/10.1155/2021/6128609

Tiwari, V., Kumar, V., Matin, M.A., Thapa, A., Ellenburg, W.L., Gupta, N. & Thapa, S. 2020. Flood inundation mapping? Kerala 2018; Harnessing the power of SAR, automatic threshold detection method and google earth engine, *PLoS ONE*, 15(8), e0237324.

Wizor, C. H., & Week, D. A. (2020). Geospatial mapping and assessment of flood-prone communities in the Core Niger Delta, Nigeria. *Asian Journal of Advanced Research and Reports*, 9, 6–20. https://doi.org/10.9734/ajarr/2020/v9i330220

Umaru, E. T., & Adedokun, A. (2020). Geospatial analysis of flood risk and vulnerability assessment along River benue basin of Kogi state. *Journal of Geographic Information System*, 12, 1–14. https://doi.org/10.4236/jgis.2020.121001

Zhou, Q., Su, J., Arnbjerg-Nielsen, K., Ren, Y., Luo, J., Ye, Z., & Feng, J. (2021). A GIS-Based hydrological modeling approach for rapid urban flood hazard assessment. *Water*, 13(11), 1483. nd indenting

Technological Innovations in Tropical Livestock Development for Environmental Sustainability and Food Security – P. Dhian Isnaeni et al. (eds)

Stock assessment to support sustainable management of Mackerel scad in Pasarwajo Bay, Buton Regency, Southeast Sulawesi

S.A. Lawelle, A. Mansyur*, R.D. Siang, A. Nurdiana & W.O. Piliana
Faculty of Fisheries and Marine Science, Fisheries Agrobusiness, Halu Oleo University, Kendari, Indonesia

ABSTRACT: This study aimed to assess the stock of Mackerel scad (*Decapterus macarellus*) in the deep-sea ecosystem of Pasarwajo Bay, Buton Regency. Mackerel scad is an important species in the fishing industry, and in-depth understanding of their population stock in this region is essential for sustainable management. The research was conducted by collecting data from field surveys that included direct observation, fish sampling, and data analysis from fishing. In addition, historical data on the Mackerel scad fishery was also analyzed to understand trends over time. The results showed that the greatest opportunity for fishermen to be able to produce a catch of Mackerel scad was at a total length size ranging from 21 cm to 23 cm. The greatest ability of Mackerel scad to spawn was at a length of 21 cm. The total mortality rate of Mackerel scad was 11.74. The population structure of Mackerel scads appears to have more survivors than total mortality. The occurrence of peak fishing mortality at this size indicates that the utilization of Mackerel scad is still relatively sustainable because of the presence of mackerel scad that are still found in all size classes (infants, juveniles and adults). These findings provide a strong basis for the management of Mackerel scad fishery resources to maintain population viability and increase catches. The results are expected to be used to aid sustainable decision-making and maintain the deep-sea ecosystem in the Pasarwajo Bay, Buton Regency.

Keywords: Stock assessment, Mackerel scad, Pasarwajo

1 INTRODUCTION

Fisheries resources are one of the country's important assets if they are managed well and provide maximum benefits for the community (Fauzi & Anna 2002). However, the fact is that Indonesia's capture fisheries production is still below that of countries that do not have fish resource potential and biodiversity as large as Indonesia. Indonesia's capture fisheries production is below China, Bangladesh, India, Myanmar, Uganda and Cambodia (FAO 2010). The condition of the capture fisheries industry in Indonesia in general is still dominated (more than 80%) by small-scale fishermen (with fleets < 10 gt) and is the livelihood of millions of households in coastal areas. Small-scale fisheries make a significant contribution to the household economy and food security (Kurien 1993).

Fishing activities carried out by humans without paying attention to the principles of sustainability and sustainability will cause many problems in the future (Gjertsen 2005). The results of the identification of fisheries potential studies can be useful for improving the economy of communities around fisheries areas by continuously preserving the fisheries environment (Hendrik 2010). Application of the concept of marine and fisheries-based development blue economy (BE) is a strategic step in implementing marine and fisheries development. The BE conception aims to create an environmentally friendly industry, so that sustainable and sustainable management of natural resources can be created (KKP 2014).

*Corresponding Author: akhmadmansyur@uho.ac.id

 DOI: 10.1201/9781003468943-34

Buton Regency's marine waters are part of the Republic of Indonesia State Fisheries Management Area 714 (WPPNRI-714). The WPP has the character of a transition area between bay waters and open waters. In this case, open waters are more dominant than the bay waters. Apart from that, the marine waters of Buton Regency are supported by general marine ecosystems such as mangrove, seagrass and coral ecosystems as well as the deep sea. The sandy beach waters are quite dominant, spreading along the coastline of this district. Furthermore, the dominant shallow water bottom topography follows the coastline in the bay area. Another characteristic of the bay waters is that the topography is sloping and increasingly open towards the outside of the bay. There are also rivers that can threaten the sustainability of aquatic ecosystems as Fishing Areas (DPI) if land use in river watersheds is not carried out with a conservative approach. Therefore, fisheries management in Buton Regency has been designed based on the concept of Integrated Fisheries Area Centers (SKPT) aims to create an environmentally friendly industry, so that sustainable and sustainable management of natural resources can be created (KKP 2014).

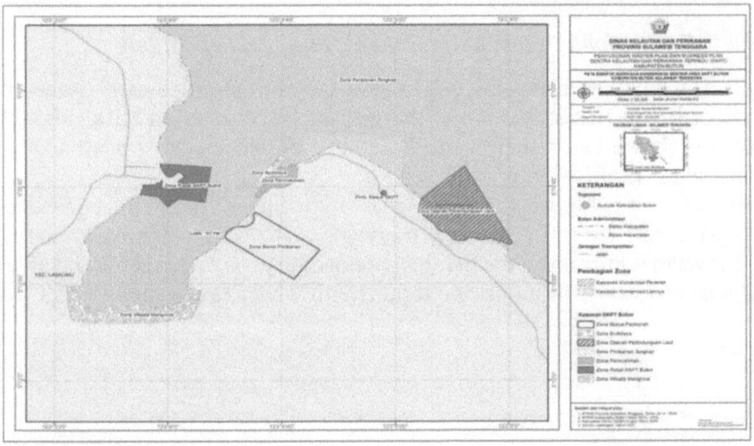

Figure 1. Development plan map of fisheries buton regency based on integrated fisheries area.

The development of the Buton Regency integrated fisheries area center (SKPT) was then confronted with conditions for the use of fisheries resources such as Moderate-exploited, Fully-exploited and over-exploited. Thus, in order to support the SKPT development framework in question, analysis of the fisheries potential of Pasarwajo Bay is considered important as basic data in future decision making. This research uses four coastal ecosystems as sources of analytical data, namely deep sea, coral, sand and seagrass ecosystems.

2 METHODS

The research uses a participatory approach through a series of activities, surveys. The activity begins with identifying potential fisheries resources, fish catches and their use, problems in handling marine fish production and processing. As well as identifying needs for assessment of fisheries resources for the development of the fisheries industry.

Scope of activities includes:

1. Survey potential fisheries resources by observing the type of fish, number and density. Potential survey activities are carried out with the aim of:
   - Obtain information on fisheries resources (especially pelagic and demersal fish)
   - Obtain information about the physical chemical conditions of waters
   - Analyze the relationship between fish density and aquatic environmental conditions

2. Survey of fish catches and their use in Buton Regency.
   The SDI potential survey will be carried out in the Buton waters area taking into account seasonal conditions. The survey will be conducted in July 2023 (representing the rainy season) and October 2023 (representing the dry season).
   Potential survey activities are carried out with the following scope:

1. Pelagic fish catch survey for 2019–2022 based on data available to fishermen (quantity and grading of pelagic types and other types of fish) in Dongkala Village – Pasarwajo District, nth Village – Pasarwajo District, nth Village – mth District – Buton Regency
2. Survey of pelagic fish catches in 2023 based on data collected during the program in Dongkala Village – Pasarwajo District, nth Village – Pasarwajo District, nth Village – mth District – Buton Regency.
3. Potential survey in the area using a fish finder instrument.

3 RESULTS AND DISCUSSION

3.1 *Frequency distribution of attendance in total length classification*

Small pelagic fish have been in status Moderate exploited since 2017. One of the small pelagic fish recorded in this status is the flying fish. In connection with this, the results of field observations showed that there were different frequencies of appearance of blue swallowtail fish in each classification of total length.

Based on Figure 2, it is known that the highest frequency of attendance (57 times) is found in mid-length (ML) 22.1 cm from the class interval 21.1 – 23 cm which occurred on September 5 2023. This shows that currently, the greatest opportunity for fishermen to be able to produce catches of Mackerel scads is found in the total length which ranges between 21 up to 23 cm.

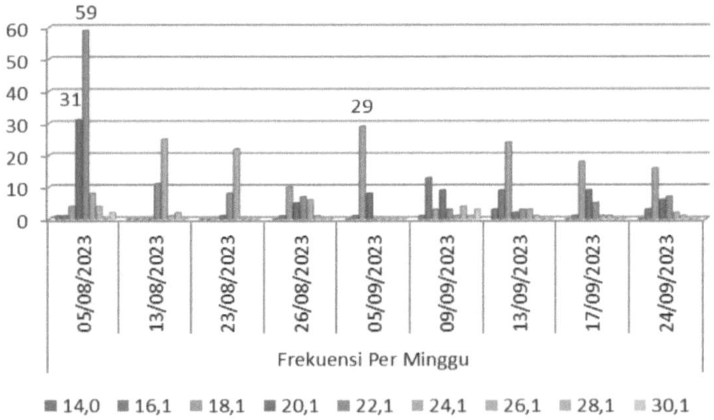

Figure 2. Frequency distribution of blue glider presence in each mid-length class of total length.

3.2 *Stock assessment based on constant growth Von Bertallanfy*

Based on the distribution of presence frequencies in each ML, a constant growth rate of 7.1 is obtained with an asymptote length of 31.5 cm. This means that the dominant longest size that fishermen can produce every time they catch is 31.5 cm. This is more clearly seen in Figure 3.

The results of stock analysis based on the conversion of catch length measurements showed that baby Mackerel scads that could be caught were at a length of 12.82 cm, while juvenile Mackerel scads were caught at a length of 13.61 cm and adult Mackerel scads were caught at a size of 14.39 cm. If this is related to the number of dominant catch frequencies

(37 times per trip), it can be seen that currently the availability of blue glider fish in the waters of Pasarwajo Bay is predominantly juveniles with a size of 13.61 cm.

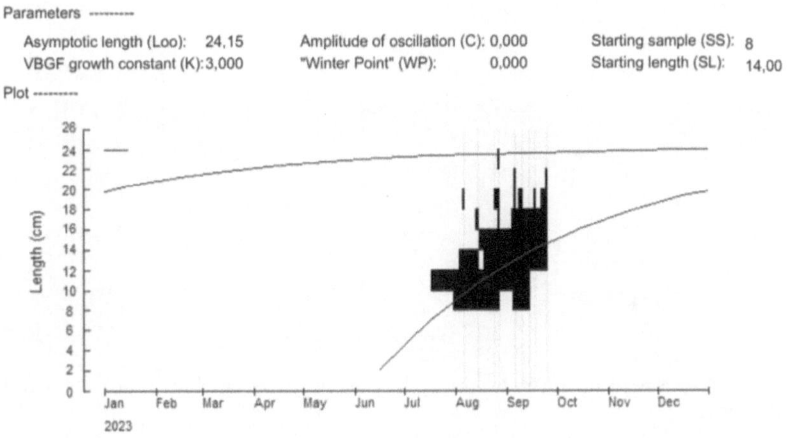

Figure 3. Stock assessment based on von Bertalanfy growth function and length frequency.

3.3 *Stock assessment is based on normal distribution separation*

The blue glider's greatest ability to spawn is 21.0 cm in length. The distribution of lengths of blue glider fish that can spawn can be seen in Figure 4.

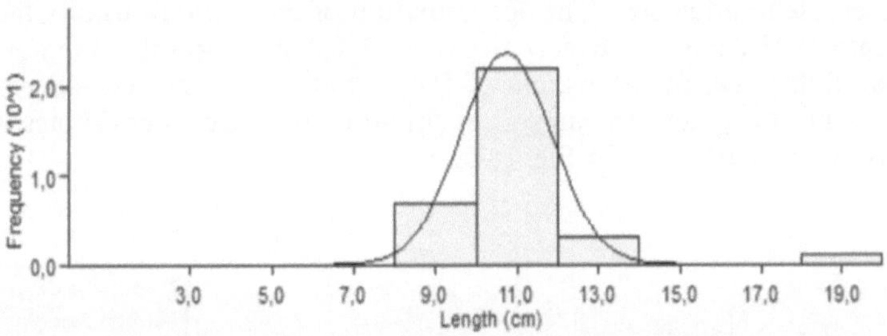

Figure 4. Stock assessment based on normal distribution separation using Bhattacharya.

3.4 *Stock assessment based on mortality*

Based on the results of the analysis of natural deaths according to Pauly, the natural death rate was 6,344 per year. This is closely related to the existence of a constant pro-growth rate of 7.1 and the existence of an asymptote length of 31.5 cm and a water temperature of around 28OC. Therefore, the analysis model for the natural death of blue swallowtail fish in Pasarwajo Bay fulfills the equation:

$$\log(M) = -0.0066 - 0.279 \log(Loo) + 0.6543 \log(K) + 0.4634 \log(T)$$

Furthermore, it is known that the death rate due to fishing (F) is 5.4 at an effort level of 0.46. Thus, the total mortality rate for blue glider fish in Pasarwajo Bay was 11.74. This can be expressed in the form of a length conversion curve for catching blue swallowtails as in Figure 5.

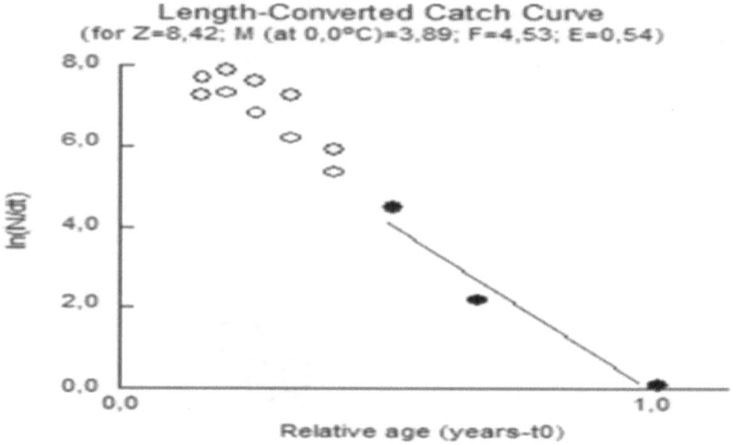

Figure 5. Stock Assessment based on total length conversion per catch of Mackerel scad fish in Pasarwajo Bay waters.

3.5 *Stock assessment based on virtual population analysis*

Based on the results of the Virtual Population Analysis (VPA), it was found that the structure of the blue swallowtail fish population in the waters of Pasarwajo Bay appears to still have many survivors compared to the total deaths. At baby size, the dominant blue glider dies naturally, but gradually decreases and even disappears when it reaches adult size. At juvenile size, blue glider fish in the waters of Pasawajo Bay have shown mortality due to fishing, then increase to adult size. The accumulation of these two mortality factors reached a peak at a length of 22.0 cm. The occurrence of peak fishing mortality at this size shows that the use of blue flying fish in the waters of Pasarwajo Bay is still considered sustainable because the presence of flying fish can still be found in all size classes (babies, juveniles and adults). This is more clearly seen in Figure 6.

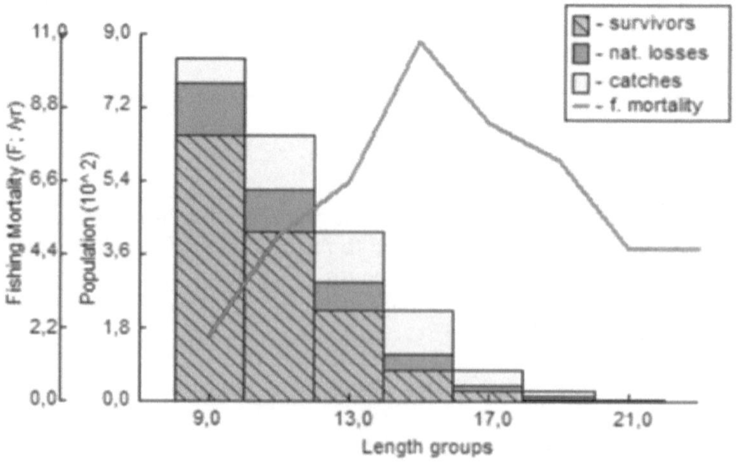

Figure 6. Stock assessment based on VPA structure.

3.6 *Stock assessment based on maximum sustainable yield and biomass*

For management purposes, the results of stock analysis based on yield/recruit (knife-edge) relativity show that the maximum sustainable yield has an effort level of 0.4 and a relative yield of 0.054 Y/R and 0.327 B/R. Furthermore, the level of effort allowed is 0.355 with a relative yield of 0.05 Y/R and 0.466 B/R. Meanwhile, utilization has just reached an effort of 0.278 with a relative yield of 0.03 Y/R and 0.626 B/R. This means that the current effort can still be increased by 21.69% to reach the permitted effort. This is illustrated by the Maximum Sustainable Yield (MSY) curve as in Figure 7.

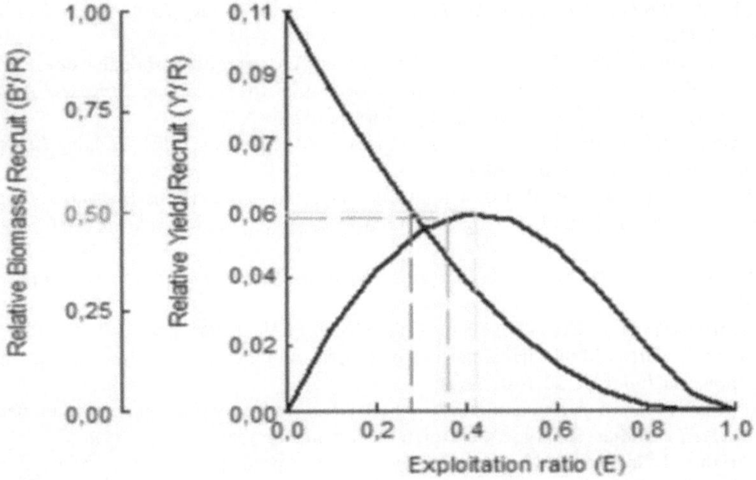

Figure 7. Maximum Sustainable Yield (MSY) curve for blue swallowtail fish in the waters of Pawasarwajo Bay, Buton Regency.

4 CONCLUSIONS

The greatest opportunity for fishermen to be able to produce a catch of mackerel scads is found in total length measurements that range from 21 to 23 cm. The constant growth rate is 7.1 and the longest dominant size that fishermen can produce each time they catch is 31.5 cm long and based on the frequency of catches, juveniles are dominant with a size of 13.61 cm. The blue glider's greatest ability to spawn is 21.0 cm in length. The total death rate for blue swallowtail fish in Pasarwajo bay is 11.74. The structure of the blue swallowtail fish population in the waters of Pasarwajo bay appears to still have many survivors compared to the total number of deaths. The mortality peaked at a length of 22.0 cm. The occurrence of peak fishing mortality at this size shows that the use of blue flying fish in the waters of Pasarwajo bay is still considered sustainable because the presence of flying fish can still be found in all size classes (babies, juveniles and adults).

REFERENCES

FAO. 2010. *The state of world Fisheries and Aquaculture 2010*. FAO Fisheries and Aquaculture Department. Food and Agriculture Organization of the United Nations, Rome. p. 17 and 21.

Fauzi A. 2004. Ekonomi Sumber daya Alam dan Lingkungan: Teori dan Aplikasi. PTGramedia Pustaka Utama. Jakarta: 98.

Fauzi A, Z Anna. 2002. Penilaian depresiasi sumber daya perikanan sebagai bahan pertim bangan penentuan kebijakan pembangunan Perikanan. *Jurnal Pesisir dan Lautan* 4(2):36–49.

Giesen W, S. Wulffraat, M. Zieren, L. Scholten. 2006. *Mangrove guidebook for Southeast Asia.* FAO and Wetlands International. Bangkok.

Gjertsen H. 2005. Can Habitat protection lead to improvements in human well-being? Evdence from Marine Protected Areas in the Philippines. *World Development*: 199–217.

Hendrik. 2010. Potensi Sumberdaya Perikanan dan Tingkat Eksploitasi (Kajian terhadap Danau Pulau Besar dan Danau Bawah Zamrud Kabupaten Siak Provinsi Riau). *Jurnal Perikanan dan Kelautan* 15(2):121–31.

Kementerian Kelautan danPerikanan. 2014. Blue economy: pembangunan kelautan dan perikanan berkelanjutan. *Kementerian Kelautan dan Perikanan.* 240hlm.

Kementerian-PPN/Bappenas. 2016. Kajian strategi industrialisasi perikanan untuk mendukung pembangunan ekonomi wilayah. *Direktorat Kelautan dan Perikanan Kedeputian Bidang Kemaritiman dan Sumber Daya Alam BAPPENAS.*

Machena C, R Kwaramba. 1997. The creation of property rights to promote sustainable development in Lake Kariba inshore fishery in Zimbabwe. In K. Remane (Ed.). *African Inland Fisheries, Aquaculture and theEnvironment* (pp. 245–254). London: Fishing News Books.

Keputusan Menteri Lingkungan Hidup Republik Indonesia No. 201 tahun 2004. *Tentang Kriteria Baku dan Pedoman Penentuan Kerusakan Mangrove.*

Mallawa A. 2006, "Pengelolaan Sumberdaya Ikan Berkelanjutan dan Berbasis Masyarakat", disampaikan dalam Lokakarya Agenda Penelitian Program COREMAP II, *Kabupaten Selayar*, 9–10 September 2006, hal. 1.

Noor, YR., M. Khazali, INN. Suryadiputra. 1999. *Panduan Pengenalan Mangrove di Indonesia.* Bogor: PHKA/Wi-IP.

Phillips M, Henriksson PJG, Tran N, Chan CY, Mohan CV, Rodriguez U-P, Suri S, Hall S dan Koeshendrajana S. 2016. Menjelajahi masa depan perikanan budidaya Indonesia. Penang Malaysia: WorldFish. *Laporan Program*: 2016–02.

Purnomo BH. 2012. Peranan perikanan tangkap berkelanjutan untuk menunjang ketahanan pangan di Indonesia. *Artikel.* Fakultas Teknologi Pertanian Universitas Jember.

Radiarta IN, Erlania, J Haryadi. 2015. Analisis pengembangan perikanan budidaya berbasis ekonomi biru dengan pendekatan analytic hierarchy process (AHP). *J. Sosek KP* 10(1): 47–59.

Rizal A, Iskandar, H Herawati, LP Dewanti. 2018. *Potret dan Review: Strategi Pembangunan Perikanan dan Kelautan.* Unpad Press. Bandung.

Sanger CLM, Jusuf A & Andaki JA. (2019). Analisis Orientasi Kewirausahaan Nelayan Tangkap Skala Kecil dengan Alat Tangkap "JUBI" di Kelurahan Batulubang Kecamatan Lembeh Selatan Kota Bitung. *Akulturasi: Jurnal Ilmiah Agrobisnis Perikanan*, 7(1): 1095–1101.

Sianturi S Jr, VAJ Masinambow, AT Londa. 2018. Dampak regulasi sektor perikanan tangkap Ikan terhadap Pertumbuhan PDRB di Kota Bitung. *Jurnal Berkala Ilmiah Efisiensi*, 18(1):103–113.

Sondita MFA. 2010. Manajemen sumber daya perikanan. Jakarta: Universitas Terbuka. Triarso I. 2012. Potensi dan Peluang Pengembangan Usaha Perikanan Tangkap di Pantura Jawa Tengah. *Jurnal Saintek Perikanan* 8 (1):65–73

Technological Innovations in Tropical Livestock Development for Environmental Sustainability and Food Security – P. Dhian Isnaeni et al. (eds)
© 2025 The Author(s), ISBN 978-1-032-74373-8

The bibliometric analysis of the studies conducted in the field of buffalo feeding

R. Rahman
Department of Animal Science, Faculty of Animal Science, Universitas Halu Oleo, Kendari, Southeast Sulawesi

N. Qomariyah*, A. Ella, A. Husni, A. Fanindi, E. Sutedi, A.M. Pongtuluran, S. Sajimin, R. Krisnan & I. Herdiawan
Research Center for Animal Husbandry, Research Organization for Agriculture and Food, BRIN, Bogor, West Java, Indonesia

M.B. Nappu
Research Center for Food Crops, Research Organization for Agriculture and Food, National Research and Innovation Agency (BRIN), Cibinong Science Center, Bogor, West Java, Indonesia

S.T. Risyahadi
Department of Nutrition and Feed Technology, Faculty of Animal Science, IPB University, Bogor, Indonesia

ABSTRACT: Feed is one of the main factors affecting the productivity of buffaloes. The present study aimed to perform a bibliometric analysis on buffalo feeding research to identify patterns and trends that have emerged recently. The bibliometric analyzes about 819 studies on feeding buffalo published between 2010 and 2023 to identify contemporary tendencies and trends. In the Scopus Collection database, a review of the terms "buffalo" AND "feeding" was conducted, and bibliometric information about the research was accessible. India, Pakistan, and The USA were the most productive nations in publishing. Wanapat M, Kamra DN, and Agarwal N have the most excellent h index and g index values among authors on feeding buffalo. The rise in bibliometrics research can significantly contribute by acting as a springboard for research in buffalo farming. The three most popular study areas in buffalo feeding are: livestock production and rumen health; rumen fermentation and growth efficiency in water buffalo; and buffalo production and nutrition for enhanced productivity. This bibliometric analysis provides an overview of the current state of research on buffalo feeding and can provide direction for future research in the development and application of more effective.

Keywords: buffalo, bibliometrics, citation, feeding

1 INTRODUCTION

Buffalo is one of the important and multipurpose types of livestock. The uses of buffalo are very diverse, ranging from ploughing fields, means of transportation, sources of meat, and milk to leather and horns used as industrial materials and manure as organic fertilizer. The development of buffalo farming is directed to support the adequacy of meat while producing milk. The pattern of buffalo rearing is still mostly done traditionally, where the rearing

*Corresponding Author: novi049@brin.go.id

DOI: 10.1201/9781003468943-35

system is carried out by cages and grazing. Pasture management is important in traditional maintenance (Barsila *et al.* 2022). According to Eisler *et al.* and Van Kernebeek *et al.* (Eisler *et al.* 2014; Van Kernebeek *et al.* 2016), the use of pastures for animal husbandry can be an appropriate strategy to increase agricultural competitiveness because there are large amounts of land called "marginal areas" where agricultural production cannot be carried out. Grazing can be a tool to improve its utilization and efficiency. This is related to some concerns raised about intensive livestock conditions, which are considered one of the causes of environmental pollution and disrespect for animal welfare, although a direct link between intensive rearing and these topics has not been provided (Gill *et al.* 2021; Van Marle-Köster & Visser 2021).

Feed represents the most significant expense in animal rearing and directly impacts profitability (Mudgal *et al.* 2022; Panda *et al.* 2018). Feed intake in quantity and quality is important in optimizing buffalo farming. Although it is rare to find thin buffalo when kept exclusively, there are obstacles in the development of buffalo with poor quality feed, such as low production and reproductivity, high first calving life, long interval calving with a long weaning period (1–2 years), and a long time to reach the specified body weight. Balanced nutrition and better management can increase buffalo productivity (Sarwar *et al.* 2009). Therefore, buffalo researchers need to consider research trends in buffalo feed to support the future development of buffalo livestock.

Bibliometric research on buffalo feeding can help find the trend latest feed research that can increase buffalo productivity. In addition, bibliometric research can also help identify gaps and deficiencies in the study that has been done to provide direction for future research related to better and effective feeding of buffalo livestock. Scientific publications, such as journal articles, conferences, and books, can be analysed to understand research trends and the country's contributions to buffalo feeding in a bibliometric study on buffalo animal feeding. The present study aimed to perform a bibliometric analysis on buffalo feeding research to identify patterns and trends that have emerged recently.

2 MATERIAL AND METHOD

2.1 *Search strategy and data collection*

Papers on buffalo feeding research were retrieved for this bibliometric study from the Scopus database (http://www.scopus.com) on October 24, 2023. Database using the keywords "buffalo" and "feeding" for bibliometric analysis. This review does not account for any changes made after that date. Figure 1 search strategy adapted from the PRISMA flow diagram comprised 891 documents. The documents include a variety of categories, including articles (n = 788) and conference papers (n = 31).

2.2 *Data analysis*

R software version 4.3.1 (R Foundation for Statistical Computing, Vienna, Austria) was used to perform the bibliometric analysis of the Scopus raw data. In particular, the Bibliometrix R package version 4.1.3 and VOSviewer carried out the study. This package includes all the primary bibliometric techniques for gauging time trends, identifying the most cited papers, and identifying the most prolific authors, journals, organizations, and nations. Specifically, the H-index (number of documents N with N or more citations), the G-index (a variant of the H-index where papers with more citations are weighted), and the M-index (the H-index divided by the number of years in active research) were used to describe the author contribution. The impact factors (IF) of the journals were also taken from the most recent Journal Citation Reports (JCR 2022) to round out the bibliometric results.

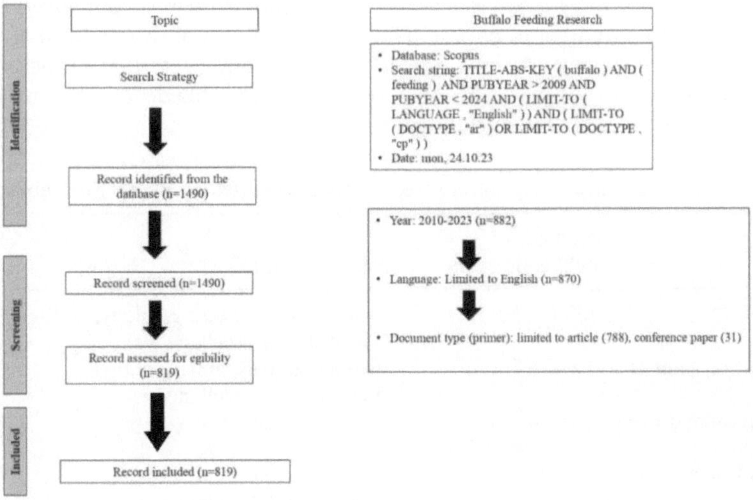

Figure 1. Search strategy adapted from the PRISMA flow diagram (Page *et al.* 2021).

3 RESULT AND DISCUSSION

3.1 *Main information*

Eight hundred nineteen papers were published, 788 were articles, and 31 were conference papers. Two thousand nine hundred seventeen authors wrote the studies; a single author wrote 24, and 2893 had various authors (Table 1). According to the records of the search made with the keywords "Buffalo" and "feeding" on October 24, 2023 in the Scopus database, there are 1,490 records found. This record comprises the 2010–2023 period.

Table 1. Main information.

Description	Results	Description	Results
Main information about the data		Authors	
Timespan	2010:2023	Authors	2,917
Sources (Journals, Books, etc)	286	Authors of single-authored docs	24
Documents	819	Authors collaboration	
Annual Growth Rate %	−2.02	Single-authored docs	24
Document Average Age	6.18	Co-Authors per Doc	4.99
Average citations per doc	7.118	International co-authorships %	19.78
References	27,198	Document types	
Document contents		article	788
Keywords Plus (ID)	4,494	conference paper	31
Author's Keywords (DE)	2,309		

3.2 *Most relevant sources*

Publications about feeding buffalo have been published in 819 journals. The ten most prolific journals are listed in Table 2. Journals were regarded as the primary source for publication because they contained most of the original recovered articles. Of the 819 papers on buffalo nutrition, 347 were published in the 10 most prolific journals, making up 42.4% of the total. Specifically, with 102 (12.5%), 66 (8.1%), and 34 (4.2%) documents, respectively, *Buffalo*

Bulletin, *Indian Journal of Animal Sciences*, and *Animal Nutrition and Feed Technology* displayed the maximum number of papers. The primary subject of five (50,0%) of the top ten most productive journals was "Animal Science and Zoology, Veterinary (miscellaneous)". Seven of the most famous journals, Animals being the top-ranked one with an IF of 0,68, had journal relevance scores higher than 0.20.

Table 2. Top 10 prolific journals on buffalo feeding research sorted by number of publications.

Source	Number of publications (% *)	Category (rank)	**2022 JCR IF
Buffalo Bulletin	102 (12.50)	Animal Science and Zoology, Veterinary (miscellaneous)	0.15
Indian Journal of Animal Sciences	66 (8.10)	Animal Science and Zoology, Veterinary (miscellaneous)	0.20
Animal Nutrition and Feed Technology	34 (4.20)	Food Animals	0.21
Indian Journal of Animal Research	31 (3.80)	Animal Science and Zoology, Veterinary (miscellaneous)	0.26
Tropical Animal Health and Production	28 (3.40)	Animal Science and Zoology, Food Animals	0.44
Revista Veterinaria	25 (3.10)	Animal Science and Zoology, Veterinary (miscellaneous)	0.14
Indian Veterinary Journal	18 (2.20)	Veterinary (miscellaneous)	0.14
Animals	17 (2.10)	Animal Science and Zoology, Veterinary (miscellaneous)	0.68
Veterinary World	14 (1.70)	Veterinary (miscellaneous)	0.43
Animal Production Science	12 (1.50)	Animal Science and Zoology, Food Science	0.41

JCR: Journal Citation Reports; IF: Impact Factor; * over 819; ** 2022 Impact Factor.

3.3 *Author impact values*

The retrieved documents (n = 819) had 2,917 authors, averaging 3.5 authors per document and 0.3 documents/author. Specifically, there were 24 single-authored articles, and the majority of the articles (n = 2893) had multiple authors. As a result, an average of 4.99 co-authors were found for each document. With a combined total of 21 published papers, Chaudhary LC and Wanapat M were the most prolific authors in buffalo feeding research (>20 articles) (Table 3).

Table 3. The top ten cited authors.

Element	h_index	g_index	m_index	TC	NP	PY_start
Wanapat M	12	19	0.857	379	21	2010
Kamra DN	10	15	0.769	242	18	2011
Agarwal N	9	14	0.692	221	18	2011
Chaudhary LC	9	14	0.692	231	21	2011
Kumar M	8	9	0.727	126	9	2013
Joshi CG	6	6	0.545	177	6	2013
Kansal VK	6	9	0.462	141	9	2011
Chanthakhoun V	5	7	0.357	111	7	2010
Cherdthong A	5	6	0.357	140	6	2010
Deka RS	5	5	0.455	90	5	2013

3.4 *Distribution by country*

The chosen papers, considering the corresponding author's affiliation, came from 55 nations on five continents. General data about the ten nations with the highest research output in buffalo feeding are shown in Table 4. Of all the published articles on buffalo feeding (n = 819), the ten most prolific countries accounted for 59.3% (n = 486). India was the most productive nation, publishing nearly 25% of all scientific production (n = 254 articles). Pakistan came in second with 66 articles, and the USA with 34. The number of multiple country publications (MCP) was extracted to calculate the MCP ratio: the MPC articles/total publications per country concerning inter-country collaboration. South Africa (MCP ratio = 0.50) was the nation with the highest proportion of MCP, followed by China (MCP ratio = 0.43) and Egypt (MCP ratio = 0.30).

Table 4. The top 10 nations for buffalo feeding research output.

No	Country	Articles	SCP	MCP	Freq	MCP Ratio	TC
1	India	254	241	13	0.310	0.051	1,354
3	Pakistan	66	54	12	0.081	0.182	314
4	USA	34	26	8	0.042	0.235	388
5	Italy	27	22	5	0.033	0.185	215
6	Brazil	25	22	3	0.031	0.120	110
7	Thailand	25	20	5	0.031	0.200	349
8	China	21	12	9	0.026	0.429	240
9	Egypt	20	14	6	0.024	0.300	121
10	South Africa	14	7	7	0.017	0.500	210

Single Country Publications (SCP); Multiple Country Publications (MCP); TC (Total Citation).

3.5 *Network visualization from co-occurrence analysis*

The co-occurrence analysis visualization shows the relationships between research topics, their popularity, and the clusters of topics that form. Consequently, co-occurrence analysis can look into the primary ideas or themes as well as the subjects of publications (Shafin *et al.* 2022). Three separate clusters of themes are visible in the network visualization produced by the cooccurrence analysis (Figure 2).

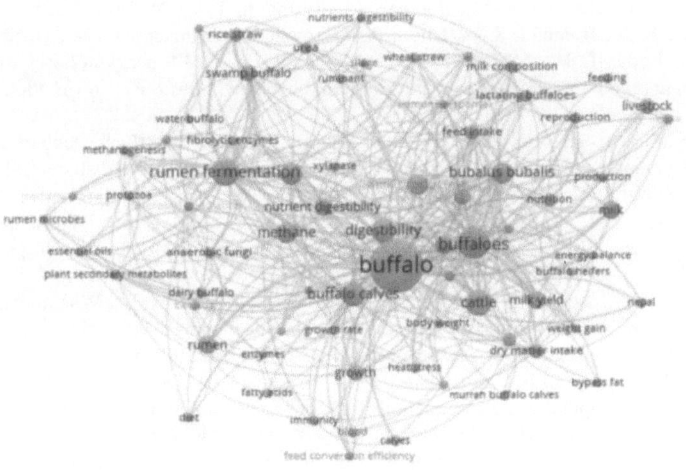

Figure 2. Co-occurrence network (keywords).

Different colors are used to represent each cluster; for example; cluster 1, 2, and 3 are represented by the red, green, and blue clusters, respectively. Through the use of data mining and cluster analysis techniques, the red cluster focuses on learning buffalo production and nutrition for increased productivity. Livestock production and rumen health are the focus of the green cluster's research. In the meantime, the blue cluster works on learning rumen fermentation and growth efficiency in water buffalo. These findings suggest that bibliometrics research could make a significant contribution by directing future studies in the husbandry field.

4 CONCLUSION

The Buffalo Bulletin journal published the highest number of studies in this area (n = 102) between 2010–2023, which proves it. According to the Scopus data platform analysis results, the ones with the highest h index value among the authors having articles on the subject of buffalo feeding are Wanapat M, Kamra DN, and Agarwal N. Bibliometric research on buffalo feeding show an increase in the number of publications over time, with most studies conducted in countries such as India, Pakistan, and the United States. The most popular research topics in buffalo feeding are buffalo production and nutrition for increased productivity; livestock production and rumen health; and rumen fermentation and growth efficiency in water buffalo.

REFERENCES

Barsila, S. R., Joshi, N. P., Poudel, T. N., Devkota, B., Devkota, N. R., & Chalise, D. R. (2022). Farmers' perceptions of grassland management in Magui Khola basin of Madi Chitwan, Nepal. *Pastoralism*, *12*(1), 40. https://doi.org/10.1186/s13570-022-00243-7

Eisler, M. C., Lee, M. R. F., Tarlton, J. F., & Martin, G. B. (2014). Steps to sustainable livestock. *Nature*, *507* (7490), 32–34. https://doi.org/10.1038/507032a

Gill, M., Garnsworthy, P. C., & Wilkinson, J. M. (2021). Review: More effective linkages between science and policy are needed to minimize the negative environmental impacts of livestock production. *Animal*, *15* (xxxx), 100291. https://doi.org/10.1016/j.animal.2021.100291

Mudgal, V., Jaiswal, P., Abraham, G., Singh, Y., Singh, P. K., & Dahiya, S. S. (2022). Azolla (Azolla microphylla) Supplementation Improves Nutrient Utilization in Lactating Murrah buffaloes. *Philippine Journal of Science*, *151*(6), 2183–2189. https://doi.org/10.56899/151.6A.10

Page, M. J., McKenzie, J. E., Bossuyt, P. M., Boutron, I., Hoffmann, T. C., Mulrow, C. D., Shamseer, L., Tetzlaff, J. M., Akl, E. A., Brennan, S. E., Chou, R., Glanville, J., Grimshaw, J. M., Hróbjartsson, A., Lalu, M. M., Li, T., Loder, E. W., Mayo-Wilson, E., McDonald, S., … Moher, D. (2021). The PRISMA 2020 statement: An updated guideline for reporting systematic reviews. *BMJ*, n71. https://doi.org/10.1136/bmj.n71

Panda, R., Sciences, F., Pawankar, K. N., Sciences, A., Laishram, M., Sciences, F., & Debbarma, A. (2018). Advances in feeding management in cattle and buffalo -A review Author Info Advances in feeding management in cattle and buffalo – A review. *Res. Environ. Life Sci.*, *11*(1), 30–32.

Sarwar, M., Khan, M. A., Nisa, M., Bhatti, S. A., & Shahzad, M. A. (2009). Nutritional management for buffalo production. *Asian-Australasian Journal of Animal Sciences*, *22*(7), 1060–1068. https://doi.org/10.5713/ajas.2009.r.09

Shafin, N., Ismail, C. A. N., Mustafa, M. Z., Ghani, N., Ahmad, A. H., Othman, Z., Wijaya, A., & Zakaria, R. (2022). Thematic analysis of multiple sclerosis research by enhanced strategic diagram. *Multiple Sclerosis Journal*, *28*(14), 2160– 2170. https://doi.org/10.1177/13524585221075542

Van Kernebeek, H. R. J., Oosting, S. J., Van Ittersum, M. K., Bikker, P., & De Boer, I. J. M. (2016). Saving land to feed a growing population: consequences for consumption of crop and livestock products. *International Journal of Life Cycle Assessment*, *21*(5), 677–687. https://doi.org/10.1007/s11367-015-0923-6

Van Marle-Köster, E., & Visser, C. (2021). Unintended consequences of selection for increased production on the health and welfare of livestock. *Archives Animal Breeding*, *64*(1), 177–185. https://doi.org/10.5194/aab-64-177-2021

Technological Innovations in Tropical Livestock Development for Environmental Sustainability and Food Security – P. Dhian Isnaeni et al. (eds)
© 2025 The Author(s), ISBN 978-1-032-74373-8

Chemical composition of chicken nugget with different levels of yellow pumpkin (*Cucurbita moschata*) substitution

A.M. Tasse, H. Hafid*, I.N. Riko & A.B. Kimestri
Department of Animal Husbandry, Faculty of Animal Husbandry, Halu Oleo University, Indonesia

S.H. Ananda
Program Study Nutrition at STIKES Karya Kesehatan Kendari, Indonesia

ABSTRACT: This study aims to evaluate the substitution of pumpkin (*Cucurbita moschata*) with different levels on the chemical properties of chicken nuggets. This research was conducted at the Animal Product Processing Technology Laboratory, Faculty of Animal Husbandry, Halu Oleo University Kendari in March 2023. The design used in this study was a completely randomized design (CRD) consisting of 4 treatments and 5 replications. The treatment used was 100% chicken meat (T0), 95% chicken meat and 5% pumpkin (T1), 90% chicken meat and 10% pumpkin (T2) and 85% chicken meat and 15% pumpkin (T3). The variables of the chemical test research included the degree of acidity (pH), crude fat, water content and crude protein. The results showed that the quality of the chemical test, chicken nuggets had a significant effect on the degree of acidity (pH), water content and crude protein, but had no significant effect on crude fat of chicken nuggets. It can be concluded that the best treatment was chicken nugget with pumpkin substitution of 5% (T1).

Keywords: Chicken meat, pumpkin, chicken nugget, chemical test

1 INTRODUCTION

Meat is defined as all animal tissues in the form of parts of the carcass, organs and glands and all products resulting from the processing of these tissues which are edible and do not cause health problems to those who eat them. Meat is often processed to increase economic value, shelf life and public consumption tastes through diversification of products such as nuggets. Nugget is a processed chicken product that is printed, cooked and frozen, made from a mixture of ground chicken meat which is given a coating material with or without the addition of permitted food ingredients. Chicken nuggets are a product of meat processing technology food made from processed boneless chicken meat which is very popular with various age groups of consumers because it is easy and fast to serve, which has good nutritional value and an affordable price when compared to processed beef products (Petracci *et al.* 2013).

The nutritional content of chicken nuggets consists of protein, fat, carbohydrates and minerals. The protein that is owned comes from chicken meat which consists of quite complete amino acids. Even though it has a fairly complete and good nutritional content, chicken nuggets contain high fat and low fiber. Therefore, many studies have been carried out to increase the nutritional content of chicken nuggets such as substitution with other food ingredients, both to reduce fat content, increase fiber content and add a nutrient so that chicken nuggets have a better nutritional content. One way to increase the nutritional content of chicken nuggets is by

*Corresponding Author: harapin.hafid@uho.ac.id

DOI: 10.1201/9781003468943-36

substituting pumpkin. Yellow pumpkin (*Cucurbita moschata*) is a vegetable that contains a lot of β-carotene as a precursor of vitamin A and has a fairly high carbohydrate, protein and several minerals such as calcium, phosphorus and iron (Kim *et al.* 2014). The nutritional content of pumpkin is quite complete and the price is relatively cheap, so this pumpkin is a very potential material to be developed as a substitute for making chicken nuggets. Pumpkin can be made into flour and has good quality because it has good gelatinization properties so that it can provide good consistency, elasticity, viscosity and elasticity to the product (Ceclu *et al.* 2020).

Substitution of pumpkin as a filler can affect the physical and chemical properties of the nugget. Where the use of non-meat components in processed meat products can improve product quality and make these products healthier and the use of pumpkin (*Cucurbita moschata*) as a substitute for making noodles is expected to provide added value for the community. Based on this description, it is necessary to study the physical and chemical tests of chicken nugget with pumpkin (*Cucurbita moschata*) substitution at different levels.

2 MATERIALS AND METHODS

2.1 *Time and location of research*

This research was conducted from March to April 2023 at the Laboratory of Animal Product Technology Unit, Faculty of Animal Husbandry, Halu Oleo University, Kendari.

2.2 *Research materials*

The tools used in this study were trays, nugget molds, labels, knives, pans, stoves, blenders, sieves, scales, filters, spoons, pots and pans, baking sheets, cutting boards, pH, water baths, ovens, autoclaves, petri dishes, thermometers and plate. The materials to be used in this study consist of main materials and supporting materials. The main ingredient is broiler chicken meat. Supporting ingredients consist of pumpkin, cooking oil, garlic, salt, flour, pepper, flavoring, eggs, ice cubes and bread flour.

2.3 *Research procedure*

The process of making chicken nuggets begins with peeling the pumpkin and washing it clean so that there is no dirt attached to it. Furthermore, it is cut into dice-like shapes, this is so that when steaming it can be cooked evenly. Steaming is done for 10 minutes. After that, crush the pumpkin until smooth and store it in the freezer. Chicken is washed then filleting, then washed again. Then grind until smooth using a meat grinder. Mixing the dough, namely ground beef with other ingredients such as steamed pumpkin, flour, eggs, garlic, ground pepper, salt, sugar, and flavoring. Then mix well until the mixture is evenly mixed. Then the dough is printed and steamed for 45 minutes at ± 100°C, cooled to room temperature for 30 minutes. Chicken nuggets before being fried were analyzed physicochemical which included moisture content, fat content and protein content. Dip the nuggets in beaten egg white (batter) and then coat with breadcrumbs. Then stored first in the freezer (freezer) before frying. After that proceed with frying using the deep-frying method. Fried chicken nuggets were subjected to sensory analysis.

2.4 *Research design*

This study used a completely randomized design (CRD) with 4 treatments 5 replications in chemical tests. The treatments given were:

T0 = 100% chicken meat;
T1 = 95% chicken meat 5% pumpkin,
T2 = 90% chicken meat: 10% pumpkin
T3 = 85% chicken meat: 15% pumpkin

2.5 *Statistical analysis*

All statistical analysis were performed using SPSS 16. In order to determine the differences in nutrient content among treatment, one-way ANOVA test was performed, followed by post-hoc test (Duncan's multiple range test) to compare means. P value <0.05 was considered significant.

2.6 *Research variable*

The parameters observed in this study were chemical quality (pH, crude fat, water content and crude protein). All of these methods are measured by the AOAC method.

3 RESULTS AND DISCUSSION

The chemical test results for pH, crude fat, water content and crude protein for substitution of chicken nugget with pumpkin (*Cucurbita moschata*) at different levels are presented in Table 1.

Table 1. Average chemical quality pH, fat content, water content and crude protein.

Variable	Treatment				Indonesian Standard
	T0	T1	T2	T3	
pH	$6.84^{a} \pm 0.05$	$6.76^{a} \pm 0.54$	$6.84^{b} \pm 0.05$	$6.86^{b} \pm 0.05$	6–7
Crude fat (%)	18.17 ± 1.38	19.56 ± 1.73	18.86 ± 1.31	19.74 ± 1.24	Max. 60
Moisture content (%)	$8.28^{a} \pm 1.05$	$10.91^{b} \pm 0.97$	$10.97^{b} \pm 1.76$	$11.40^{b} \pm 2.00$	Max. 9
Crude protein (%)	$12.15^{b} \pm 0.05$	$11.96^{b} \pm 0.84$	$11.93^{b} \pm 0.37$	$9.13^{a} \pm 0.17$	Max. 20

Note: Different superscripts in the same line show a significant difference (P<0.05).

3.1 *pH*

Table 1 shows that the mean degree of acidity (pH) of chicken nugget with the addition of pumpkin in treatment T0 was significantly different from treatment T1 but not significantly different from treatment T2 and T3. The pH value of chicken nugget with pumpkin substitution at different levels showed a normal pH value of 6.76–6.86. This is in accordance with the SNI ranged from 6–7. Kariang *et al.* (2023) in his research said that the pH value of chicken nuggets with the addition of broccoli ranged from 6.30 to 6.85. The pH value of the basic ingredients used can affect the pH value in each different treatment. The pH value of the basic ingredients results in a change in the pH value of the nuggets (Laksmi *et al.* 2012). This occurs due to a change in the hydrogen balance in the nuggets as a result of the pH value of the base material used in making the nuggets. Mixing the ingredients creates a new hydrogen balance point in the nugget. Yashari *et al.* (2019) also added that changes in the structural composition of restructuring meat in its function as meat protein have been shown to affect the pH of the resulting product.

3.2 *Crude fat*

The average crude fat obtained in this study ranged from 18.71–19.74%. The 15% pumpkin substitution treatment showed high crude fat, namely 19.74%, while the treatment without the addition of pumpkin showed low crude fat, namely 18.71%. This is due to the fact that pumpkin contains fat of 0.18% so substituting a certain amount of pumpkin for chicken nuggets will further increase the fat content of the resulting nuggets (Gumolung 2019). The fat that can be contained in chicken nuggets is a maximum of 20% (Lestario *et al.* 2012). From Table 1. the fat content in the chicken nugget produced from all treatments is lower than the SNI quality standard.

The high fat content can be expected because of the basic ingredients used in making nuggets. In addition, the decrease and increase in fat content is thought to be influenced by the processing process. The fat on the nuggets will melt during the steaming process. steaming meat can use medium or moderate heating, namely a temperature of 58°C to 75°C. This is what causes the fat content to have a real difference. Yuliana *et al.* (2013) explained that fat melts during cooking. During cooking, not much marbling fat is separated from the muscles because shrinkage of the meat is minimal, while meat juices and flavors are maximally released during mastication along with some of the free water from the meat.

3.3 *Moisture content*

The average moisture content of chicken nuggets with the addition of pumpkin in treatment T0 was significantly different from treatment T3 but not significantly different to treatments T1 and T2. For each nugget mixture added with pumpkin, it can be seen that the water content produced has a high value compared to the nugget mixture without addition. One of the factors that affect the increase in water content in a product is the nutrient content of the main ingredients and additional ingredients such as pumpkin. According to Rif'an *et al.* (2017), the increased water content in chicken nuggets was caused by pumpkin containing pectin which is able to bind water better than starch in wheat flour. Even though it has been made into flour, the pectin in pumpkin is not damaged, it can even bind water well. In addition, the increase in water content in chicken nuggets is also influenced by the high fiber content in pumpkin. Apart from that, the length of boiling time is also an aspect that can affect the water content of the nuggets. Shamsuri and Ahmad (2019) states that the water content from administering (*C. Maxima*) in 10 minutes of steaming produces a high moisture content, namely 82.11%.

3.4 *Crude protein*

Table 1 shows that the mean crude protein value of chicken nugget with pumpkin substitution in treatment T0 was significantly different from treatment T3 but not significantly different from treatment T1 and T2. The average crude protein obtained in this study ranged from 9.13–12.15%. There was a tendency to decrease protein levels with increasing pumpkin substitution. This is because pumpkin contains quite high protein, which is equal to 4.28% Dewi and Minah (2020) so that with increasing levels of substitution, the protein content also increases. The use of ingredients with high protein content can increase the protein content of food stuffs (Lestario *et al.* 2012). A small amount of animal protein can improve the quality of vegetable protein in large quantities (BSN 2014). According to Widyastuti *et al.* (2010) the protein content that can be contained in chicken nuggets is at least 9%, so that chicken nuggets with the addition of pumpkin in this study met SNI standards.

4 CONCLUSION

The chemical composition of chicken nuggets with 5% -15% substitution of yellow pumpkin (*cucurbita maxima*) meets SNI 6683-2015 concerning chicken nuggets, and the best result were found in the 5% treatment (T1).

ACKNOWLEDGEMENT

The authors send their gratitude to Halu Oleo University for the funding of this research.

REFERENCES

AOAC International. 2000. *Official Methods of Analysis of AOAC International*. 17th ed. Arlington: AOAC International: google scholar.

Badan Standarisasi Nasional. 2014. Syarat Mutu nugget. *SNI* 7758. Badan Standarisasi Nasional, Jakarta.

Ceclu L., D.G. Mocanu, O.V. Nistor. 2020. Pumpkin-Health Benefits. *Journal of Agroalimentary Processing and Technologies*. 26(3):241–246.

Dewi RK dan FN Minah. 2020. Penentuan kadar protein pada spirulina platensis menggunakan metode lowry dan kjeldah. *Jurnal Teknik Kimia*. 15(1): 40–45.

Gumolung D. 2019. Analisis proksimat tepung daging buah labu kuning (Cucurbita moschata). *SS Fullerene Journal of Chemistry*. 4(1): 8–11.

Kim M.Y., E.J. Kim, Y.N. Kim, C. Choi, B.H. Lee. 2012. Comparison of The Chemical Composition and Nutritive Value of Pumpkin (*Cucurbitaceae*) Species and Parts. *Nutr Res Pract*. 6(1):21–27. doi:10.4162/nrp.2012.6.1.21.

Laksmi RT, AM Legowo dan K Kusrahayu. 2012. Daya ikat air, pH dan sifat organoleptik chicken nugget yang disubstitusi dengan telur rebus. *Animal agriculture journal*. 1(1): 453–460.

Lestario LN, M Susilowati dan Y Martono. 2012. Pemanfaatan Tepung Labu Kuning sebagai Bahan Fotifikasi Mie Basah. *Prosiding*. 18:182–189.

Petracci M., M. Bionchi, S. Mudalal, C. Cavani. 2013. Functional Ingredients for Poultry Meat Products. *Trends Food Sci. Technol*. 33(1):27–39.

Rif'an, Nurrahman dan S Aminah. 2017. The influence of kind of dryer instrument to physical characteristics, chemistry and organoleptic of pumpkin soup instant. *Jurnal Pangan dan Gizi*. 7(2): 104–116.

Shamsuri N.M., & F.T. Ahmad. 2019. Effect of Different Cooking Methods and Time Interval on Phisico-Cemical and Antioxidant Properties of Golden Pumpkin (*Cucurbita maxima*). *Malays. Apple. Biol*. 48 (1):221–227.

Widyastuti ES, AS Widati, RD Hanjariyanto dan MY Avianto. 2010. Kualitas nugget ayam dengan penambahan keju gouda. *Jurnal Ilmu dan Teknologi Hasil Ternak*. 1–10.

Yashari R, N Nurhaedah, F Fitriani dan I.D Novieta. 2019. Uji organoleptik dan nilai ph bakso daging kerbau yang ditambahkan karagenan (Eucheuma cottonii). In *Prosiding Seminar Nasional Sinergitas Multidisiplin ILmu Pengetahuan dan Teknologi*. 2: 267–271.

Yuliana N, YB Pramono dan A Hintono. 2013. Kadar lemak, kekenyalan dan cita rasa nugget ayam yang disubstitusi dengan hati ayam broiler. *Animal Agriculture Journal*. 2(1): 301–308.

Technological Innovations in Tropical Livestock Development for Environmental Sustainability and Food Security – P. Dhian Isnaeni et al. (eds)

The contribution of *Lactobacillus acidophilus* in improving the antimicrobial ability of bifidus milk

Yurliasni*, E. Mariana, Z. Hanum, R.R.B. Pasaribu & D. Pratiwi
Laboratory of Milk Science and Technology, Faculty of Agriculture, Syiah Kuala University, Darussalam-Banda Aceh, Indonesia

ABSTRACT: Indigestion is one of the health problems that is still often encountered in society. Using fermented goat's milk containing probiotics is one alternative to overcome digestive problems. This research aimed to look at the contribution of *Lactobacillus acidophilus* in improving the antimicrobial ability of Bifidus milk as a probiotic milk to the growth of *Salmonella sp and Escherichia coli.* This research was conducted using a completely randomized design (CRD) consisting of 5 (five) treatments, namely P1 = 1%: 4%, P2 = 2%: 3%, P3 = 2.5%: 2.5%, P4 = 3%: 2%, P5 = 4%: 1%. Each treatment consisted of 4 replications so 20 were obtained from the experimental unit. Parameters measured are pH, total plate count (TPC), and the ability of antimicrobials to inhibit *Salmonella sp* and *Escherichia coli.* The results show that the pH and TPC of bifidus milk, namely 4.08–4.18 and 8.52 to 8.89 log CFU/ml respectively, are still within the SNI range. The width of the resulting zone of inhibition that the antimicrobials contained in bifidus milk are weak in inhibiting *Salmonella* and *E. coli.* It can be concluded that the contribution of *L. acidophilus* is not significant

Keywords: Bifidus milk, antimicrobial, fermented milk, zone inhibition

1 INTRODUCTION

Improper lifestyle and eating habits have a significant impact on a person's quality of life. It is closely associated with the development of several diseases that can affect the productivity of affected people, such as Indigestion, high cholesterol, and colon cancer. Based on information from the World Health Organization (WHO), statistically 68% of deaths worldwide are caused by cancer, heart disease, respiratory diseases, and diabetes (WHO 2020). One way to prevent this disorder is by consuming healthy foods and drinks, such as probiotic drinks.

A probiotic drink is a functional health drink that contains live microorganisms (probiotics) and has health benefits. Probiotics themselves are live bacteria that can impact health by balancing the microbiome in the gut, and preventing and selecting dysfunctional microorganisms (Primurdia & Kusnadi 2014).

Bifidobacterium milk is a type of probiotic milk that is currently in high demand as a healthy alternative beverage with beneficial effects on the gastrointestinal tract. Antibacterials of bifidus milk can be differentiated based on their mechanism of action, namely antibacterials that inhibit cell wall growth, antibacterials that cause changes in cell membrane permeability or inhibit active transport through the cell membrane, antibacterials that inhibit protein synthesis, and antibacterials that inhibit cell nucleic acid synthesis (Hanum *et al.* 2017). The mechanism of antibacterial action can occur in five ways:

*Corresponding Author: yurliasni@usk.ac.id

 DOI: 10.1201/9781003468943-37

inhibition of cell wall synthesis, changes in cell permeability, changes in nucleic acid molecules, inhibition of enzyme action, and inhibition of nucleic acid and protein synthesis. However, based on early studies (Yurliasni 2021), the antibacterial capacity of bifidus milk against some pathogens appears to be still suboptimal. Therefore, this study aims to optimize the antibacterial ability of Bifidobacterium milk by cooperating with *L. acidophilus* in a multistep combination.

2 MATERIALS AND METHODS

2.1 *Acidity (pH) of bifidus milk*

Acidity (pH) tests are performed using a pH meter pre-calibrated with pH 4, 7, and 9 buffers. Next, clean the electrode with an aqueous solution and dry air. Add 10 ml and insert the pH meter electrode into the sample's beaker. The pH value displayed on the pH meter is then recorded, after which the electrode is cleaned with distilled water and dried with a tissue before the next sample is inserted (Wahyudi2006).

2.2 *Total Plate Count (TPC)*

The TPC test was performed using the cast plate method (Wahyu *et al.* 2012). A 1 mL sample was taken and added to 9 ml of distilled water (10^{-1}). The dilution is then performed aseptically. Dilutions from 10^{-1} to 10^{-7} were made, then 1 ml of the suspension from the 10-7 dilution was inoculated into Petri dishes and MRSA medium was added. The Petri dish was then rotated clockwise to homogenize the bacterial suspension and agar medium. After the agar solidified, the petri dishes were incubated for 48 h at 37°C in an inverted position. The colony count by

$$\text{TPC (CFU/mL)} = (\text{Number of colony bacteria grown X1})/(\text{Dilution}).$$

2.3 *Antimicrobial test*

Antibacterial tests were conducted using the disk diffusion method. Collect one loop of *E. coli* and one loop of Salmonella using a loop needle. A dose of E. coli was then added to the 10^{-1} to 10^{-2} dilution and Salmonella was added to the 10^{-1} to 10^{-2} dilution. in a dilution of 10^{-1} to 10^{-3} (Pelczar and Chan 2008). Next, 1 ml of each bacterial suspension was inoculated into NA (nutrient agar), homogenized by gently rotating the beaker, and allowed to stand until the medium solidified. Paper discs were immersed in the samples for 30 min. Place the soaked paper disc onto the agar surface using sterile tweezers. Stick the disc paper to the agar by pressing lightly with tweezers. Antibiotics like chloramphenicol discs and tetracycline discs were also used as positive controls. It was then incubated at 37°C for 24 hours. The area of the formed inhibition zone is measured with a ruler and calculated using the following formula

Inhibition zone area = $(DV + DH) / ((2) - X)$

Description: DV: Vertical diameter

DH: Horizontal diameter

X: Diameter of the paper disc.

2.4 *Data analysis*

The data obtained were analyzed using ANOVA, and if there were differences, continued with Duncan's multiple range test. Descriptive analysis is used for antimicrobial ability on pathogens.

3 RESULTS AND DISCUSSION

3.1 *pH of bifidus milk added with lactobacillus acidophilus*

Analysis of variance showed that the combination of starter cultures *Bifidobacterium longum* and *Lactobacillus acidophilus* had no significant effect on the pH of fermented milk (P~0.05). These two bacteria are thought to be able to optimally hydrolyze lactose as an energy source during the fermentation process. Rochman and Fardiaz (1990) stated that acidity can increase during the fermentation process, resulting in a decrease in pH. This is confirmed by Chou and Weimer (1999) who found that increased lactic acid production by LAB affected the acidity (pH) of fermented milk products. The acid produced by lactic acid bacteria converts lactose into glucose and galactose, lowering the pH of milk. The addition of the starter *Bifidobacterium longum* tends to further reduce the pH value. The addition of an additional *Bifidobacterium longum* starter resulted in a lower pH of 4.098. This is probably because Bifidobacteria produce multiple organic acids, namely lactic acid and acetic acid. *Bifidobacterium longum* also produces other flavor compounds such as acetaldehyde, formic acid, acid, succinate, acetone, acetoin, and diacetyl. These may play a role in lowering pH.

Table 1. Average of bifidus milk composition with *Lactobacillus acidophilus*.

	Comparison Level of *B. longum and L. acidophilus*				
Parameter	1:4	2:3	2.5:2.5	3:2	4:1
pH	4.12 ± 0.06	4.14 ± 0.04	4.18 ± 0.05	4.11 ± 0.06	4.09 ± 0.06
TPC CFU/mL	8.53 ± 0.18	8.52 ± 0.025	8.59 ± 0.17	8.75 ± 0.09	8.89 ± 0.21
Zone of inhibition (mm)					
Salmonella sp	0.70 ± 0.00	0.70 ± 0.00	1.06 ± 0.71	0.70 ± 0.00	0.99 ± 0.58
E. coli	0.99 ± 0.33	1.36 ± 0.16	1.23 ± 0.00	1.27 ± 0.09	1.33 ± 0.10

Note: different superscripts in rows and columns are significantly different (P < 0.05) of the mean of pH (P < 0.01), Total Plate Count of Bifidus Milk.

The number of LAB populations measured in this study exceeded the minimum standard for fermented milk. The minimum requirement for a good total LAB value in fermented milk is 1.0 x 10^6 CFU/ml (SNI 7552: 2018). According to Fuller (1992), the number of lactic acid bacteria good for health and consumption is 10^6-10^9 CFU/ml. Based on the results of a study on goat milk fermentation using a combination of *Bifidobacterium longum* and *Lactobacillus acidophilus*, all LABs obtained have been shown to meet the minimum standards of SNI 7552: 2018. Proliferated total BAL ranged from 8.52 to 8.89 log CFU/mL. An indicator of the microbiological quality of fermented milk can be seen from the increase in the number of LAB populations. Positive interactions occur with some strains of probiotic bacteria, such as *Lactobacillus acidophilus* and *Bifidobacterium longum* (Tamime 2005). This indicates that *Lactobacillus acidophilus* and *Bifidobacterium longum* do not inhibit each other. The growth of the maximum number of bacterial cells is influenced by the availability of nutrients in the medium. The starter combination of *Bifidobacterium longum* and *Lactobacillus acidophilus* did not affect TPC due to the limited nutrient content of each treatment.

Bifidobacterium longum and *L. acidophilus* utilize only the nutrients in goat milk. According to Aziza *et al.* (2013): The successful growth of lactic acid bacteria in fermented milk depends on the availability of nutrients in the growth medium. Another reason why the combination of starters from *Bifidobacterium longum* and *Lactobacillus acidophilus* does not affect the TPC of fermented goat milk. According to Jundi *et al.* (2015) combining *Bifidobacterium longum* and *Lactobacillus acidophilus* starter at a ratio of 1: 4 to 10% had a real effect on the total bacterial count in fermented goat milk. Mahdian and Tehrani (2007) also explained that bacterial growth is influenced by several factors such as milk composition, temperature, inoculum amount, incubation time, and milk cooling time. Afidah and Trimulyono (2019) stated that to produce good quality fermented milk, proper starter culture, availability of nutrients in the fermentation medium, and milk quality should be considered.

3.2 *Antimicrobial on Salmonella sp and E. coli*

Fermented goat milk, which is a combination of *Bifidobacterium longum and Lactobacillus acidophilus* starter, has a weak antibacterial effect. The area of the inhibition zone formed is 0.707 to 1.061 mm. Antimicrobial metabolites produced by *Bifidobacterium longum* and Lactobacillus acidophilus have a relatively weak ability to damage the cell walls of Salmonella spp., and therefore cannot optimally kill these pathogens. This weak antibacterial power is supported by the very strong composition of the Salmonella cell wall, which increases its resistance to the bioactive compounds produced. Differences in the susceptibility of Gram-negative bacteria to antibiotics may be influenced by the structure of the bacterial cell wall. According to Syarifah *et al.* (2018), the cell walls of Gram-negative bacteria such as Salmonella are more complex and layered and do not contain teichoic acids, one of the bacteriocin receptors, making them more resistant. In addition, the outer cell membrane is protected and acts as an effective barrier against certain bacteriocins.

The combined treatment with *Bifidobacterium longum* and *Lactobacillus acidophilus* did not significantly affect the area of the inhibition zone formed by *E. coli,* as shown by the area of the inhibition zone from 0.99 to 1.36 mm. This indicates that the antibacterial inhibitory effect of fermented goat milk is in the weak category. According to Alakomi *et al.* (2006), this weak inhibitory effect is because E. coli is a Gram-negative bacterium with a polysaccharide cell wall that acts as a protection, and the activity of metabolic compounds that degrade the cell wall of this pathogen is not optimal. The activities of *Bifidobacterium longum and Lactobacillus acidophilus* act synergistically and exhibit antibacterial activity against *Escherichia coli.*

The inhibition zone formed indicates whether the pathogenic bacteria are resistant to the compounds produced by her LAB. When inhibiting *E. coli*, the combination of all starters forms an inhibition zone. This means that *E. coli* cannot grow or is prevented from growing due to the presence of antibacterial compounds made from a combination of probiotic bacterial acids, one of the bacteriocin receptors, makes *E. coli* is more resistant as it is unable to grow or is prevented from growing.

Another reason why the starter combination of *Bifidobacterium longum* and *Lactobacillus acidophilus* lacks antibacterial inhibitory effect against E. coli is that the LAB metabolism has not yet reached the stationary phase due to the suboptimal incubation time of fermented goat milk. The incubation time of fermented goat milk in this study was 18 h. This means that the metabolites produced from the starter combination are suboptimal and the resulting inhibitory effect is relatively weak. According to Hadadji and Bensoltane (2006), the peak number of starter combinations appeared after 24 h of incubation. Rahmiati and Mumpuni (2017) found that the size of the inhibition zones that lactic acid bacteria form against pathogens depends on the ability of the bacterial isolate to produce hydrolytic enzymes, the age of the bacterial culture, the number of enzymes produced, and the composition of the medium, and incubation time.

4 CONCLUSION

It can be concluded that fermented goat milk (Bifidus milk) combined with *Bifidobacterium longum* and *Lactobacillus acidophilus* starters does not affect the total bacterial count and the ability to stimulate *Salmonella sp* growth but inhibits *E. coli*. The inhibitory effect caused by the starter formulation in Bifidus milk falls into the weak category.

REFERENCES

Af'idah, F. and Trimulyono, G. 2019. Uji aktivitas antioksidan dan kadar asam laktat yoghurt tempe kedelai (*glycine max*) dan yoghurt tempe kacang hijau (*Vigna radiata*). *LenteraBio*, 8(1), pp. 17–24.

Alakomi, H. L., Paananen, A., Suihko, M. L., Helander, I. M. and Saarela. 2017. Weakening effect of cell permeabilizers on gram-negative bacteria causing biodeterioration. *Environmental Microbiology*, 72(7), pp. 4695–4703.

Azizah, N., Pramono, Y. B. and Abduh, S. B. M. 2013. Sifat Fisik, Organoleptik, dan kesukaan yogurt drink dengan penambahan ekstrak buah nangka. *Jurnal Aplikasi Teknologi Pangan*, 2(3), pp. 148–151

Fuller, R. 1992. *Probiotics*. London: Champman and Hill.

Hadadji, M. and Bensoltane, A. 2006. Growth and lactic acid production by *Bifidobacterium longum* and *Lactobacillus acidophilus* in goat's milk. *African Journal of Biotechnology*, 5(6), pp. 505–509.

Hadiwiyoto, S. 2009. *Teori dan Prosedur Pengujian Mutu Susu dan Olahannya: Teknik Uji Mutu Susu*. 2 ed. Yogyakarta: Liberty.

Hanum, Z., Rastina dan Wanniatie, V. 2017. Kemampuan antibakteri susu fermentasi terhadap *Escherichia coli* dan Shigella flexneri. *Agripet*, 17(1), pp. 24–30.

Mahdian, E. and Tehrani, M. M. 2007. Evaluation the effect of milk total solids on the relationship between growth and activity of starter cultures and quality of concentrated yoghurt. *American-Eurasian J. Agric and Eviron Sci*, 2(5), pp. 587–589

Pelczar, M. J. and Chan, E. 2008. *Dasar-Dasar Mikrobiologi* 1. Jakata: Universitas Indonesia Press.

Rahmiati and Mumpuni, M. 2017. Eksplorasi Bakteri Asam Laktat Kandidat Probiotik dan Potensinya dalam Menghambat Bakteri Patogen. *Journal of Islamic Science and Technology*, 3(2), pp. 141–150.

Standar Nasional Indonesia. 2018. *SNI 7552:2018 Minuman Susu Fermentasi*, Badan Standardisasi Nasional.

Steel, R. G. and Torrie, J. H. 1995. *Prinsip dan Prosedur Statistika*. Jakarta: PT Gramedia Pustaka Utama.

Syarifah, R., Harris, F. A. Erina, A. S. and Winaruddin, 2018. Uji daya hambat ekstrak biji buah pala (*myristica fragrans houtt*) terhadap pertumbuhan bakteri *Escherichia coli*. *Jurnal Ilmiah Mahasiswa Veteriner*, 2(3), pp. 361–372.

Tamime, A. 2005. *Probiotic dairy products*. Ayr: Blackwell Publishing.

Wahyu, S. S., Julaikha, S., Suranto, Lorentina, Y., Sopian, Y. and Arfah, Z. Y., 2012. *Pengujian total bakteri/ total plate count (TPC)*, Jakarta: Departemen Pendidikan Nasional.

Yurliasni, Novita, C. I., Hanum, Z. and Latif, H. 2021. *Optimizing the quality and antimicrobial ability of yogurt through a combination of starter and dates puree at different levels*. IOP Conference Series, Earth, and Environmental Science.

Technological Innovations in Tropical Livestock Development for Environmental Sustainability and Food Security – P. Dhian Isnaeni et al. (eds)

Added value analysis of aren sugar and granulated aren sugar processing in Rejang Lebong regency, Bengkulu province

F. Rosbarnawan, Y. Evendi, N. Gultom, Harwindah & R. Wati
Development Planning Agency at Sub-National Level Province of Bengkulu, Indonesia

T. Hidayat, E. Fauzi*, T. Rahman, Afrizon & A. Ishak
National Research and Innovation Agency of Indonesia

ABSTRACT: Sugar aren plants from male bunches in the form of sap are generally processed into aren sugar which produces added value for processors. This research aims to compare the added value obtained from processing aren sugar and granulated aren sugar. The research was carried out from August to September 2023 in Rejang Lebong Regency, Bengkulu Province. Data was collected through interviews regarding input, labour, output, and selling prices for small and medium businesses of aren sugar and granulated aren sugar processing in "Kampung Aren" Rejang Lebong. The analysis was carried out descriptively using the Hayami value-added method. The analysis results show that the added value from the production process in the sap processing business into aren sugar is IDR 950 -/kg. Meanwhile, the added value of processing aren sugar into granulated aren sugar is IDR 10,000/kg. The comparison of the increase in added value between processing sap into aren sugar and processing granulated aren sugar into granulated aren sugar is 1.052,63%. This shows that the increase in added value will be greater if derivative products are produced from a commodity.

1 INTRODUCTION

Aren (*Arenga pinnata Mer.*) is a type of palm that has high economic value because all parts of the aren plant ranging from roots to leaves can be utilized (Fatsan *et al.* 2020). Aren sap or Nira is the main product of the aren palm plant. Nira productivity differs based on the type of aren plant. Aren Dalam has a trunk height $\geq$ 10 m, a production age of 8 – 10 years, with nira production > 20 litres/mang per day and produces 10–15 mayangs/tree. While the Genjah Aren has a stem height of 3 – 4 m, with a production age of 5 – 6 years, and nira production of $\pm$ 12 l/mayang/day with mayang production of 6 – 8/tree (Laksananny & Pujirahayu 2017).

Down streaming is very important because it can increase the added value of products and provide wider market opportunities. By processing products to become more valuable, the selling price of products can be increased and provide greater profits for producers. Value added is the increase in the value of a commodity because it undergoes processing, transport, or storage in production. Processing will change the shape and composition of raw materials. In the processing process, value-added can be defined as the difference between the value of the product and the cost of raw materials and other inputs, excluding labour. Meanwhile, the

*Corresponding Author: emlan.81@gmail.com

DOI: 10.1201/9781003468943-38

margin is the difference between the value of the product and the price of raw materials only. This margin includes the components of the production factors used, namely labour, other inputs, and processing entrepreneur fees (Hayami *et al.* 1989).

The greater added value of a product can certainly play a role in economic growth. Large economic growth certainly has an impact on increasing business opportunities and community income which leads to an increase in community welfare (Zaini *et al.* 2019). Various research results show that the added value of processed aren products is obtained from aren sugar and granulated aren sugar products. The added value of aren sugar is high with a ratio of 41.00% to 79.96% (Bustam & Sabrab 2021; Faliha *et al.* 2022; Gobel *et al.* 2022; Marpaung & Siburian, 2023; Putra *et al.* 2020). The high added value of processing nira into aren sugar shows that the price of nira harvested by farmers from aren plants is low compared to the price of aren sugar. The production process of aren sugar is relatively cheap so it becomes the main product of aren trees that are widely cultivated by the community. Meanwhile, granulated aren sugar has a relatively smaller added value. The added value of granulated aren sugar reaches 18.18% (Miftah *et al.* 2018).

The processing of aren products is still carried out with simple technology which results in the quality of the 'technology. Improvements in technology will increase added value (Simarmata 2019). Production continuity is also one of the factors that affect price fluctuations of aren processing products. The processing of aren products at the farm level has not been able to maintain production continuity because there is no partnership with the business/industry world so it increases business risk (Melly *et al.* 2019). Partnerships will increase market opportunities that positively affect the innovation of aren products (Sultan *et al.* 2020). The role of the government in the development of aren sugar marketing is needed to improve product quality to produce added value (Astuti *et al.* 2019).

The processing of aren sugar into granulated aren sugar in Rejang Lebong Regency has not yet developed, while the source of raw materials is quite available. Currently, aren sap is only processed into aren sugar, so it does not provide significant added value. Processing to increase added value is not easy to do. Large investments and careful research are required to process the product into more valuable products. In addition, infrastructure and supportive government policies are also important factors in the process. For this reason, it is necessary to study the added value and margin of aren products in small and medium industries in the Rejang Lebong district to obtain information related to processed aren products that have the best potential for downstream. This study was conducted to identify the processing process and analyse the income of aren sugar and granulated aren sugar processing business actors and determine the added value generated from processing nira into aren sugar and aren sugar into granulated aren sugar in the Sari Aren group of Air Meles Atas village, North Curup subdistrict, Rejang Lebong Regency.

2 MATERIALS AND METHODS

The research was carried out from August to October 2023 in Rejang Lebong Regency, Bengkulu Province. The data collected includes primary data and secondary data. Data collection was carried out through individual interviews involving 5 palm sugar processors and 1 granulated aren sugar processor. Primary data taken regarding aren sugar processing business data includes input, output, production costs, product prices, labour and profits for industrial players/small and medium businesses who process sap into aren sugar and granulated aren sugar. Meanwhile, secondary data was obtained from literature books, journals and agencies related to this research.

The data analysis method used in this research is a value-added analysis using the Hayami method, then descriptively analysed to explain the added value and profit margin of the aren products produced. The procedure for calculating the added value of products using the Hayami method is presented in Table 1.

Table 1. Procedure for calculating the value added of products using the Hayami method (Hayami *et al.* 1989).

Variable	Code
I. Output, Input and Price	
1. Output (Kg)	(1)
2. Input (Kg)	(2)
3. Labour (DPW)	(3)
4. Conversion factor	(4) = (1)/(2)
5. Labour coefficient (DPW)	(5) = (3)/(2)
6. Output Price (Rp/Kg)	(6)
7. Direct labour cost (Rp/ DPW)	(7)
II. Revenue and Profit	
8. Raw material price (Rp/Kg)	(8)
9. Other Input Contributions (Rp/Kg)	(9)
10. Output Value (Rp/Kg)	(10) = (4) × (6)
11. a. Added Value (Rp/Kg)	(11a) = (10) – (9) – (8)
b. Added value ratio (%)	(11b) = (11a)/(10) × 100%
12. a. Direct labour revenue (Rp/Kg)	(12a) = (5) × (7)
b. Labour share (%)	(12b) = (12a)/(11a) × 100%
13. a. Profit (Rp/Kg)	(13a) = (11a) – (12a)
b. Profit rate (%)	(13 b) = (13a)/(11a) × 100%
III. Return for production factors owner	
14. Margin (Rp/Kg)	(14) = (10) – (8)
a. Direct labour income (%)	(14a) = (12a)/(14) × 100%
b. Other Input Contributions (%)	(14b) = (9)/(14) × 100%
c. Company Owner's Profit (%)	(14c) = (13a)/(14) × 100%

Source: Hayami *et al.* (1989).

The analysis model used to determine the income of aren sugar processing agroindustry business is (Soekartawi 2006):

$$\pi = TR - TC \tag{1}$$

where:

$$TR = P \times Q \tag{2}$$

$$TC = FC + VC \tag{3}$$

Π = Revenue (Rp)
TR = Total revenue (Rp)
TC = Total cost (Rp)

3 RESULTS AND DISCUSSION

3.1 *Aren product processing business in "Kampung Aren"*

Kampung aren is an aren processing centre located in Air Meles Atas Village, Selupu Rejang Sub-district, Rejang Lebong Regency. The source of raw materials in the aren village is very abundant because more than 80% or around 350 people have aren plantations and process the juice into aren sugar. The average production of aren sugar is 10 kg/kk/day, with a total production of 10,500 kg/month. Since 2010, in this aren village, an aren processing business group named Sari Aren has been established with various aren products such as aren sugar and granulated aren sugar. The Sari Aren processing business group currently consists of 60 members of aren sugar processors in the aren village with a production capacity of 600 kg of aren sugar per day so that in one month 18,000 kg is produced. Meanwhile, the production of granulated aren sugar is 2,520 kg/month.

Aren agribusiness in the aren village increases the added value of the products produced. Aren sugar is processed from nira and granulated aren sugar is processed from high quality aren sugar. The aren sugar produced in the aren village is marketed to meet the demand both in the local market in Bengkulu Province, as well as the regional markets of neighbouring provinces such as South Sumatra Province, Jambi Province, Riau Province, and Lampung Province. Meanwhile, granulated aren sugar is marketed to almost all provinces in Indonesia. Product marketing is adjusted to customer demand. The aren sugar processing business is carried out by each group member, while the granulated aren sugar processing is carried out by the Sari Aren group. The Sari Aren group was formed to increase the scale of production, product diversification, and improve the quality of aren products following market demand.

The market prospect of aren sugar is very potential with prices that tend to be stable. The price of aren sugar from farmers is sold from Rp. 12,000/kg to 14,000/kg according to the quality of the sugar product produced. Improvements in the quality of aren sugar have led to an increase in prices at the level of aren sugar processors by Rp. 2,000/kg to Rp. 3,000/kg. While in the market, the average price of sugar is Rp. 15,000/kg to Rp. 18,000/kg, even in certain months it can even reach a price of Rp. 22,000/kg. The increase in the price of aren sugar is determined by the length or shortness of the marketing channel (Prihantini *et al.* 2022).

3.2 *Processing of aren sugar and granulated aren sugar in Kampung Aren*

The processing of high-quality aren sugar starts from the nira tapping process. The average aren farmer produces 10 kg of aren sugar per day from 70 litres of nira tapped from 12 aren trees. The processing of aren sugar is done by family farmers who on average have 15–20 aren trees. Nira tapping is done in the morning and afternoon, while aren sugar processing is done in the morning after tapping in the morning. The process of aren sugar processing by farmers in the aren village is shown in Figure 1.

The sap that is processed into aren sugar is the result of previous tapping. The nira is filtered and then put into a cauldron which is then cooked in a furnace using wood fuel. Cooking is carried out for 5–6 hours until the nira water thickens. After saturation, it continues to be stirred while cooling and then inserted into the mould. Generally, the mould used is coconut shell. The moulded aren sugar is packed in plastic sacks before being sold. The thing that needs to be considered in the process of processing nira into aren sugar is that during the cooking and cooling process, the cooking temperature is controlled in such a way that it burns.

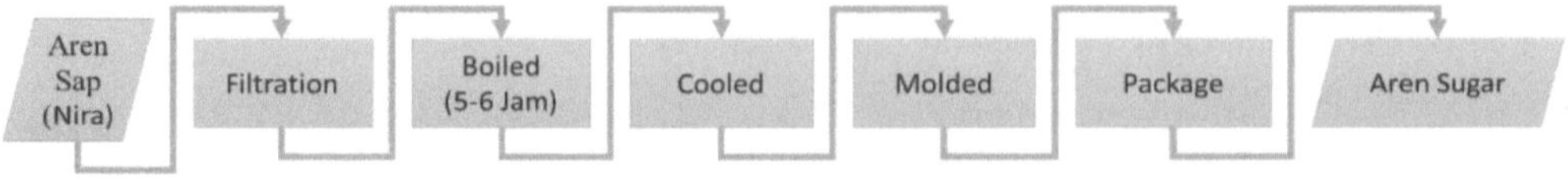

Figure 1. Aren sugar processing process.

Granulated aren sugar is processed from high-quality aren sugar. The raw material is selected from aren sugar with a brownish colour and crumb texture. The quality of aren sugar is determined by various factors, namely the quality of the nira used, the cooking temperature and the cooking time of the nira (Haloho & Susanto 2015; Winarno 2002). The processing of aren sugar uses tools and machines as shown in Figure 2

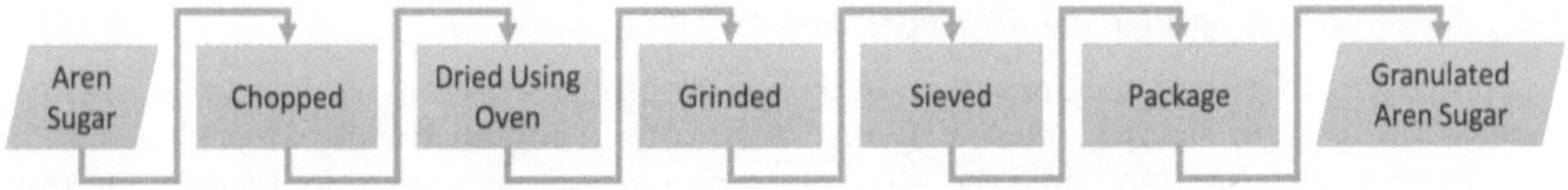

Figure 2. Processing of granulated aren sugar.

The Sari Aren business group uses high-quality aren sugar as raw material. The aren sugar from group members is selected and then chopped using a chopping machine. After chopping, the aren sugar is spread on a drying rack and then baked for approximately 1 hour. After that, it is cooled, then mashed using a grinding machine then sieved and packaged in the form of 7 g sachets, 250 g, 400 g and 1,000 g pouches.

3.3 *Added value of aren sugar processing*

The results of the calculation of the added value of aren sugar processing business in the aren village of Rejang Lebong Regency, Bengkulu Province with the raw material of nira is harvested on the farmer's land. The number of workers in one production process is 1 person with 70 litres of nira raw material that can produce 10 kg of aren sugar. The output value generated from processing nira into aren sugar is Rp 2,000/kg. This output value is obtained by multiplying the conversion factor of 0.14 with the output price of Rp.14,000/kg. The results of the value-added analysis of aren sugar can be seen in Table 2.

From Table 2, the added value obtained from processing nira into aren sugar is Rp. 950/kg with a value-added ratio of 48%. Thus, there is an increase in the added value of nira through the application of aren sugar processing technology. This follows the statement in a study conducted previously (Putra *et al.* 2020) that the application of technology will affect the costs and revenues of farmers. The margin obtained from aren sugar processing was Rp. 1,300/kg. Direct labour income to the margin of 44%, the contribution of other inputs of 27% and profit for the owner of capital/company of 29%.

Table 2. Value-added analysis of processing sap into aren sugar.

No	Description	Value
A	Output, Input, and Price	
1	Output (kg aren sugar)	10
2	Input ((Aren sap) Liter)	70
3	Labour (DPW)	0.50
4	Labour coefficient	0.14
5	Labour cost	0.01
6	Output Price (Rp/Kg)	14,000
7	Direct labour cost (Rp/ DPW)	80,000
B	Revenue and Profit	
8	Raw material price (Rp/Liter)	700
9	Other input value (Rp/Kg)	350
10	Output value (Rp/Kg)	2,000.00
11	A. Added value (Rp/Kg)	950.00
	B. Added value ratio (%)	0.48
12	A. Direct labour revenue (Rp/Kg)	571
	B. Labour share (%)	0.60
13	A. Profit (Rp/Kg)	378.57
	B. Profit rate (%)	0.40
C	Return for production factors owner	
14	Margin (Rp/Kg)	1,300
	A. Direct labour income (%)	0.44
	B. Other input contributions (%)	0.27
	C. Company Owner's Profit (%)	0.29

3.4 *Added calue of granulated aren sugar processing*

The processing of granulated aren sugar in the Sari Aren business is carried out by using raw materials from aren sugar produced by members in the Selupuh Rejang aren village with prior quality selection. One time the production process of granulated aren sugar, the raw material used was 300 kg of aren sugar which produces 210 kg of granulated aren sugar. The output value generated from processing aren sugar into granulated aren sugar is IDR 24,500/kg. This output value is obtained by multiplying the conversion factor of 0.70 with the output price of IDR 35,000/kg. The added value obtained from processing aren sugar into granulated aren sugar is IDR 10,000/kg with a value-added ratio of 41%. The margin obtained from processing granulated aren sugar is Rp. 10,500/kg. Direct labour income to the margin of 0.8%, the contribution of other inputs by 0.5% and the profit for the owner of the capital/company by 88%. The results of the analysis of the added value of granulated aren sugar can be seen in Table 3.

The yield of the aren sugar production process carried out by the Sari Aren Group was 14.29%. Meanwhile, the production of aren sugar with raw materials of 300 kg/production process produces 210 kg of aren sugar with a yield of 70%. The yield is calculated based on the ratio of the final weight to the initial weight multiplied by 100% (Sani *et al.* 2014). The total production cost in one of aren sugar production processes is Rp. 115,820, – and the total revenue obtained is Rp. 140,000, – so that the income obtained in one production process per day is Rp. 24,150, -. While the total production cost of granulated aren sugar in one production process is Rp. 4,503,000, – with a revenue value of Rp. 7,350,000, – so that the income earned is 2,847,000, -/ production process. The calculation of revenue from aren sugar and granulated aren sugar processing is presented Calculation of income from aren sugar and granulated aren sugar processing in Sari Aren farmer group in Table 4.

Table 3. Value-added analysis of aren sugar processing into granulated aren sugar.

No	Description	Value
A	Output, Input, and Price	
1	Output (kg) (granulated aren sugar)	210.00
2	Input (aren sugar) (kg)	300.00
3	Labour (DPW)	3.00
4	Conversion factor	0.70
5	Labour coefficient	0.01
6	Output Price (Rp/Kg)	35,000.00
7	Direct labour cost (Rp/ HOK)	80,000.00
B	Revenue and Profit	
8	Raw material price (Rp/Liter)	14,000.00
9	Other input value (Rp/Kg)	500.00
10	Output value (Rp/Kg)	24,500.00
11	A. Added value (Rp/Kg)	10,000.00
	B. Added value ratio (%)	0.41
12	A. Direct labour revenue (Rp/Kg)	800.00
	B. Labour share (%)	0.08
13	A. Profit (Rp/Kg)	9,200.00
	B. Profit rate (%)	0.92
C	Return for production factors owner	
14	Margin (Rp/Kg)	10,500.00
	A. Direct labour income (%)	0.08
	B. Other input contributions (%)	0.05
	C. Company Owner's Profit	0.88

Table 4. Calculation of income from aren sugar and granulated aren sugar processing in Sari Aren farmer group.

Materials/Components	Unit Price (Rp)	Cost per process (Rp)	Production Cost per Month (Rp)
Aren Sugar			
-. Aren sap (70 liter)	700	49,000	1,470,000
-. Palm Oil (0,001 liter)	20,000	20	600
-. Firewood (0,25 m^3)	100,000	25,000	750,000
-. Labour (0,5 DP)	80,000	40,000	1,200,000
-. Packaging and other cost	180	1,800	54,000
A. Total Cost (TC)		115,820	3,474,600
B. Aren Sugar Product (10 kg)	14,000	140,000	4,200,000
Granulated Aren Sugar			
-. Aren Sugar (300 kg)	14,000	4,200,000	126,000,000
-. Labour (3 OH)	80,000	240,000	7,200,000
-. Packaging and other costs	63,000	63,000	1,890,000
A. Total Cost (TC)		4,503,000	135,090,000
B. Granulated aren sugar product (210 kg)	35,000	7,350,000	220,500,000

4 CONCLUSIONS

(a) Processing aren sugar from nira produces an added value of IDR 950/kg with a value-added ratio of 48%.
(b) Processing ants from aren sugar produces an added value of Rp. 10,000/kg with a value-added ratio of 41%
(c) The more processed the aren products from nira to aren sugar and granulated aren sugar will increase the added value and decrease the ratio of added value.
(d) The margin on granulated aren sugar processing received by the company owner is higher than that on aren sugar processing.

ACKNOWLEDGEMENT

We would like to thank the Chairman of Bengkulu Province Regional Research and Development Planning Agency, who has approved funding for this research in the 2023 fiscal year through the independent research collaboration.

REFERENCES

Astuti, W., Sulistyaningsih, T., & Prastiyanto, D. (2019). Peningkatan kualitas gula aren tradisional (Produksi Desa Jawisari Kabupaten Kendal). *Jurnal Puruhita, 1*(1), 66–70. https://journal.unnes.ac.id/sju/index.php/puruhita/

Bustam, & Sabrab, M. A. (2021). Analisis nilai tambah produk gula aren di desa Ogowele Buga Kabupaten Tolitoli. *Insight Management Journal, 2*(1), 20–26. https://journals.insightpub.org/index.php/imj

Faliha, S. H., Purwandari, I., Kurniawati, F., & Kifli, F. W. (2022). Analisis nilai Tambah dan efisiensi agroindustri gula Aren di Desa Gonoharjo Kecamatan Limbangan Kabupaten Kendal Jawa Tengah. *AGRIFITIA: Journal of Agribusiness Plantation, 2*(1), 42–50. https://doi.org/10.55180/aft.v2i1.198

Fatsan, A., Dinarti, D., & Maskromo, I. (2020). Potential yield and diversity of phenotypic of Palm Sugar (Arenga pinnata (Wurmb) Merr.) in Southeast Sulawesi. *Jurnal Berkala Penelitian Agronomi, 8*(2), 7–15.

Gobel, Z., Boekoesoe, Y., Agribisnis, J., Pertanian, F., Gorontalo, N., Prof, J., Habibie, I. B. J., Bone, K., & Bolango, K. B. (2022). Analisis pendapatan dan nilai tambah gula Aren pada usaha iIndustri rumah tangga di Kecamatan Atinggola Kabupaten Gorontalo Utara. *Jurnal Agrinesia, 7*(1), 17–24.

Haloho, W. F., & Susanto, W. H. (2015). Effect the addition of lime and Sodium Tripolyphosphate (STPP) to quality palm sugar. *Jurnal Pangan Dan Agroindustri*, *3*(3), 1160–1170.
Hayami, Y. T., Kawagoe, Y., Maraoka, & Siregar, M. (1989). *Agricultural marketing and processing in up land java a perspective from a sunda village*. CEPRT.
Laksananny, S. A., & Pujirahayu, N. (2017). Analisis kelayakan usahatani tanaman Aren (Arenga pinnata Merr) genjah pada sistem agroforestri di kawasan tahura Nipa-Nipa Kendari. *Ecogreen*, *3*(1), 33–39.
Marpaung, P. H. P., & Siburian, F. (2023). Analisis nilai tambah pengolahan nira aren menjadi gula aren Desa Buluh Awar, Kecamatan Sibolangit. *Jurnal Regionomic*, *5*(1), 21–35.
Melly, S., Hadiguna, R. A., Santosa, S., & Nofialdi, N. (2019). Manajemen risiko rantai pasok agroindustri gula merah tebu di kabupaten agam, provinsi sumatera barat. *Industria: Jurnal Teknologi Dan Manajemen Agroindustri*, *8*(2), 133–144. https://doi.org/10.21776/ub.industria.2019.008.02.6
Miftah, H., Yoesdiarti, A., & Maulana, D. M. (2018). Analisis nilai tambah olahan gula aren di Kelompok Usaha Bersama (KUB) Gula Semut Aren (GSA). *Jurnal Agribisains*, *4*(2), 8–14.
Prihantini, C. I., Purbaningsih, Y., Sari, A., Joka, U., Taufik, M. I., & Hardina, S. (2022). Marketing channel analysis of palm sugar business (Case study: Puudongi Village, Polinggona District, Kolaka Regency). *REVENUE: Jurnal Ekonomi Pembangunan Dan Ekonomi Syari'ah*, *5*(2).
Putra, W. E., Firison, J., Harta, L., & Ishak, A. (2020). Analisis nilai tambah pengolahan gula Aren (Kasus di Desa Gunung Kembang, Manna – Bengkulu Selatan). *Jurnal AGRIBIS*, *11*(2), 1573–1578.
Sani, R. N., Nisa, F. C., Andriani, R. D., & Maligan, J. M. (2014). Analisis rendemen dan skrining fitokimia ekstrak etanol Mikroalga laut (Tetraselmis chuii). *Jurnal Pangan Dan Agroindustri*, *2*(2), 121–126.
Simarmata, T. (2019). *Percepatan Transformasi Teknologi dan Inovasi dalam Era Smart Farming dan Petani Milenial Untuk Meningkatkan Produktivitas, Nilai Tambah dan Daya Saing Pertanian Indonesia. Makalah disampaikan pada rangkaian seminar/kuliah umum.*
Soekartawi. (2006). *Agribisnis Teori dan Aplikasi.* Rajawali press.
Sultan, Rianda, L., & Herdhiansyah, D. (2020). The influence of market orientation on product innovation in the palm sugar industry in the Watchunu Sub-District and North Poleang Bombana District. *Jurnal Teknologi Dan Manajemen Industri Pertanian*, *1*(1), 21–28.
Winarno, F G. (2002). *F.G. Winarno, Kimia Pangan dan Gizi.* PT. Gramedia Pustaka Utama.
Zaini, A., Palupi, N. P., Pujowati, P., & Emmawati, A. (2019). *Nilai Tambah dan Daya Saing Produk Unggulan di Kutai Barat* (A. D. Nabila, Ed.; Pertama, Vol. 1). Deepublish.

Technological Innovations in Tropical Livestock Development for Environmental Sustainability and Food Security – P. Dhian Isnaeni et al. (eds)
© 2025 The Author(s), ISBN 978-1-032-74373-8
Open Access: www.taylorfrancis.com, CC BY-NC-ND 4.0 license

A study of hazard analysis critical control point method to secure the food safety honey production

F.S. Nastain
Doctoral Program Animal Science, Faculty of Animal Science, Brawijaya University, Malang, Indonesia

L.E. Radiati* & K.U. Al Awwaly
Department of Animal Products Technology, Faculty of Animal Science, Brawijaya University, Indonesia

D. Masyithoh
Animal Husbandry Program, Faculty of Animal Husbandry, Islamic University of Malang, Indonesia

ABSTRACT: Honey contamination is the biggest factor that can affect honey quality. The hazard of honey contamination can come from implementing hygiene and sanitation management from the arrival of honey raw materials to the finished goods being inappropriate. PT Kembang Joyo Sriwijaya is an industry that operates in honey processing. In carrying out the company's operational activities, it refers to the management system to produce the best quality honey. The study aims to observe and determine the implementation of the HACCP system in honey production at PT Kembang Joyo Sriwijaya. The HACCP (Hazard Analysis Critical Control Point) method can be used as a food quality and safety assurance system. The HACCP method is used to identify all possible hazards (biological, chemical, and physical), analyze them based on risk and severity, and control actions to avoid hazards that occur in the honey processing process. In conducting a HACCP study, refer to the 7 principles in the guidebook for the preparation of a HACCP plan. The results of the HACCP implementation study at PT Kembang Joyo Sriwijaya showed that the determination of CCP in honey processing was filtering, pasteurization, and evaporation. CCP has received good supervision on all lines. In carrying out the implementation of HACCP, verification procedures have been carried out, namely, periodic reviews of the entire production process to ensure that the HACCP program has been implemented following the HACCP design and is still effective and correct. A HACCP program that has been implemented well is a guarantee of the results of the HACCP verification procedure. Conformity in implementing HACCP helps identify, prevent, and reduce hazards to acceptable limits by establishing critical control points to improve the quality and safety of honey.

Keywords: Honey, food safety, quality, HACCP

1 INTRODUCTION

Honey is an organic compound derived from the nectar of flowering plants, which is collected and processed by the apidae (bees) of the genus Apis (family: Apidae). The composition is highly variable, depending on the botanical and geographic origin of the plant (Tafere 2021). The production of honey and bee products has traditionally been associated with a sense of naturalness, healthiness, and purity. Honey is not commonly referred to as a nourishing food, but rather as a complex combination of sugars (including monosaccharide, glucose, and fructose) and other ingredients, including proteins, minerals, vitamins, organic compounds, and enzymes (Guerzou *et al.* 2021). Despite its biological activity, honey does not remain free

*Corresponding Author: lilik.eka@ub.ac.id

DOI: 10.1201/9781003468943-39

from contaminants and the chemical safety monitoring of honey is still of paramount importance today, not only for the quality of the product and the protection of consumer health but also for the preservation of the landscape and biodiversity (Massous *et al.* 2003).

Contamination of honey is currently one of the top concerns for the global honey market. The main reasons for poor quality are high temperature, high moisture, adulterations, inadequate packaging, and storage conditions (Lomiso 2019). This is because honey quality deteriorates during harvesting, processing, and marketing (Klutse *et al.* 2021). The sources of contamination of honey can be roughly categorized as environmental, apicultural (Bogdanov 2006), and beekeeping practices (Al-Waili *et al.* 2012).

The food industry is a vital and rapidly expanding sector in the world, due to the rapid expansion of the human race and the growing preference of consumers for the consumption of superior products (Rahman *et al.* 2014). Hazards, as defined by the Codex 1997, are contaminants that could render a food product unsafe for human consumption (Dias *et al.* 2012). Food can be contaminated at any time during the process of harvesting, processing, storing, distributing, transporting, and preparing.

The Hazard Analysis and Critical Control Point (HACCP) system is an effective and efficient method of producing food that is safe to consume. In the food production process, HACCP is a systematic, scientific-based system that identifies specific food safety risks and establishes the necessary food safety control measures (FAO and WHO 2003). In addition, a well-designed HACCP program can help food companies enhance their management effectiveness and increase employee safety awareness (Shuvo *et al.* 2019). The CAC has approved the HACCP principles and application guidance can be found in the Annex to the General Principles of Food Hygiene (FAO). Therefore, the objective of this study was to observe and determine the implementation of the HACCP system in a honey processing plant to identify CCPs by using the 7 HACCP principles so that the production process can be controlled and produce products that meet consumer demands (safe and quality). This will be useful for process engineers as well as quality control experts to design and implement controls in the honey industry. The method is designed for use in honey production when more control is required for wider application. The implementation of HACCP can effectively guarantee the quality and security of the final product.

2 METHODS

This study was conducted at PT Kembang Joyo Sriwijaya, Malang, East Java on October 2023. The method used in this research is descriptive, namely a method that describes and explains conceptual theoretical studies through literature searches, collecting literature from various secondary library sources such as books, research journals, and articles accessed from the internet. Apart from that, primary data collection was also carried out by observing and conducting interviews with company management and employees at PT Kembang Joyo Sriwijaya. HACCP studies of the honey production process at PT Kembang Joyo Sriwijaya using the HACCP Plan Preparation Guide followed the five basic requirements and Seven principles of the HACCP system Based SNI CXC 1:1969 including:

Five basic requirements: 1) Establishment of a HACCP Team, 2) Description of product type, 3) Identify product uses, 4) Creation and development of flow charts, 5) Flowchart of verification actions. Meanwhile, the seven main principles in HACCP are: 1) Hazard analysis and prevention, 2) Identify Critical Control Points (CCP), 3) Establish critical limits (CP), 4) Establish monitoring, 5) Determine corrective action (correction action), 6) Develop verification procedures, 7) Establish recording procedures (documentation).

3 RESULTS AND DISCUSSION

The Hazard Analysis and Critical Control Point (HACCP) system is a management approach that focuses on the prevention and management of food safety risks associated with the production, procurement, and handling of raw materials, as well as the production, distribution, and consumption of finished products. To ensure the successful implementation of a Hazard Analysis and Critical Control Point (HACCP) plan, management needs to demonstrate a strong commitment to the concept of HACCP. A strong dedication to HACCP from senior management will instill in company personnel a sense of the significance of producing food that is safe to consume.

3.1 *Implementation of the HACCP system at PT Kembang Joyo Sriwijaya*

PT Kembang Joyo Sriwijaya implemented the HACCP system in 2023 to obtain a HACCP certificate. Implementation of the HACCP management system PT Kembang Joyo Sriwijaya adheres to the rules in 12 steps for implementing the HACCP system. The implementation steps can be seen in Figure 1.

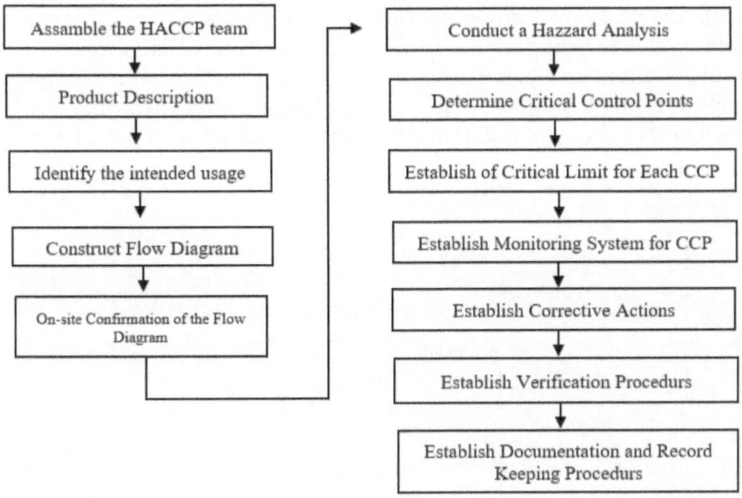

Figure 1. HACCP implementation flow diagram.

3.2 *Initial steps to enable hazard analysis*

3.2.1 *The HACCP team*

The team was intended to consist of six individuals (Jubayer *et al.* 2022): 1) Members must possess the necessary qualifications and experience to be proficient in their respective areas of expertise, 2) A team leader should be in charge of the team and lead the activities, 3) The team will be responsible for creating, setting up, and keeping the HACCP up and running, 4) All members of the team are required to undergo training, 5) All documents must be developed and maintained by the team following HACCP, 6) In addition, if the process changes, the team will need to assess the suitability of HACCP system

Thus, the team HACCP was involved as follows: HACCP Team Leader, Manufacturing Manager, Head of Warehouse, Head of Quality Assurance, HACCP Team Members, Maintenance (Electrical and Mechanical), Purchasing Manager and Marketing Supply Chain Manager.

3.2.2 *Product descriptions*

The honey produced by PT Kembang Joyo Sriwijaya has been described in detail. Access information can be obtained clearly and included in the packaging. The product description was followed by BSN regulations which contain information about the product name, scientific name, origin of raw materials, method of receipt, final product, additional ingredients, origin of additional ingredients, process steps, packaging, storage, shelf life, labels/specifications, how to use, customer instructions, product sales system until it reaches the user or consumers (BSN 2005).

3.2.3 *Identifications of the intended usage*

After the product descriptions are identified, the next stage is further identification in the form of product use, for whom the product is used, and how the product is used. So, it is necessary to identify who and where the products produced are used. More important is the user or consumer segment. The products produced by PT Kembang Joyo Sriwijaya are intended for all consumers, except for babies.

3.2.4 *Construction of flow diagram*

The HACCP team prepared and determined flow diagrams by grouping stages in the production process. The purpose of grouping each process stage was to make it easier to identify hazards. Similarly, it has been proposed that only a flowchart that's well-structured, clear, and well-thought-out makes it easier to understand what's going on in the production process, which makes it much simpler to spot any potential issues (Marques *et al.* 2012). The flowchart showing the whole manufacturing process of honey is shown in Figure 2.

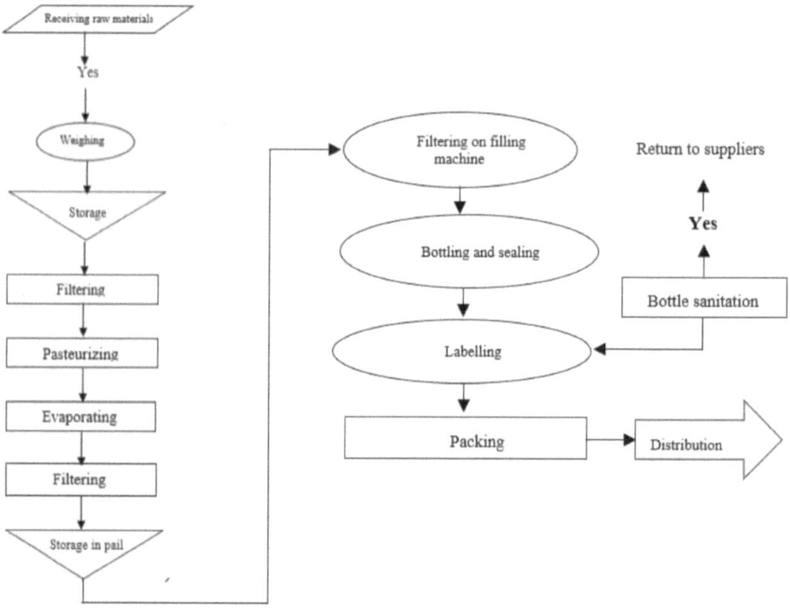

Figure 2. Flowchart manufacturing process of honey.

3.2.5 *Flow chart verification*

The verification activities are carried out by the HACCP team to see the totality of facts/actualities in honey production activities to produce the desired final product. The flow diagram verification method can be used by interview systems, observation, and laboratory testing. If the production process, there are deviations or discrepancies between the flow diagram that has been created and the resulting product, the Team will take corrective action according to the needs or level of failure and have to be added to complete the process flow diagram or flow chart in production of honey processing.

3.2.6 *Analysis of hazard (principle 1)*
All hazards at PT Kembang Joyo Sriwijaya were assessed and categorized into three groups: biological, chemical, and physical hazards. Based on the HACCP manual PT Kembang Joyo Sriwijaya for the honey production process, significant hazards exist in the filtering, pasteurizing, and evaporating processes. In the production process stage of filtering raw honey, a significant hazard that often arises is the presence of physical contamination related to wood, parts of bees, and hive debris, which are hazards that can reduce food safety factors. The presence of physical contamination in honey can come from the apiary due to substandard equipment used during the harvest process and postharvest handling. Similarly, it has been confirmed by Eissa and Taha (2022), that the presence of numerous types of foreign materials in honey depends on the type of hive, extraction method, post-extraction cleaning, and packaging. The majority of foreign material present in honey consists of dead bees, larval parts, hair, and beeswax. The process of pasteurization and evaporation decreases the amount of moisture present in the honey, resulting in the destruction of yeast cells and the liquefaction of crystals.

3.2.7 *Determination of critical control point (principle 2)*
Determining critical control points starts with ensuring and looking at the significance of the manual, which contains hazard analysis in the production process. Based on the HACCP manual PT Kembang Joyo Sriwijaya for the honey production process, significant hazards exist in the filtering, pasteurizing, and evaporating processes (PT. Kembang Joyo 2023). The CCP determination of honey filtering includes dusk, wood, parts of bees, and hive debris, while the CCP is in pasteurization and evaporation is yeast and molds. All those included in the CCP group must be identified and developed appropriately and carefully. It should be monitored continuously and documented.

3.2.8 *Establishment of critical limits (principle 3)*
The determination of critical limits by the PT Kembang Joyo HACCP team refers to the rules or Indonesian National Standard CXC 1-1969 (2020). The critical limit in the honey filtering process was honey is free from physical contamination. This filtering aims to remove physical contamination related to dust, wood, parts of bees, and beehive debris. To remove physical contamination, PT Kembang Joyo Sriwijaya used a filter of 200 mash fine nylon fabrics. Meanwhile, the critical limit in the process of pasteurization and evaporation of honey is a category of hazard in the aspect of microbiological hazard/contamination (mold and yeast). Based on the Indonesian National Standard (2013), the maximum TPC value for honey is 1×10^3 cfu/g and the maximum total yeast value is 1×10^1 cfu/g. The temperature for the pasteurization and evaporation process was 60°C–70°C in 30 minutes and cooling quickly. This temperature can eliminate microbial contamination and effectively to delay the granulation in honey. The pasteurization process not only removes the spoilage organisms but also removes the risk of fermentation as it reduces the moisture content down to a safe level and delays the crystallization process (Sing and Singh, 2018).

3.2.9 *Establishment of a monitoring system (principle 4)*
The monitoring system is an act of observation and/or measurement carried out to provide an assessment of whether the CCP is under control. A critical limit monitoring method or system that has been carried out by PT Kembang Joyo Sriwijaya, especially by the HACCP Team, is to carry out sequential and planned measurements and observation or monitoring to determine whether a CCP (critical control point) is in a stage of the production process honey under monitored and controlled conditions. The PT Kembang Joyo Sriwijaya HACCP team created monitoring procedures to ensure that the critical limits or threshold limits that had been set had been implemented. The methods or procedures used by the HACCP team carry out observations and monitoring that provide valid and accountable values, such as using appropriate and appropriate sampling methods, sufficient

frequency, having qualified and trained personnel or teams, calibrated monitoring equipment, and being Able to work together in a team-oriented manner.

3.2.10 *Establishment of a corrective actions (principle 5)*

PT Kembang Joyo Sriwijaya in implementing a food safety system, or HACCP, designs or prepares an activity or action that is mandatory and must be carried out if a hazard has exceeded the critical limit previously determined by the HACCP Team. If deviations occur, for example, levels of physical contamination exceeding the specified limits, then the raw materials used for sampling will be rejected before receiving them, and if they have already been processed, they will not be processed further. An action taken by a company if a hazard of physical and biological contamination is found in a product with a size that exceeds the specified limits is to withhold the product. Moreover, if physical and microbiological contamination can be neutralized (cleaned up) and it can be confirmed that its presence was not detected in laboratory tests, then the product can be reused or reprocessed (PT Kembang Joyo 2023).

3.2.11 *Establishment of verification procedure (principle 6)*

In implementing HACCP principles, the PT Kembang Joyo Sriwijaya HACCP Team accomplished several verification actions as part of the implementation effort. Verification was the attempt to test whether a HACCP plan that has been created meets process conditions or still requires a new system to modify the previous plan. Furthermore, system validation can be executed. The HACCP Team went through HACCP validation activities, evaluated the results of monitoring the production process (a monitoring system), tested the products produced, and followed through with internal audits of the production process. The verification process or activity carried out by PT Kembang Joyo Sriwijaya was analyzed by each of the processed stages identified and declared as a CCP. Attery (2016) stated that the validation involves the identification and documentation of the scientific evidence to support the adequacy of food safety hazards to be controlled through prevention measures. An "Initial Validation" occurs during the development and initial implementation of a food safety system.

3.2.12 *Establishment of documentation (principle 7)*

The documentation system referred to was not only needed when the HACCP system can be implemented but it was also followed through for the process activities of the verification system and review system of the HACCP plan carried out or implemented by the company. The records should be taken from a particular logbook in which they have been recorded: 1) Monitoring activities; 2) The corrective actions were eventually adopted; and 3) The verification procedures adopted.

In fulfilling documentation activities, PT Kembang Joyo Sriwijaya carried out standard documentation and followed the guidelines and planning written in the HACCP manual. The documentation activities through PT Kembang Joyo Sriwijaya were timely targeted, effective, and easy to understand for all PT Kembang Joyo Sriwijaya employees. The documentation system implemented is internal and controlled.

4 CONCLUSION

PT Kembang Joyo Sriwijaya has been able to implement a food safety system in terms of an HACCP program as a commitment to creating food safety for consumers. The honey production process follows the plans made in the manual by the HACCP teams, so it can be ensured that the product produced by the company affords a guarantee of food safety. The HACCP system at PT Kembang Joyo Sriwijaya is deliberately implemented to protect the consumers when consuming food through food safety quality control throughout the production process, involving various personnel from various scientific disciplines.

ACKNOWLEDGEMENTS

The authors are grateful to PT Kembang Joyo Sriwijaya for affording financial and resource support.

REFERENCES

Al-Waili, N., K. Salom, A. Al-Ghamdi, and M. J. Ansari. 2012. Antibiotic, pesticide, and microbial contaminants of honey: human health hazards, *The Scientific World Journal* Vol. 2012, 2–9. DOI:10.1100/2012/930849

Bogdanov, S. 2006. *Contaminants of bee products, Apidologie*, 2006, 37(1): 1–18. DOI: 10.1051/apido:2005043

D.P. Attrey. Role of risk analysis and risk communication in food safety management. *Food Safety in the 21st Century*. 2016:53–68. DOI: 10.1016/B978-0-12-801773-9.00005-4. Epub 2016 Oct 14. PMCID: PMC7150068

Dias, M.A.C., A.S. Sant'Ana, A.G. Cruz, J.A.V Faria, C.A.V. Oliveira, E. Bona. 2012. On the implementation of good manufacturing practices in a small processing unity of mozzarella cheese in Brazil. *Food Control*. 2012, vol. 24, Page. 199–206.

Eissa, F. and E.A. Taha. Contaminants in honey: an analysis of EU RASFF notifications from 2002 to 2022. *Journal of Consumer Protection and Food Safety*. Springer page. 1–10. DOI://doi.org/10.1007/s00003-023-01460-

FAO & WHO. 2003. *Recommended international codex of practice. General principles of food hygiene, CAC/RCP 1 – 1969, Rev. 4-2003, including "annex on hazard analysis critical control point (haccp) system and guidelines for its application"*, FAO & WHO, Geneva, Switzerland, 2003

Guerzou, M., H.A. Aouissi, A. Guerzou, J. Burlakovs, S. Doumandji, A.E. Krauklis,. 2012. From the beehives: identification and comparison of physicochemical properties of algerian honey. *Resources*, 2021, vol. 10(94), page 1–11. DOI: https://doi.org/10.3390/resources10100094.

Indonesian National Standards. general principles of food hygiene (CXC 1-1969 Rev. 2020, IDT).

Jubayer, M.F., M.S. Hossain, M. Al-Emran, M. N. Uddin. 2022. Implementation of HACCP management system in a cake manufacturing company in Dhaka, Bangladesh: A Case Study, *Journal of Food Quality*, 2022, Page: 1–12, DOI: https://doi.org/10.1155/2022/5321333

Klutse, C.K., D.A Larbi, D. K. Adotey, Y. Serfor-armah. 2021. Assessment of effect of post-harvest treatment on microbial quality of honey from parts of Ghana. *Radiation Physics and Chemistry*, 2021, Vol.182. DOI: https://doi.org/10.1016/j.radphyschem.2021.109368.

Lomiso, D.F. 2019. Assessment on postharvest handling practices of honey in Chena District, Southwestern Ethiopia, *Food Science and Quality Management*, 2019, vol. 89. DOI: 10.7176/FSQM.

Marques N., J. Matias, R. Teixeira, and F. Brojo. 2012. Implementation of hazard analysis critical control points (HACCP) in a SME: case study of a bakery," *Polish Journal of Food and Nutrition Sciences*, 2012, vol. 62, no. 4, pp. 215–227.

Massous, A., T. Ouchbani, V. Lo Turco, F. Litrenta, V. Nava, A. Albergamo, A. G. Potortì, G. Di Bella. 2023. Monitoring moroccan honeys: physicochemical properties and contamination pattern. *Foods*, 2023, vol.12.969. DOI:.https://doi.org/10.3390/foods12050969

National Standardization Agency, BSN. 2005. RSNI 01-2705-2005, Frozen Shrimp. *National Standardization Council, Jakarta*, 2007. [Indonesian]

National Standardization Agency, Honey. Indonesian national standard (SNI), 2013, 01-3545- 2013. *Honey*. Indonesian Standardization Council, Jakarta.

PT Kembang Joyo Sriwijaya. 2023. PT Kembang Joyo Sriwijaya HACCP Manual. *Malang. East Java*.

Rahman, M., S.H. Gan, M. Khalil. 2014. Neurological effects of honey: Current and future prospects. *Evid. Based Complement. Altern. Med.* 2014 DOI: 10.1155/2014/958721

Shuvo, S. D., M. S. K. Josy, R. Parvin, M. A. Zahid, D. K. Paul, and M. T. Elahi. 2019. Development of a HACCP-based approach to control risk factors associated with biscuit manufacturing plant, Bangladesh," *Nutrition & Food Science*, 2019, vol. 49, no. 6, pp. 1180–1194.

Singh I, and Singh S. Honey moisture reduction and its quality. *J Food Sci Technol*. 2018, vol. 55(10):3861–3871. doi: 10.1007/s13197-018-3341-5

Tafere, D. A,. 2021. Chemical composition and uses of honey: A review, *J Food Sci Nutr Res*, 2021, vol. 4 (3): 194–201. DOI: 10.26502/jfsnr.2642-11000072

Technological Innovations in Tropical Livestock Development for Environmental Sustainability and Food Security – P. Dhian Isnaeni et al. (eds)

Humic compounds: formation, compositions and applications

P.H. Maharani*, E. Maftu'ah, A. Noor, R.D. Ningsih & K. Napisah
Research Center for Food Crops, National Research, and Innovation Agency (BRIN), Cibinong, Bogor Regency, Indonesia

N. Yuliani
Research Center for Horticultural and Estate Corps, National Research, and Innovation Agency (BRIN) Cibinong, Bogor Regency, Indonesia

ABSTRACT: Organic material is defined as a series of carbon compounds that originate from living organisms and have been stored on or within the structural components of the earth. Organic matter in soil is distinguished in uncompostable materials such as fresh pine and uncomposed components from old pine, and humus as a result of the transformation of fresh organic material. Humic compounds are irregular, polymerized, brown-to-black organic compound with different solubility: humic acid (AH), fulvate acid (AF), humin, and hematomelanic acid. The presence of humus compounds in the soil in the form of insoluble macromolecular complexes, macro-molecule complexes bound together with Ca^{2+}, Fe^{3+}, and Al^{3+} and combinations with platinum minerals, hydrogen bridges or van der Waals with cations. Humic compounds in the soil are formed through lignin modification, quinon fusion and sugar-amine condensation. The result of the fractionation of organic material will be obtained humic acid, fulvate acid, humin and hematomelanin acid. Humic acid is characterized by lower levels of carboxyl group than fulfate acid. Humate compounds have broad roles in agriculture, industry, and health.

Keywords: organic material, lignin modification, fractionation, humic acid, fulvatic acid

1 INTRODUCTION

The process of soil formation from ancient sedimentary rocks or deep-sea sediments typically involves mineral materials devoid of organic content with varying levels of sand, silt, clay, and carbonate. Although fluctuating temperature and humidity support the transformation of minerals, living organisms and organic products created by living creatures are most involved in the mineral transformation into soil. The pedosphere is the canvas, the lithosphere is the supporting pillar, and the biosphere is the painting on the canvas (Hardjowigeno 1993). The biosphere and organic compounds produced by living organisms have both direct and indirect impacts on soil minerals. For example (a) Microorganisms transform organic materials and lead to the formation of CO_2, which is quantitatively the most aggressive weathering agent. This occurs because of the formation of carbonic acid with water ($H_2O + CO_2 \rightarrow H_2CO_3$); (b) Many water-soluble organic compounds are created in the biosphere, which have the ability to complex and mobilize metal ions, and can reduce the metal ions; (c) Strong energy is generated through the uptake of specific elements by plants and microorganisms, resulting in the release of these elements into the soil; (d) Many

*Corresponding Author: puspitaharummaharani@gmail.com

 DOI: 10.1201/9781003468943-40

microorganisms can accelerate catalytic reactions, oxidation, and reduction of minerals in the soil that would otherwise be slow (Stevenson 1982).

Soil organic matter includes the remains of plants and animals that have fallen or become buried beneath the Earth's surface, as well as organic pesticides synthesized by humans. Soil organic matter also encompasses a range of carbon compounds originating from living organisms and stored in the structural components of the Earth. Most of the organic material in neutral and alkaline soils consists of humic and humin acids; in acidic conditions, soils with high sand content experience significant leaching (Tipping 2004).

In mineral soils with high organic horizons, such as Spodosols, Mollisols, and Andisols, the role of humic compounds in soil pedology has been extensively studied because the content of these compounds in the soil is relatively higher than non-humified organic compounds. Humic compounds are highly effective in mineral dissolution, complexing metal ions, creating mineral humus complexes, precipitating, and crystallizing aluminum, and forming iron oxides, among other functions (Kumada 1987). The purpose of this paper is to gain an understanding of the processes of formation, compositions, and applications of humic acids.

2 MATERIALS AND METHODS

2.1 *Humic compounds*

Soil organic matter is initially created by living organisms (plants or animals) and is then returned to the soil through the process of decomposition. Many materials that make up soil organic matter come from the decay of plant tissues, which contain about 60–90% water. Other dry materials consist of carbon, oxygen, hydrogen, and small amounts of sulfur, as well as elements such as nitrogen, phosphorus, potassium, and magnesium (Bot and Benites 2005). Many variables influence the content of organic matter in soil, but climate has the most significant impact on the decomposition process, as moisture and temperature increase with decomposition. Rainfall, temperature, pH, and clay content are all environmental components that affect the rate of decomposition.

The dark-colored nature of organic matter in soil can increase soil temperature by retaining up to twenty times its weight in water. Organic matter has the ability to form complexes with clay minerals and aggregate soil particles by cementing them. Because of its association with clay, organic matter is not soluble, and leaching removes only a small amount of organic matter. To help maintain uniform reactions in soil, organic matter demonstrates buffering capacity within a moderately acidic, neutral, and alkaline range. Organic matter contributes 20–70% of soil CEC (cation exchange capacity) and the total acidity of the humus fraction ranges from 300–1400 cmol/kg. The decomposition of organic matter results in CO_2, NH_4^+, NO_3^-, PO_4^{3-}, and SO_4^{2-}, which serve as nutrient sources for plants. Organic matter can react with other organic chemicals, influencing the bioactivity, presence, and biodegradation capacity of other organic chemical pesticide compounds.

Organic matter in soil is divided into two main categories. The first is non-decomposed organic matter, such as fresh litter and undecomposed components of aged litter. The second category is humus, which results from the transformation of fresh organic matter and has a different morphological structure from its source material. Characteristics of humic compounds include dark brown color, amorphous structure, hydrophilicity, high molecular weight, and resistance to microbial degradation. Humus also comprises about 40–60% of soil organic matter. Humified material is the product that has formed during the decomposition process and consists of complex compound groups-comprising humic and non-humic substances and can be subdivided as (i) Humic acids (HA), fulvic acids (FA), humin, and humatomelanin are polymer humic substances that are typically irregular in shape and range from brown to black in color; (ii) Non-humic substances consist of biochemically known compound groups, such as polysaccharides, polypeptides, modified lignin, amino acids, glucose, and low molecular weight organic acids like acetic acid, oxalic acid, citric acid, tartaric acid, and so on. These components can be produced by microbes or can be generated from similar parts in the original litter.

The higher content of humic compounds compared to non-humic compounds indicates that humic substances are a major component of soil organic matter and play a crucial role in the decomposition of soil minerals. Humic compounds are natural organic compounds found in sediments, water, and soil, serving to support plant growth and maintain the biogeochemical stability of organic carbon in ecosystems. To date, there are many questions about the significant role of humic substances, particularly regarding their reactivity and chemical properties. However, since 1826, our understanding of humic substances has improved, with suggestions that they play a vital role in the dissolution of rocks and minerals.

2.2 *The formation of humic compound*

There are several fundamental theories about how humic compounds form in soil. While Stevenson (1982) suggested that lignin modification leads to the formation of humic substances, most researchers believe that quinone breakdown precedes humic formation and condensation of sugar-amines is involved. The presence of humic compounds in soil can manifest in three main forms (a) insoluble macromolecular complexes: insoluble components are primarily found in peat soils and sediment rich in other organic matter, where clay and metal complexes are scarce to form bonds with humus components; (b) macromolecular complexes bonded with Ca^{2+}, Fe^{3+}, and Al^{3+}; (c) combination with clay minerals, hydrogen bridges, or van der Waals forces with cations (clay-metal-humus).

In all types of soils, the pathways for humic substance formation can function, but the extent and sequence of these pathways may vary. In dry soils and wet sediments (marshes, etc.), the lignin pathway may dominate, but polyphenol synthesis can be more prevalent in some forest soils. The synthesis of humus through sugar-amino acid solutions can be influenced by abrupt changes in terrestrial soil surface conditions such as temperature, humidity, and radiation.

(a) The Path 3 (polyphenol theory) suggests that lignin still plays a significant role in humus synthesis. In this scenario, phenolic aldehydes and acids are released from lignin during microbiological attack through enzymatic conversion to quinones, which polymerize with or without the presence of amino compounds to form humic-like macromolecules.
(b) Path 2 (polyphenol theory) is somewhat similar to Path 3 except for the difference that polyphenols are synthesized by microorganisms from non-lignin carbon sources (e.g., cellulose). The polyphenols are then enzymatically oxidized into quinones and converted into humic substances. As mentioned earlier, the classical Waksman theory is now considered outdated by many researchers. The concept of quinones originating from lignin, along with those synthesized by microorganisms, is seen as the primary building blocks of the humic substances formed.
(c) The theory of sugar-amino condensation. This theory suggests that non-enzymatic polymerization is used to form brown-colored nitrogenous polymers, similar to those produced when certain food products are dehydrated at moderate temperatures. The reactants (sugars, amino acids, and others) produced in abundance through microbial activity are an intriguing feature of this theory. One of the primary challenges with this theory is that the reaction results are rather slow at temperatures below normal soil conditions. However, significant environmental changes in the soil, such as freezing and thawing, wetting, and drying, and the interaction of reactants with mineral substances possessing catalytic properties, can facilitate condensation.

Humic compounds have been shown to consist of various molecular components. Some common components include polysaccharides and fatty acids, such as polypeptides, lignin, esters, phenols, ethers, carbonyls, quinones, lipids, and peroxides. They involve various combinations of benzene, acetals, ketals, lactols, as well as furan ring compounds and aliphatic (carbon chain) compounds. In addition to n-alkanes and n-alkanoic acids, oxidative degradation produces some aliphatic, phenolic, and benzene carboxylic acid humic substances. The carboxyl group content in humic acids is lower than that in fulvic acids. The nitrogen content in humic acids is twice that of fulvic acids in temperate and tropical soils. The total acidity of fulvic acids is also double that of humic acids, arising from carboxyl and phenolic hydroxyl groups due to complex cation exchange activity. As a result, fulvic acids can surpass humic acids in chelation and cation exchange (Tan 1991). In the characterization of humic acids, three types of hydroxyl groups are typically distinguished: (i) total hydroxyl groups: OH groups measured through acetylation, related to all functional groups; (ii) phenolic OH groups: OH groups bound to benzene rings and calculated based on the difference between total acidity (mEq) and carboxyl acidity (mEq); (iii) alcoholic OH groups: OH groups associated with alcoholic functional groups, calculated as the difference between total OH (mEq) and phenolic OH (mEq) (Tan 1991).

Compared to FA (1) HA contains approximately 10% more carbon but 10% less oxygen than AF; (2) the hydrogen content in HA is lower than in AF, while the nitrogen content in HA is higher than in AF, and the sulfur content in HA is lower than in AF; (3) the total acidity in terms of COOH is higher in AF, (4) both materials contain approximately the same concentration of phenolic OH, total C=O groups, and OCH_3 groups, but AF has more alcoholic OH groups compared to HA; (5) about 74% of the oxygen in HA is present as functional groups, while all of the oxygen in AF is dispersed in similar groups (Huang and Schnitzer 1997).

The content of AF and HA varies in different soils. In Alfisols and Mollisols, the highest content is found, with HA dominating in Alfisols. In Ultisols, the humic fraction is primarily composed of AF (Huang and Schnitzer 1997). Humic substances are responsible for various chemical activities that occur in the soil and interact with soil clays. Clays and humic compounds participate in complex reactions and can directly affect plant growth. Humic compounds also play a crucial role in soil formation, particularly in the translocation or mobilization of clays, aluminum, and iron, leading to the development of horizons like spodic and argillic (Tan 1991).

Fractionation is performed to simplify analysis by reducing the heterogeneity of isolated materials. Humic acid, fulvic acid, humin, and humatomelanin are the results of fractionating organic matter. The solubility of humic substances in alkali, acid, or ethyl alcohol determines the type of humic material produced. Fractionation alters the color of the compound solution. Fulvic acid is yellowish brown to bright yellow, humic acid is dark brown to deep gray-black, and humin is deep black (Stevenson 1982).

3 RESULT AND DISCUSSION

3.1 *Application of humic compound extract*

Humic compounds are relatively resistant to stress and represent one of the largest carbon reservoirs on Earth. The industrial application of humus and derivative products has been quite rare so far. In contrast, the use of coal increased during the late 19th and early 20th centuries. The four main categories of humic substance applications are agriculture, industry, environment, and biomedicine.

3.1.1 *Agricultural applications*

The quality and productivity of soil are greatly influenced by humic substances. Additionally, humic substances enhance soil CEC (cation exchange capacity) (Zhang and Dia 2004). To improve soil fertility, calcium humate is used (Buckau *et al.* 2000). There is an explanation about how sodium humate affects leaf plant fertilization. Moreover, it has been found that ammonium humate plays a significant role in promoting growth (Lotosh 1991). The properties and use of humic acids extracted from various composts have also been studied.

Factors like height, wet weight, dry weight, shoots and roots, the number of lateral roots, root initiation, seedling growth, nutrient uptake, and flowering were influenced by the amount of humic acid provided. The extraction of humic compounds from Andisol and Peatland soil can increase soil CEC and enhance phosphate availability in soils rich in reactive iron and aluminum oxides (Oxisols and Ultisols) (Selvi 2010). Minardi (2010) stated that soybean plants experience improvements in various aspects, including growth, above-ground and root dry weight, P uptake, and yield (number of pods and seed weight per plant). Furthermore, humic acid significantly reduces the available lead content in the soil. This organic acid, which can enhance membrane permeability and help facilitate nutrient penetration through cell walls, enhances photosynthesis and chlorophyll production, increases hormone stimulation, and boosts enzyme activity, playing a vital role in supporting soil microorganism life. Humic acid's ability to enhance nutrient uptake in *Agrostis stolonifera* L. plants (Cooper *et al.* 1998). However, Olk and Cassman (1995) found that the application of humic acid could reduce potassium fixation in vermiculite soil, increasing potassium availability in the soil. Ayuso's research (1996) indicated that the addition of humic acid enhances the nutrient uptake capacity for macronutrients (N, P, K). However, the amount of nutrients absorbed differs for each element. Leoniy (2011) noted that compost enriched with humic acid and activator bacteria increased seedling vigor and reduced Fusarium sp. infection, which causes damping-off in tomato plants, by 60.24% to 69.52%.

3.1.2 *Industrial application*

Humus and humic materials have been used as additives to control the setting rate of concrete in large construction projects. The leather industry also utilizes humic substances. According to Mendez (2005), they were first used as leather dyes, then as materials for tanning leather, and finally as finishing agents for leather. In the ceramic industry, humic substances are used as additives to enhance the mechanical strength of processed ceramics and improve their casting properties. They are also used in pottery preparation. Furthermore, humic materials are employed in the production of plastics, especially as colorants for coloring Nylon 6 or PVC plastics, polyurethane foam hardeners, or plasticizers for PVC-based materials (Majakova and Proskurjakov 1972). Industries use humic compounds as ion exchangers and as sources of synthetic hydrocarbons and fuel. The ability of humic compounds to retain transition metals results in the formation of metal-organic complexes, making metals more available to plants.

Interesting research involves the production of humic substances from industrial waste processing. Research results indicate that the conversion of cellulose into humic acid clearly occurs in the production of liquid packaging board (LPB) recycling (Koivula and Hanninen 1999). Saleh (2014) conducted an experiment by mixing sodium humate and sodium sulfate in a 1:1 ratio at temperatures between 80°C to 90°C. A certain amount of sulfinated Na-humate solution was then mixed with cement mixtures. The experiment showed that adding 0.10 g of sulfinated Na-humate solution to 50 g of cement mixture increased the compressive strength of the cement without the solution mix. However, mixing cement with an excess of sulfinated Na-humate, for example, up to 1 gram in 50 grams of cement, would decrease the compressive strength of the cement. Operational exploration drilling activities generally use bentonite mud with specific viscosity as the flushing fluid. To overcome difficulties in drilling, the viscosity of drilling mud needs to be adjusted, either by dilution or thickening with specific additives. Na-humate extracted from peat has been tested as a dilution additive. Saleh's experiment (2014) showed that Na-humate can restore the viscosity of thickened bentonite mud.

3.1.3 *Environmental application*

Natural organic colloids, such as humic and fulvic acids, can form solutions in water that are complex with many metals, including radionuclides. This makes them important as carriers of radionuclides, and humic compounds play a significant role in this regard (Ghabbour *et al.* 2001; Pacheco and Havel 2001). It is known that the presence of humic compounds in natural waters can influence the adsorption of radionuclides by natural solids. As a result, radionuclides cannot migrate to the surface or groundwater because natural solids prevent the adsorption of radionuclides (Samanidou *et al.* 1991). In the environment, the function of humic compounds is to remove heavy metals like iron, nickel, mercury, cadmium, copper, and others from water. Calcium humate can also be used to remove radioactivity from nuclear waste disposal. They also utilize their selective binding ability to neutralize ammunition and chemical warfare agents (Ghabbour and Davies 1999).

Humic-based filters have been developed for wastewater purification and have many benefits. They can clean up chromium smelter effluents, remove oil and dyes from wastewater and water systems, eliminate pesticides from wastewater, and remove phenols from water. Humic compounds are also used to filter gases, such as waste gas emissions from fish processing plants. To remove sulfur dioxide and hydrogen sulfide from urban air pollution, humic compounds are modified (Green and Manahan 1981). Considered environmental pollutants, various types of compounds such as herbicides, fungicides, insecticides, nematicides, dioxins, and some pharmaceutical products like estrogenics are used to remove contamination from water, soil, and sludge because of humic compounds' ability to absorb organic pollutants from the environment (Lofredo *et al.* 2000).

3.1.4 *Biomedical application*

Humic compound is produced commercially and used in human and animal medicine. There is some research on the medicinal properties of compounds containing humic substances (Brzozowski *et al.* 1994). When tested on rats with duodenal and gastric ulcers, humic acid given as a preventive measure significantly reduced ethanol-induced stomach damage (Brzozowski *et al.* 1994). Preincubation of cell cultures with ammonium humate can prevent herpes virus infection, confirmed the role of humic substances as microorganism protectors (Thiel *et al.* 1981). In a two-year treatment with humic extract solution, patients suffering from cancer caused by tumors in the esophageal tract were completely cured from the development of larger tumors (Yuan 1993). As a highly potent natural antioxidant, humic extracts usually only halt the growth and spread of cancer, but not all humic extracts destroy cancer cells. In the fields of medicine and biology, the use of humic compounds continues to grow. Research is ongoing regarding the extraction of humus from soil containing amino acid complexes and analogs of vitamin B, which serve as the basis for cosmetic and pharmaceutical products. Due to its interactions with developed antivirals, profibrinolytic, anti-inflammatory, and estrogenic activities, humic substances are still under investigation (Yamada *et al.* 1998). Because of humic acid's ability to form chelates containing heavy metals such as cadmium, it can be used to remove metal toxins from living organisms (Klöcking 1992).

4 CONCLUSION

Humic compounds, natural organic compounds found in sediments, water, and soil, play a role in supporting plant growth and maintaining the biogeochemical stability of organic carbon in ecosystems. To this day, the significant role of humic substances continues to raise many questions regarding their reactivity and chemical properties. A humic compound has been shown to have various molecular components. Some common components include polysaccharides and fatty acids, such as polypeptides, lignin, esters, phenols, ethers, carbonyls, quinones, lipids, and peroxides. Various combinations of benzene, acetals, ketals, and lactols, as well as cyclic furan compounds and aliphatic compounds (carbon chains), can be found in humic compounds. All types of soils have four pathways for forming complex humic compounds, but the levels and sequences may vary. In arid soils and wet sediments (marshes, etc.), the lignin pathway may dominate, but polyphenol synthesis may dominate in some forest soils. In extreme climates, sharp fluctuations in land surface conditions such as temperature, humidity, and radiation can aid in the synthesis of humus through the sugar-amino acid pathway. The chemical properties of humic allow them to be used in various industries, agriculture, environmental applications, and biomedicine.

REFERENCES

Ayuso M., Hernandez T., Garcia C, and Pascual A. 1996. *Biosecure Terchnology Journal* (57:3):251–257. https://doi.org/10.1016/S0960-8524(96)00064-8

Bot, A. Dan J. Benites. 2005. The Importance of Soil Organik Matter, Key to Drought-Resistant Soil and Sustained Food Production. FAO Soils Bulletin. *Dalam Munawar, A. 2011. Kesuburan Tanah Dan Nutrisi Tanaman.*IPB Press. Bogor

Buckau G, Artinger R, Geyer S, Wolf M, Fritz P, Kim J.I. 2000. Groundwater In-Situ Generation of Aquatic Humic and Fulvic Acids and The Mineralization Of Sedimentary Organic Carbon. *Applied Geochemistry Journal* (15): 819–832 https://Doi.Org/10.1016/S0883-2927(99)00078-5

Cooper R.J., Chunhua Liu and Fisher D.S. 1998. Influence of humic substances on rooting and nutrient content of creeping betgrass. *Crop Science Journal* (38):6. https://doi.org/10.2135/cropsci1998.0011183X003800060037x

Ghabbour E.A. and Davies G. 1999. *Understanding Humic Substances: Advance Methods, Properties and Applications.* The Royal Society of Chemistry. Cambridge. UK.

Ghabbour E.A., Davies G., Ghali N. K. and Mulligan M.D. 2001. The effect of temperature on tight metal binding by peat and soil derived solid humic acids. *Canadian Journal of Soil Science* 81(3): 331–337. https://doi.org/10.4141/S00-065

Hardjowigeno, S. 2003. *Ilmu Tanah.* Akademika Presindo. Jakarta

Huang, P.M. and M. Schnitzer. 1997. *Interaksi Mineral Tanah Dengan Organik Alami Dan Mikroba.* UGM Press. Yogyakarta.

Klöcking R. 1992. Interaction Of Humic Acids and Humicacid-Like Polymers with Herpes Simplex Virus Type 1. *Humanic Substances in The Aquatic and Terrestrial Environment.* Berlin.

Koivula N. and K. Hanninen. 1999. Biodeterioration of Cardboard-Based Liquid Containers Collected for Fibre Reuse. *Chemosphere* (38): 1873–1887

Kumada, K. 1987. Chemistry Of Soil Organik Matter. *Japan Scientific Societies. Tokyo.*

Leoniy, Alfian. 2011. Keefektifan Kompos yang Diperkaya dengan Asam Humat dan Bakteri Aktivator untuk Mengendalikan Penyakit Rebah Kecambah (Damping Off) yang Disebabkan oleh *Fusarium sp.* pada Tanaman Tomat. Skripsi. IPB

Lotosh T.D. 1991. *Experimental Bases and Prospects for The Use of Humic Acid Preparations from Peat In Medicine And Agricultural Production.* (In Russian) *Naucn.* Dokl. Vyss. Skoly. *Biol. Nauki* (10): 99–103

Majakova E.F. and Proskurjakov V.A. 1972. *Some ways of complex chemical processing of peat.* Peat congress. Finland

Mendez, Eladia, Joff Havel, Dan Jiri Patocks. 2005. Humic Substances. Compounds Of Still Unknown Structure: Applications in Agriculture, Industry, Environment, And Biomedicine. *Appl. Biomed.* (3): 13–24

Munawar, Ali. 2011. *Kesuburan Tanah Dan Nutrisi Tanaman.* IPB Press, Bogor

Olk D.C., and Cassman K.G. 1995. Reduction of Pottasium Fixation by Two Humic Acid Fractions in Vremiculitic Soil. *Soil Science Society of America Journal* (58:5): 1250–1258. https://doi.org/10.2136/sssaj1995.03615995005900050007x

Pacheco M. and Havel J. 2004. Capillary zone electrophoretic (CZE) study of uranium (VI) complexation with humic acids. *Journal of Radioabalitical and Nuclear Chemistry* (248:3): 565–570

Prasad R, Power JF. 1997. *Soil Fertility Management for Sustainable Agriculture.* New York: CRC Lesi Publisher

Saleh, Rahmat. 2014. Ekstraksi Asam Humat Dari Gambut Untuk Industri. *Pusdiklat Mineral Dan Batubara*

Samanidou V., I. Papadoyannis, G. Vasilikiotis. 1991. Mobilization of Heavy-Metals from River Sediments Of Northern Greece, By Humic Substances. *J. Environm. Sci. Health* (A26):1055–1068

Selvi A. 2010. Karakteristik Erapan Dan Desorpsi P Pada Rhodic Eutrudox Dan Typic Paleudult, Kuaro Dari Kalimantan Timur. Skripsi. IPB

Stevenson, F.J. 1982. *Humus Chemistry. Genesis, Composition, Reactions.* Jhon Wiley & Sons. Canada

Tan, K.H. 1991. *Andosols.* Van Nostrans Reinhold Company. England

Tipping, Edward, 2004. *Cation Binding by Humic Subtances.* Cambidge University Press, USA.

Yamada E., T. Ozaki, M. Kimura: Determination and Behavior of Humic Substances as Precursors of Trihalomethane in Environmental Water. *Anal. Sci.* (14): 327–332

Yuan, Shenyuan. 1993. *Application of Fulvic Acid and Its Derivatives in The Fields of Agriculture and Medic.* First Edition: June.

Zhang M. and Z. He. 2004. Long-Term Changes in Organik Carbon And Nutrients Of An Ultisol Under Rice Cropping In Southeast China. *Geoderma* (118): 167–179

Technological Innovations in Tropical Livestock Development for Environmental Sustainability and Food Security – P. Dhian Isnaeni et al. (eds)
© 2025 The Author(s), ISBN 978-1-032-74373-8
Open Access: www.taylorfrancis.com, CC BY-NC-ND 4.0 license

Community perceptions of village innovation development using the pentahelix approach in Central Bengkulu regency

W.E. Putra*, H. Subagio, D. Wamaer, V. Siagian, A. Ishak, E. Fauzi, Yahumri, Afrizon & S. Rosmanah
National Research and Innovation Agency, Jakarta Selatan, Indonesia

ABSTRACT: The development of village innovation has become unsustainable and village funding support from the Government each year has become less effective in encouraging the development of innovation. This research aims to determine the factors that influence the development of village innovation from a community perspective. Research locus in two villages in Talang Empat Subdistrict, Central Bengkulu Regency, Bengkulu Province, Indonesia. The research locations were determined deliberately at Air Sebakul Village (has village assets) and Panca Mukti Village (does not have village assets). Data collection was carried out through a survey of 60 respondents representing the village community according to the results of identification with the village government. The survey was conducted from July to September 2023, involving 30 respondents in each village. The data variable is in the form of community perceptions using the Pentahelix approach (the role of social institutions, government programs, market support, innovation sources, and communication media) in developing village innovation with 22 indicators. Data analysis was carried out descriptively using Importance Performance Analysis (IPA). All aspects of the pentahelix have an important role in developing village innovation, but the performance of several indicators still needs to be improved. Strengthening the role of village-owned enterprises and empowering existing economic institutions in villages to support the implementation of village innovation is very necessary through support from village communities and assistance from relevant stakeholders from outside the village.

Keywords: innovation, pentahelix, village

1 INTRODUCTION

The development of rural areas in Indonesia is one of the things that the Government really pays attention to. Indonesia has 84,096 villages/sub-districts with various unique characteristics as potential for economic development and community welfare. The government encourages village community participation in development through the allocation of village funds amounting to IDR 70 trillion in 2023 (BPS 2023). Village funds began to be distributed in 2015 amounting to IDR 20.8 trillion which continues to increase every year by an average of 21.3% until 2023 (Kompas 2023). Poverty is one of the problems in the village. The percentage of poor people in Indonesia in September 2022 will average 9.57%, higher in rural areas (12.36%) compared to rural areas (7.53%). In fact, of Indonesia's total population of 275,773,774 people, only around 44% live in rural areas (BPS 2023). The ability of village communities to develop innovations in accordance with village potential is one of the challenges in village development and poverty alleviation.

Innovation as a new idea and practice in society to solve certain problems (Kristiawan *et al.* 2018). The development of village innovation essentially aims to empower the community by involving the roles of all relevant stakeholders. Therefore, the innovation

*Corresponding Author: wawan_ekaputra@ymail.com

DOI: 10.1201/9781003468943-41

development approach must be carried out comprehensively by involving all actors in an innovation system. The pentahelix approach can be used to understand the framework of the innovation system. This approach involves academics, companies, society, media, and government in tourism development (Yasir *et al.* 2021), small and medium businesses (Rosyadi *et al.* 2020), digital technology development (Novani *et al.* 2022), and developing programs. empowerment of village communities (Yusnita *et al.* 2022).

Central Bengkulu Regency has enormous potential for developing village innovation. Its location near Bengkulu City as the capital of Bengkulu Province means that villages in the city border area have greater opportunities to involve various parties in developing innovation. This research aims to determine the community's perspective regarding the development of village innovation using the pentahelix approach in Central Bengkulu Regency.

2 RESEARCH METHODS

This research was carried out from July to September 2023 in two peri-urban villages in Central Bengkulu Regency, namely Air Sebakul Village and Panca Mukti Village, Pondok Kelapa Subdistrict (Figure 1).

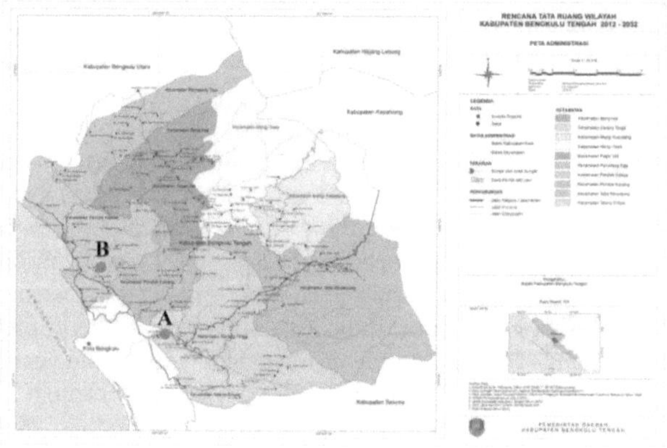

Figure 1. Research location (A. Air Sebakul Village; B. Panca Mukti Village).

These two villages are peri-urban areas where most of the population's economic activities are directly related to urban areas, without abandoning community activities in the field of agriculture as a traditional business. Data was collected through a survey involving 60 respondents, each village was represented by 30 respondents were chosen deliberately to represent village stakeholders consisting of village government and community leaders. Determination of survey respondents was carried out together with the village government. The variables collected include five pentahelix variables consisting of 22 indicators (Table 1).

Table 1. Variables and indicators for village innovation development.

Variables	Indicators
Social institutions	(1) Public awareness; (2) Community participation; (3) Economic institutions; (4) Community compliance with norms; (5) Application of technology
Government program	(1) The existence of village funds; (2) The role of Village-Owned Enterprises; (3) The role of village assistant officers
Market support	(1) Local markets; (2) Regional markets; (3) Marketing of superior village products
Innovation sources	Universities; (2) Research institutions; (3) Private companies; (4) non-governmental organizations; (5) Local governments; (6) Innovator figures
Communication media	(1) Interpersonal communication; (2) Communication in groups; (3) Communication with village assistant officers; (4) Communication via social media; (5) Communication via mass media

Respondents' perceptions about the indicators of the pentahelix variable are made on a Likert scale with a score of 1–5. This perception is divided into 2 categories, namely the importance and performance categories of all indicators for the development of village innovation. Data analysis was carried out descriptively using Importance Performance Analysis (IPA). Measurement of the level of importance and level of performance is shown in Table 2.

Table 2. Importance and performance assessment guide.

Score	Level of importance	Performance level
5	Very important	Very good
4	Important	Good
3	Quite important	Pretty good
2	Not too important	Not good
1	Not important	Very not good

The indicator values for each variable are then averaged based on the respondents' answers to obtain a value for the level of importance and performance of each indicator using the following formula (Tjiptono and Chandra 2019):

$$\overline{X} = \frac{\sum_{i=1}^{k} Xi}{n} \text{ and } \overline{Y} = \frac{\sum_{i=1}^{k} Yi}{n} \quad (1)$$

where:

$\overline{X}$ = The average value of the i-th indicator performance assessment level
$\overline{Y}$ = The average value of the level of importance assessment of the i-th indicator
n = Number of respondents

Based on the calculation results in equation (1), the Level of Conformity (LCi) between performance levels and interests is calculated as follows:

$$LCi = \frac{\overline{Xi}}{\overline{Y}} \times 100\% \quad (2)$$

Next, the average value of the level of importance and performance for all indicators is calculated using the formula:

$$\overline{\overline{Xi}} = \frac{\sum_{i=1}^{k} \overline{Xi}}{n} \text{ and } \overline{\overline{Yi}} = \frac{\sum_{i=1}^{k} \overline{Yi}}{n} \quad (3)$$

where:

$\overline{\overline{Xi}}$ = The average value of the performance assessment level of all indicators of the i-th variable $\overline{\overline{Yi}}$ = The average value of the level of importance assessment of all indicators of the i-th variable n = Number of variables.

This $\overline{\overline{Xi}}$ value cuts perpendicular to the horizontal axis, namely the axis that reflects the performance level of all performance indicators. Meanwhile, the $\overline{\overline{Yi}}$ values cut perpendicular to the vertical axis which reflects the level of importance of all indicators. These values are then plotted on a Cartesian diagram (Figure 2). The indicators that need to be paid attention to are the indicators in the second quadrant (Q2) because their performance is still low and on the contrary, they are very important in developing village innovation.

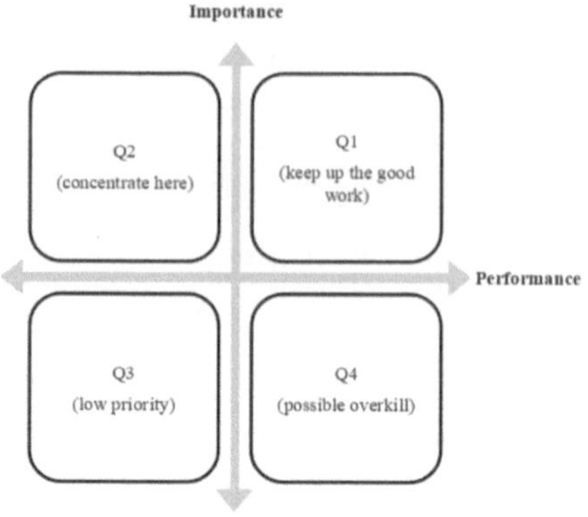

Figure 2. The four IPA quadrants (Wu 2021).

3 RESULTS AND DISCUSSION

3.1 *Village innovation development opportunities*

Air Sebakul and Panca Mukti Villages are located on the border with Bengkulu City (the capital of Bengkulu Province). The livelihoods of the residents are diverse, no longer relying solely on agricultural businesses. Some residents still grow food crops such as rice and secondary crops, grow oil palm and rubber plantations, and raise cows, goats or chickens. Most residents work as daily laborers or sell processed agricultural products. It is still difficult to develop technological and institutional innovations by exploiting village potential because community economic efforts are still small scale, carried out by each household. Therefore, innovation should be developed on a village scale by utilizing government programs in the form of village funds provided annually by the Central Government to be managed by the Village Government.

The potential that can be developed in these two villages is tourism and agriculture. The Air Sebakul Village Government is developing a check dam which will become a village asset for water tourism, in addition to processing various agricultural products such as kalamansi orange syrup, banana chips, and smoked catfish. Meanwhile, in Panca Mukti Village, the main agricultural product that is a source of income for the community is processing cassava into *tapai* and chips, while a tourist attraction that can be developed is *Batik* Village. Therefore, the Village Government has developed a tourist car that will make it easier for visitors to tour the village to see culinary processing and batik making businesses during holidays. Based on the survey results in the two research locus villages, the innovations proposed to be developed as village innovations are shown in Table 3.

Table 3. Proposals for developing village innovation.

	Air Sebakul		Panca Mukti	
No.	Innovation	%	Innovation	%
1.	Check dam tourism	80.00	Coconut cultivation	86.67
2.	Fishing pond	63.33	Culinary	33.33
3.	Culinary	56.67	Tourist car	30.00
4.	Floating net cages	43.33	Batik marketing	30.00

Table 3 shows that the proposed innovation in Sebakul Water Village is more directed at utilizing check dams which are village assets for water tourism activities, fishing ponds, culinary preparations, and floating net cage cultivation. This proposal is in accordance with the utilization of village potential. In Panca Mukti Village, the community proposed that innovation be directed towards developing coconut cultivation in yards that would be managed by the village.

3.2 *Level of conformity of innovation supporting variables*

The level of conformity in developing innovation is influenced by five variables that can support innovation (pentahelix). Figure 3 shows the results of a survey of community perceptions regarding the level of suitability of the pentahelix variable in developing innovation in the two research villages.

The comparison between the level of importance and the level of innovation performance in the two villages is relatively good because all of them are above the average value, namely 60%. However, the level of suitability for all variables supporting innovation in Panca Mukti Village is relatively higher than in Air Sebakul Village, except for the government program support variable. The level of suitability of the communication media variable has the highest value compared to other variables, respectively 96.85 for Air Sebakul Village and 99.36% for Panca Mukti Village. The difference in suitability levels is only 2.51%. This means that the gap between the importance and performance of the communication media support variable is relatively low. The two villages close to urban areas have relatively good access to information and communication technology services, making it easier to support interpersonal communication, group communication, communication with village assistant officers, communication via social media, and communication via mass media.

Apart from the communication media support variable, the variable which also has a low difference in the level of suitability in the two villages is support for government programs in village development, namely 79.80% (Air Sebakul) and 75.75% (Panca Mukti) with a difference of 4.05%. The distribution of village funds, which began in 2015, has become the main supporting factor for village development, resulting in relatively low levels of performance and importance. Even though village funds are not entirely directed towards developing village innovation, all work plans have been prepared jointly by community components through village development planning meetings which are held every year. The use of village funds for the development of check dams in Air Sebakul Village has started in 2021, while the development of coconut cultivation in Panca Mukti Village is supported by village funds, so that the community's perception of the level of suitability of government programs is higher in Air Sebakul Village.

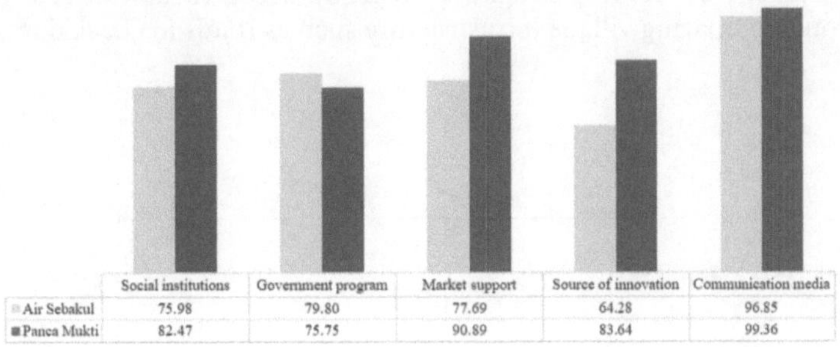

Figure 3. Percentage of pentahelix variables conformity in developing village innovation.

The social institutional variables that support the development of coconut cultivation innovation in Panca Mukti Village are relatively high (82.47%) because the community is used to planting coconuts in their yards. A strategy is only needed to develop village innovation by involving community participation. On the other hand, the social institutions variable does not support the development of check dam tourism in Air Sebakul Village (75.98%) because existing institutions in the community have not been formed to support these tourism activities. The difference in the level of innovation suitability between the two villages is 6.49%.

Market support for the development of coconut cultivation innovation in Panca Mukti Village (90.89%) is higher than market support for the development of checkdam tourism in Air Sebakul Village (77.69%) with a difference of 13.20%. Coconut products have a higher market potential compared to tourism development because coconuts have been used for various needs in society, especially for cooking. Meanwhile, the performance of check dam tourism in Air Sebakul Village is still relatively low because this tourist attraction only started to open in 2022.

The highest gap in the level of variable suitability between the two villages is found in the innovation source variable, namely 19.36%. The level of suitability of the innovation source variable in Panca Mukti Village in coconut cultivation is quite high (83.64%) because it is relatively easier for the community to obtain innovation from various sources (assistant staff, related agencies, universities, the private sector, even the internet). On the other hand, innovation in developing checkdam tourism has a lower level of suitability for the innovation source variable (64.28%) because the community has not been able to identify sources of innovation that can be accessed regarding the development of checkdam tourism.

3.3 *Recommendations for village innovation development*

3.3.1 *Air Sebakul village*

Innovation in Air Sebakul Village is directed at developing check dam tourism which is an asset owned by the village. The recommendations given for the development of innovation are arranged based on the Science Quadrant in Figure 4. There are several indicators whose performance needs to be improved for the development of innovation in Air Sebakul Village, namely the development of economic institutions or BUMDES, the development of technological innovation, the growth of local markets, and the role of Regional Government as a source of innovation in developing checkdam tourism. These five indicators are located in quadrant 2 of the IPA diagram whose performance needs to be encouraged in order to move towards quadrant 1. The role of the Check dam tourism management institution is very important in developing innovation in Air Sebakul Village. Collaboration between BUMDES and community groups is able to increase community income through productive economic development (Sara *et al.* 2020). The initiation of a village market is needed to support the development of check dam tourism in Air Sebakul Village. Therefore, the Regional Government of Central Bengkulu Regency needs to take a role in supporting innovation through preparing village infrastructure such as roads to check dams and tourism promotion.

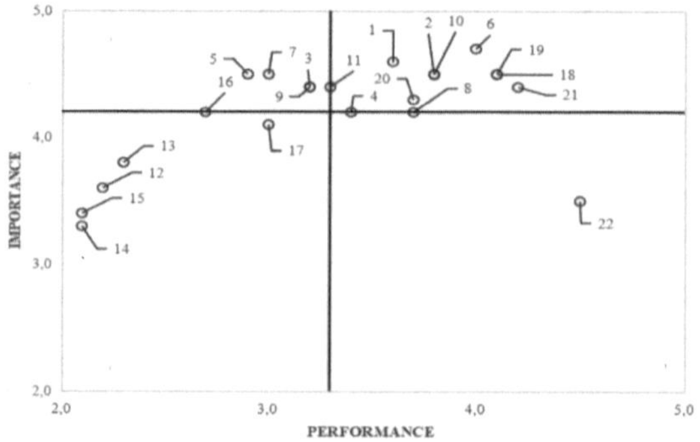

Figure 4. IPA quadrant for the development of tourism innovation at the Air Sebakul Village.

3.3.2 *Panca Mukti village*

Coconut cultivation is a village innovation proposed by the community in Panca Mukti Village. Recommendations for developing coconut cultivation innovations are shown in Figure 5. There are 8 pentahelix indicators in the development of coconut cultivation innovation in Panca Mukti Village which is in quadrant 2 which needs to be encouraged to increase its performance towards quadrant 1. These indicators are community awareness to develop coconut cultivation innovation, community participation, the role of economic institutions community, support from village funds, the role of BUMDES, support from village assistants, provision of innovation from universities, and support from community leaders. Community collaboration in building a shared vision for progress and business partnerships are the keys to developing village innovation (Suryani and Soedarso 2021).

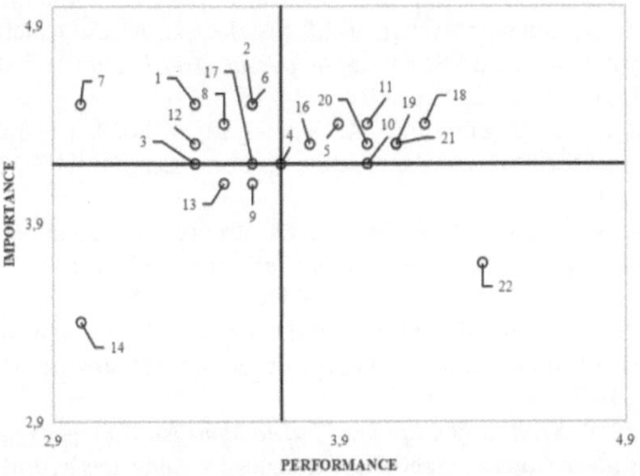

Figure 5. IPA quadrant development of coconut cultivation innovation in Panca Mukti Village.

Coconut cultivation by utilizing residents' yards is a new innovation that really needs the support of the Panca Mukti Village community. Therefore, there is a need for awareness and participation of citizens as well as support from community leaders. Collaboration between villages and communities in coconut cultivation needs to be built by utilizing capital facilities sourced from village funds through empowering community groups and strengthening the role of BUMDES Panca Mukti Village. Coconut cultivation requires a process of several years before the people of Panca Mukti Village get the benefits of increasing income. Therefore, the coconut cultivation innovation assistance program needs to be designed with a clear road map.

4 CONCLUSION

Analysis of the development of village innovation using the pentahelix approach in Air Sebakul Village is directed at developing check dam tourism by utilizing village assets. Meanwhile, the direction of village innovation in Panca Mukti Village is coconut cultivation. Strengthening the role of BUMDES and empowering community economic institutions are very important indicators to encourage improved performance in these two villages in the context of developing village innovation. These processes really need internal support from the village community as well as external support from various stakeholders from outside the village.

ACKNOWLEDGEMENT

We would like to thank the the Chairman of Research Organization for Governance, Economy, and Community Welfare, National Research and Innovation Agency, who has approved funding for this research in the 2023 fiscal year through the Economic and Community Welfare Program Scheme.

REFERENCES

BPS-Statistics Indonesia. 2023. *Statisticak Yearbook of Indonesia*. Jakarta.

Kompas.id, Dana Desa dan Peningkatan Desa Mandiri. 2023. https://www.kompas.id/baca/riset/2023/07/26-dana-desa-dan-peningkatan-desa-mandiri.

Kristiawan, M., Suryanti, I., Muntazir, M., Ribuwati, Areli A. J., Agustina, M., Kafarisa, R. F., Saputra, A. G., Diana, N., Agustina, E., Oktarina, R., Hisri, T. B. 2018. Inovasi Pendidikan, *WADE Group*, Ponorogo.

Novani, S., Cyntiawati, C., Kijima, K., Trianto, A. S., Mayangsari, L., Alamanda, D. T., Anggadwita, G. 2022. Empowering digital creative ecosystem using problem structuring method and a service science perspective: A case study in Cimahi and Bandung, *Indonesia, Asia Pacific Management Review* 28 (2): 215–228, https://doi.org/ 10.1016/j.apmrv.2022.09.003.

Rosyadi, T., Kusuma, A. S., Fitrah, E., Haryanto, A., Adawiyah, W. 2020. The multi-stakeholder's role in an integrated mentoring model for SMEs in the creative economy Sector, *SAGE Open* 10(4). https://doi.org/ 10.1177/2158244020963604.

Sara, I. M., Saputra, K. A. K., Utama, I. W. K. J. 2020. Improving economic development through the establishment of village-business enterprises, *Journal of Advanced Research in Dynamical and Control Systems*, 12(6):3032–3039. https://doi.org/105373/JARDCS/V12I6/ S20201269.

Suryani, A., Soedarso. 2021. Community-based development and collective learning: How does a local community engage and learn to initiate a smart village development?. *Journal ff Development Research*, 5 (1):39–49. https://doi.org/10.28926/jdr.v5i1.127.

Tjiptono, F., Chandra, G. 2019. *Service, Quality and Satisfaction*. Andi Press, Yogyakarta.

Wu, C. H. 2021. Exploring green hotel competitive strategies by using the hybrid method for complex data analysis, *Mathematical Problems in Engineering*. https://doi.org/10.1155/ 2021/9982387.

Yasir, F., Firzal, Y., Sulistyani, A., Yesicha, C. 2021. Penta Helix communication model through community based tourism (CBT) for tourism village development in Koto Sentajo, Riau, Indonesia. *Geo Journal of Tourism and Geosites*, 37(3): 851–860. https://doi.org/10.30892/gtg.37316-718.

Yusnita, V., Tresiana, N., Meutia, I. F. 2022. Economic empowerment through community village. *Przegląd Politologiczny*, (4):111–124. https://doi.org/10.14746/PP.2022.27.4.9.

Technological Innovations in Tropical Livestock Development for Environmental Sustainability and Food Security – P. Dhian Isnaeni et al. (eds)
© 2025 The Author(s), ISBN 978-1-032-74373-8
Open Access: www.taylorfrancis.com, CC BY-NC-ND 4.0 license

Potential development of Balinese cattle breeding in the seedling source area of Palangga sub-district, South Konawe district

M. Abadi*, L.O. Nafiu, T. Saili, M.A. Pagala & L.O.A. Sani
Faculty of Animal Husbandry, Halu Oleo University, Kendari, Indonesia

L. Yunus, R.M. Iswandi, L. Rianda & L.O. Alwi
Faculty of Agriculture, Halu Oleo University, Kendari, Indonesia

ABSTRACT: This study aims to determine and analyze the development potential of Bali cattle breeding in the seedling source area of Palangga Sub-district, South Konawe Regency. Variables related to technical aspect support include maintenance system, maintenance pattern, feed source, seedling source, production and reproduction, disease management, availability of field officers, availability of farmer groups, availability of financial institutions, and marketing. Variables related to technical aspect support include Animal Health Service Center, AI posts, Agricultural Training Center, pasture, water source, and slaughterhouse. The data obtained were analyzed using descriptive qualitative analysis, which describes the potential carrying capacity of Bali cattle breeding development in the Palangga Sub-district. The results showed that the Palangga Sub-district of South Konawe Regency has the potential to develop Bali cattle breeding as a source area for Bali cattle seedlings, this can be seen from the availability of the carrying capacity of technical aspects and non-technical aspects.

Keywords: Development, Breeding, Bali Cattle, Technical Aspects, Non-Technical Aspects, *Andrographis paniculata*, immunomodulator, spleen, infection

1 INTRODUCTION

Animal husbandry is part of the agricultural subsector that continues to be developed to meet animal protein needs (Talakua *et al.* 2022). One of the livestock businesses that can help support these needs is Bali cattle. Bali cattle itself is one of the original Indonesian cattle breeds originating from the Bali area which is currently spread to almost all parts of Indonesia with a high ability to convert feed, have good meat quality, adapt to the tropics (Nindhia *et al.* 2021).

South Konawe is one of 17 regencies/cities in Southeast Sulawesi Province with an area of 4514.20 Km^2 which has the potential for agricultural development, one of which is the livestock sector (Abadi *et al.* 2021). The livestock sector that is widely developed by the community independently is Bali cattle, but the number of livestock populations raised by the community is still low when compared to the available resources (Abadi *et al.* 2022; Abadi *et al.* 2023).

According to Abadi *et al.* (2023b), Ibrahim & Hadiana (2023) raising cattle requires adequate resources, namely place, capital, human resources and natural resources. Where natural resources are also a supporting factor in fulfilling the needs of livestock regarding the availability of feed and land while human resources will help the pattern of farming that will be formed. Based on data from 2022, the total cattle population was 69,274 heads with meat production of 1,108,850kg. While Palangga sub-district is one of the sub-districts with the highest population compared to other sub-districts, namely 5,804 heads and 57,787.50kg of meat production. This shows that Bali beef production in Palangga Sub-district in 2022

*Corresponding Author: musram.abadi79@uho.ac.id

contributes around 19.18% of the total Bali beef production in South Konawe Regency (BPS Konawe Selatan 2022).

The level of population in South Konawe District illustrates that this region has the potential to develop Balinese cattle breeding business, one of which is Palangga Subdistrict, but its development efforts require support related to technical potential which has a very important role such as the application of systems and maintenance patterns carried out by farmers, availability and sources of feed, origin and source of seeds, appearance of production and reproduction, how to handle diseases, as well as the availability of field officers, farmer groups, financial institutions, livestock unit prices, and marketing, while non-technical aspects consist of the availability of health posts, AI posts, Agricultural Training Centers, pastures, water sources, and slaughterhouses. These technical and non-technical aspects greatly influence the success of the Balinese cattle breeding business in the Palangga Sub-district Balinese cattle breeding area of South Konawe District, which is still managed simply with the community farming model.

Therefore, it is necessary to know what potentials can support the development of Balinese cattle breeding in the seedling source area, most of which still apply to the smallholder farming system(Abadi *et al.* 2023), so that this research can be used as a reference for government policy and for Balinese cattle breeding business actors who still apply the smallholder breeding pattern in the seedling source area of Palangga District, South Konawe Regency and in other areas.

2 MATERIALS AND METHODS

This research was conducted in September-December 2022, in Palangga District, South Konawe Regency. Respondents in this study were determined by the census, namely all farmer households (RTP) in Palangga District, South Konawe Regency, totalling 758 RTP. Variables related to technical aspect support include respondent characteristics, rearing system, food sources, population structure, calving interval, estrus duration, disease management and prevention. The data analysis used in the research is descriptive qualitative analysis, namely by describing the potential carrying capacity of Bali cattle farming business development in Palangga District which aims to describe systemically and accurately the situation or events in a particular field/region.

3 RESULTS AND DISCUSSION

3.1 *Farmer age and education level*

Age is one of the factors that greatly affect the management and productivity capabilities of a person in carrying out cattle-raising activities because age will be closely related to the mindset in their livestock business activities. In other words, those who are older tend to be stronger than those who are older. The age of Bali cattle farmers in Palangga Sub-district, South Konawe Regency is presented in Figure 1.

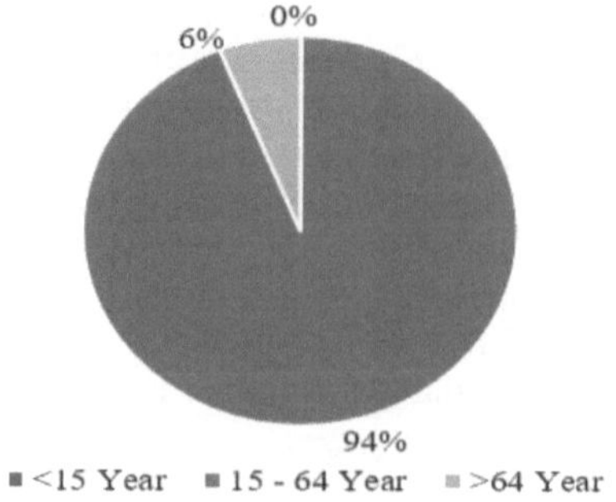

Figure 1. Age of cattle Balinese farmers.

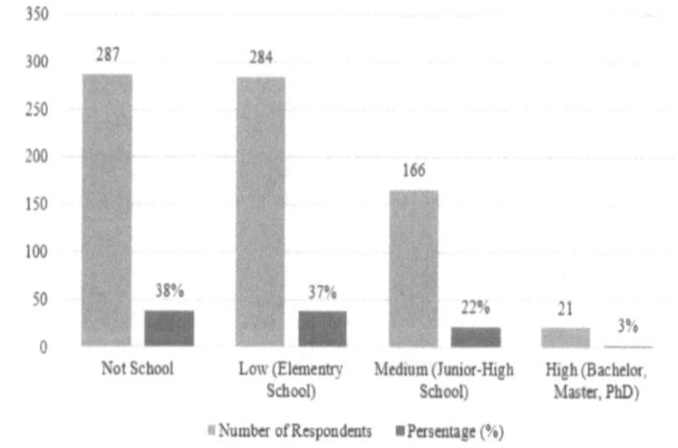

Figure 2. Education level of Balinese cattle farmers.

Figure 1 shows that farmers in Palangga Sub-district are predominantly aged 15–64 years with a presentation of 94% (713 people). At this age most farmers have high motivation in working, especially raising cattle. The age level of farmers, which is dominated by 15–64 years, is something that supports the potential for the development of Bali cattle farming in Palangga District because the age of farmers is classified as productive making cattle enterprise development programs easier to accept and implement. According to Nalle *et al.* (2023), the productive age is 35–55 years in an area because at that age they can know their social situation and the condition of the population in their area. So, it is very productive in running and developing their business. Data from Kemenkes RI (2017) that people who are categorized as productive age with an age range (of 15–64 years).

3.2 *Education level*

The level of education is an important indicator for running a business, including the Bali cattle business because it will be the main capital in increasing the productivity of the livestock itself. This means that the higher the education of the farmer, the higher the level of quality of resources subsequently the higher/increased productivity of the work done. Therefore, based on the higher level of education of farmers, it can be expected that livestock business activities will grow. The education level of Bali cattle breeders in Palangga Sub-district, South Konawe Regency is presented in Figure 2.

Figure 2 shows that farmers in Palangga sub-district are highly dominated by farmers with no schooling and primary school education. As many as 38% did not attend school and 37% had an elementary school education. This level of education is expected to continue to support the potential for Bali cattle business development even though they are still dominated by those with low education levels. This is because farmers in Palangga Subdistrict still have high motivation in farming and the results of livestock sales are very profitable so education that is still classified as low does not affect Bali cattle farming. According to Irwanto *et al.* (2023)one of the perception-forming factors is the length of formal education. Concerning this study, an example of such perception is the development of their livestock or progress in the livestock business. Other research states that the development of the livestock business itself will be greatly influenced by those with higher levels of education(Omelia *et al.* 2023). Nurdiyansah *et al.* (2020) the development of animal husbandry is supported by their education, meaning that innovations in animal husbandry are the impact of their higher education, because their thinking power is broader and more insightful to always progress.

3.3 *Maintenance system*

The husbandry system of Bali cattle farming will greatly impact the livestock production process. In general, Bali cattle farming in the study area is intensive. However, some farmers choose to raise their cattle extensively and semi-intensively. Balinese cattle are kept in cages and grazed in grazing areas and on the edge of rice fields. In addition, some farmers in the study area raise their cattle by tying them to the house area or on the fields. The husbandry system of Bali cattle farmers in Palangga Subdistrict, South Konawe Regency is presented in Figure 3.

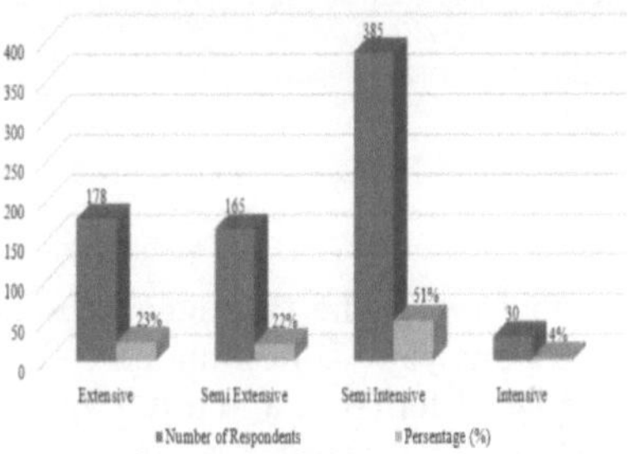

Figure 3. Balinese cattle rearing system.

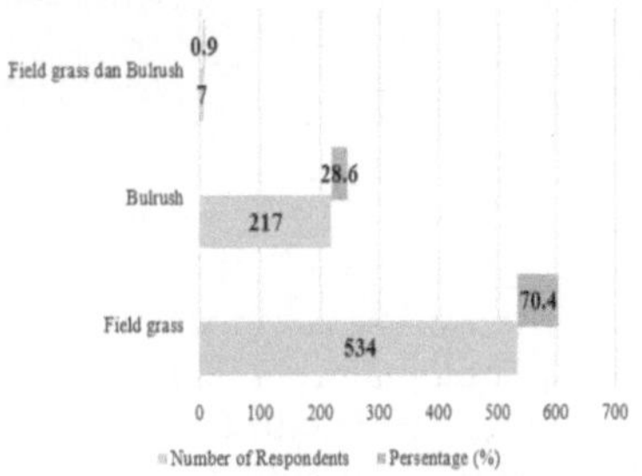

Figure 4. Types of forage for Bali cattle.

Figure 3 shows that the Bali cattle rearing system model in Palangga Subdistrict is dominated by semi-intensive rearing as much as 51%. Bali cattle are grazed during the day and stabled at night. This is chosen because it is relatively easy and cost-effective, but on the other hand, this kind of maintenance often has a large risk such as the safety factor of livestock that cannot be controlled. Cattle are housed and receive more regular treatment in terms of feeding drinking water and cleaning the cage. According to Sani *et al.* (2018), the various livestock-rearing systems applied by farmers will greatly impact their own Bali cattle production activities.

3.4 *Type of fodder forage*

Feed is a basic requirement in the maintenance of Bali cattle in this case forage feed, because all forms of feed ingredients come from fresh forage through several processes (Akoso, 1996). Types of forage for Bali cattle in Palangga Subdistrict, South Konawe Regency are presented in Figure 4. Figure 4 shows that the type of feed used by farmers in Palangga Subdistrict is dominated by field grass as much as 70%. Farmers who provide forage grass generally have more than 2 Bali cattle, therefore in fulfilling their feed needs farmers provide other types of grass besides natural grass. A combination of grass species (natural grass, cultivated grass and rice straw) is used as a low fresh feed supply, such as during the dry season. The availability of cultivated grass feed and agricultural by-products (rice straw) is needed by farmers during the dry season to support the supply of feed for Bali cattle in Palangga District. Utilizing combination feed is a potential carrying capacity for the development of Bali cattle in Palangga District, South Konawe Regency. According to Bilyaro *et al.* (2023), the provision of forage in the process of raising ruminants is very important.

3.5 *Population structure of Bali cattle*

Livestock population structure is the structure of the origin of a herd of livestock, for example, Bali cattle. The population structure of Bali cattle in this study can be divided by age, where the age of cattle consists of adults (Bali cattle that have been producing, generally aged 2 years or more), young (Bali cattle weaned between one and two years old and not yet producing), and calves (Bali cattle calves aged 0 months to one year or calves that are still breastfeeding on their mothers). The population structure of Bali cattle in Palangga Subdistrict, South Konawe Regency is presented in Figure 5.

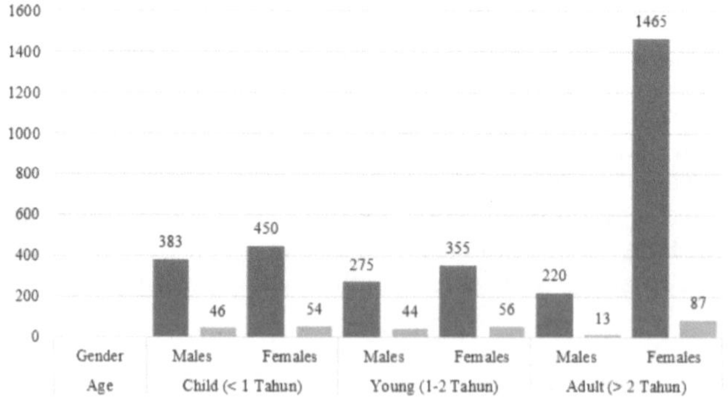

Figure 5. Population structure of Bali cattle.

Figure 5 shows the composition of the Bali cattle population in the Palangga sub-district based on age and male and female sex. Child age (less than one year) is dominated by 54% of females, young age (one to two years) is dominated by 56% of females, and adult age (more than two years) is dominated by 87% of females. From this research data, it can be concluded that females dominate the existing population both at the child, young and adult levels. On the other hand, Balinese cattle in the area have relatively good reproduction because they have adequate males and females.

3.6 *Calving interval and length of estrous*

The calving interval is the difference in months/days from one birth to the next. The calving interval is an illustration of livestock facilities. This means that the shorter the calving interval, the better. The calving interval can also be measured through the lactation period plus the dry period or the empty period plus the gestation period. The calving interval of Bali cattle in Palangga subdistrict, South Konawe district is presented in Figure 6.

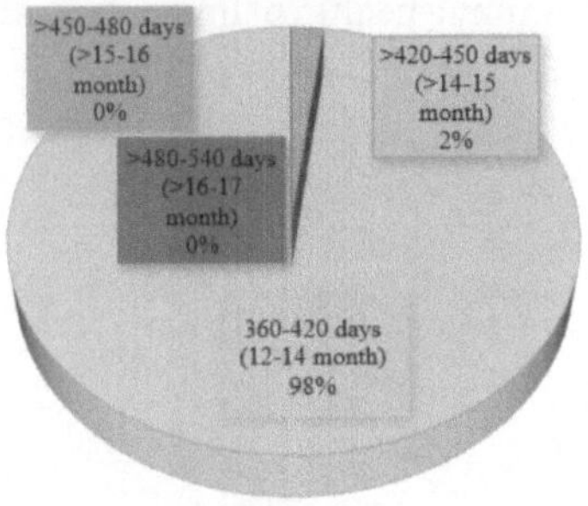

Figure 6. *calving interval* of Bali Cattle.

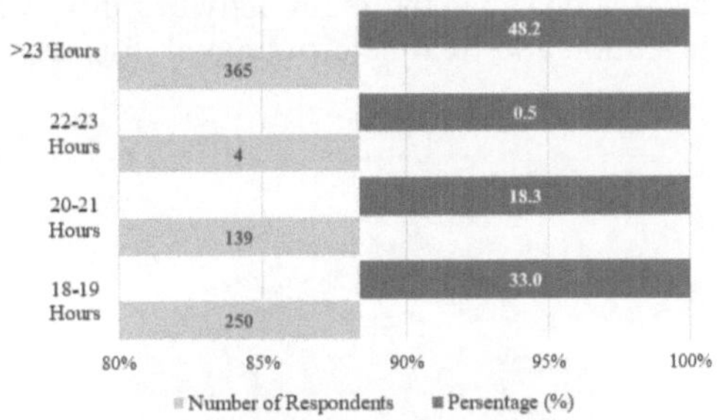

Figure 7. Length of estrous of Bali cattle.

Figure 6 shows that Bali cattle reproduction is dominated by a lambing distance between 12–14 months or 360–420 days as much as 98%. The shorter the distance between the birth of one livestock and the previous or subsequent livestock reveals the better the reproductive activity of the livestock itself. So, the short birth spacing of livestock in the Palangga Subdistrict is very supportive of the development of Bali cattle in the reproductive process. A good birth spacing is 365 days/12 months (Ananda *et al.* 2020). According to Kristyari *et al.* (2021) 12.64 $\pm$ 1.48 months is a fairly good calving interval value.

Length of lambing is a condition where female cattle have shown signs of asking for mating. The length of estrous of Bali cattle in Palangga Subdistrict, South Konawe Regency is presented in Table 7. Figure 7 shows that the reproductive performance of cattle, especially in the length of oestrous, is dominated by more than 23 hours as much as 48%. This time reveals that after cattle experience oestrous, this cycle will occur after more than 23 hours. Dhayanti *et al.* (2021) the shortest post-partum estrus time is 1 month, and long estrus is > 24 hours (Adinda *et al.* 2023).

3.7 *Disease and disease management*

The success of cattle farming is not only in the efforts to develop the existing cattle population but also in the prevention and control of diseases that keep the health of livestock maintained. The way to prevent disease can be done by maintaining the health of livestock so that sick cattle are separated from healthy cattle and immediately treated and regular livestock health checks and vaccinations are carried out according to instructions. The types of Bali cattle diseases in Palangga Subdistrict, South Konawe Regency are presented in Figure 8.

Figure 8 shows that diseases that occurred in livestock were dominated by diarrhoea diseases commonly called worms. This disease was experienced by about 10%, of which 76% of farmers did not experience disease in their livestock. Based on these results, it is necessary to improve maintenance management to support the development of Bali cattle breeding in Palangga Subdistrict, South Konawe Regency so that diseases that interfere with livestock such as worms/diarrhoea can be resolved as early as possible. Islami *et al.* (2022) in raising Bali cattle must pay attention to several things so that their livestock are not threatened, one of which is livestock health problems such as types of livestock diseases.

Preventive measures taken to protect cattle health include keeping cages and equipment clean, separating sick cattle from healthy cattle, treating them, and conducting regular cattle health checks and vaccinations as required. Disease management of Bali cattle in the Palangga subdistrict is presented in Figure 9. Figure 9 shows that farmers in the Palangga subdistrict dealt with disease to prevent diseases affecting their Bali cattle. The dominant handling is reporting the disease to the officer, which is 29%. This means that on the other hand, the majority or 70% did not handle the disease. Meanwhile, the remaining 1% handled the disease with their own medicine. Many farmers do not handle diseases of their livestock due to the low incidence of diseases that occur, which is 76% (table 9). Putra & Simanjuntak, (2023) stated that the main activities in this aspect of animal health management are the prevention and treatment of animal diseases.

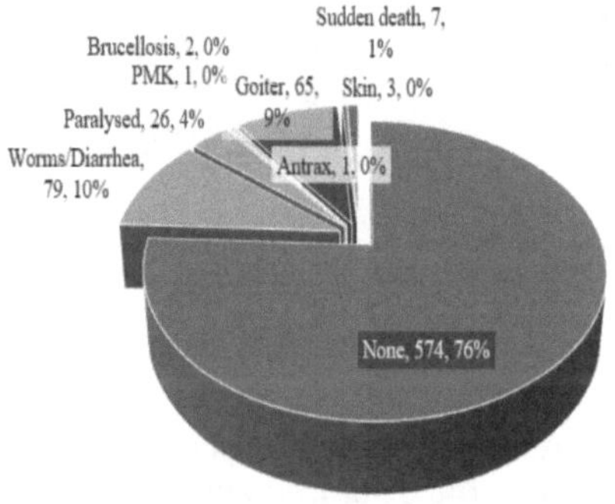

Figure 8. Types of diseases in Bali cattle.

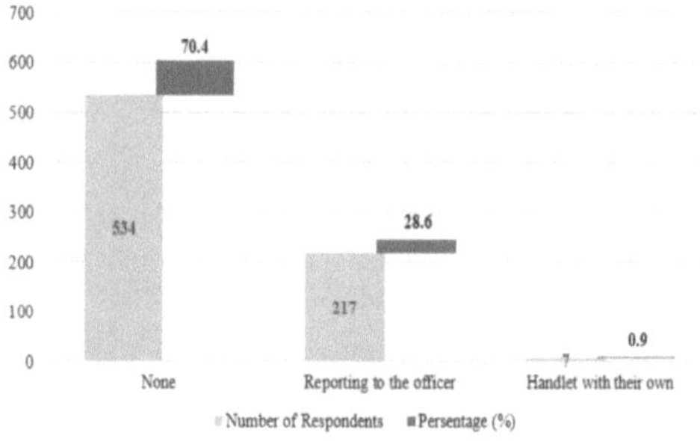

Figure 9. Disease management of Bali cattle.

4 CONCLUSION

Based on the results of the study, it is concluded that Palangga District of South Konawe Regency has the potential for the development of Bali cattle breeding as seen from technical aspects including the maintenance system carried out by farmers, availability and sources of feed, calving interval, length of lambing, handling and prevention of disease. The carrying capacity of technical aspects can support the breeding of Bali cattle by the ideal breeding system and can be used as a reference in the development of a Bali cattle breeding business with a community breeding pattern.

REFERENCES

Abadi, M., Libriani, R., Nafiu, L. O., Hadini, H. A., Rizal, A., Gerhana, & Surahmanto. 2023a. Development potential of bali cattle in baito sub-district South Konawe Regency. *Chalaza Journal of Animal Husbandry*, *8*(1). https://doi.org/10.31327/chalaza.v8i1.1904

Abadi, M., Nafiu, L., Libriani, R., Rahman, & Gerhana 2023b. Analysis of regional carrying capacity for bali cattle development in Baito District, South Konawe Regency. *Jurnal Peternakan Terapan (PETERPAN)*, *5*(2).https://doi.org/10.25181/peterpan.v5i2.2944

Abadi, M., Nafiu, L. O., & Karim, J. (2019). Mapping the potential of bali cattle fodder forage land resources in Tinanggea District, South Konawe Regency. *Journal of Tropical Livestock Science and Technology*, *6*(1), 124. https://doi.org/10.33772/jitro.v6i1.8203

Abadi, M., Saili, T., Hijrawati, H., & Rizal, A. 2021. Capacity to increase bali cattle population in Mowila District, South Konawe Regency. *Musamus Journal of Agribusiness*, *4*(1), 35–46. https://doi.org/10.35724/mujagri.v4i01.4184

Abadi, M., Nafiu L. O., Yunus, T., Saili, T., & Rizal, A. 2022. Supportability of bali cattle development in the bali cattle breeding center area of South Konawe Regency. *Musamus Journal of Livestock Science*, *5*(2), 25–24.

Abadi, M., Nafiu, L., Saili, T., & Yunus, L. 2023c. Sustainable bali cattle breeding and the future of smallholder farming in South Konawe District, Indonesia. *Journal Of Law And Sustainable Development*, *11* (12), 1–17. e844. https://doi.org/10.55908/sdgs.v11i12.844

Adinda, D., Yuandry, S., Fitri, A. I., & Atifah, Y. 2023. Literature review: analysis of failure factors of artificial insemination in cattle. *Proceedings of SEMNAS BIO. UIN Raden Fatah Palembang*, 571–580.

Ananda, H. M., Wurlina, W., Hidajati, N., Hariadi, M., Samik, A., & Restiadi, T. I. 2020. The relationship between age and calving interval, days open, and service per conception of sapifriesian Holstein (fh). *Ovozoa: Journal of Animal Reproduction*, *8*(2), 94. https://doi.org/10.20473/ovz.v8i2.2019.94-99

Akoso, T. B. 1996. *Cattle Health*. Kanisius: pp: 157–160, Yogyakarta.

Bilyaro, W., Lestari, D., Putra, B. A., Mahardika, A. I., & Alfahri, A. 2023. Development of feed processing technology to increase the productivity of beef cattle in farmer groups in Sawojajar village, KotabumiUtara Sub-district, North LampungUtara Regency. *Lumbung Innovation: Journal of Community Service*, *8*(2), 224–231. https://doi.org/10.36312/linov.v8i2.1171

BPS. 2022. South Konawe Regency in Figures 2022. BPS-Statistics of Konawe Selatan Regency. Andoolo.

Dhayanti, N. L. E., Laksmi, D. N. D. I., & Sampurna, I. P. 2021. Postpartum breeding in balinese cattle in several livestock groups in the working area of Puskeswan Sobangan, Badung, Bali. *Indonesia Medicus Veterinus*, *10*(4), 576–588. https://doi.org/10.19087/imv.2021.10.4.576

Ibrahim, & Hadiana, M. H. 2023. Farm resources utilization on the integrated system of bali cattle-palm oil. *Journal ofAnimalScience, PadjadjaranUniversity,23*(1), 42. https://doi.org/10.24198/jit.v23i1.44401

Irwanto, Prayoga, A., Mahfud, K., & Indrayanti, T. 2023. Analysis of farmers' perceptions of alsintan service business (Upja) in Upja Tirtosari, Gunungkidul, D.I. Yogyakarta. *Journal of Agricultural Extension*, *18*(1), 10–18.

Islami, R., Zahra, S. F., Yuniastuti, P., Pranata, P. E. A., Sefi, M., & Widianingrum, D. C. 2022. Knowledge, policies, and control of anthrax disease in livestock in Indonesia. *Sriwijaya Journal of Animal Husbandry*, *10*(2), 1–8. https://doi.org/10.36706/JPS.10.2.2021.12191

Kristyari, N. P. G., Trilaksana, I. G. N. B., & Laksmi, D. N. D. I. 2021. Calving distance for bali cattle raised in galungan village, Sawan District, Buleleng Regency, Bali Province. *Indonesia Medicus Veterinus*, *10*(4), 553–563. https://doi.org/10.19087/imv.2021.10.4.553

Nalle, M. N., Asa, M. L. M., & Indrasti, R. 2023. The Role of farmer groups in increasing of rice farmers in lakekun village, kobalima sub-district, malaka district east Nusa Tenggara Province. *IOP Conference Series: Earth and Environmental Science*, *1153*(1), 012022. https://doi.org/10.1088/1755-1315/1153/1/012022

Nindhia, T. G. T., McDonald, M., & Styles, D. 2021. Greenhouse gas mitigation and rural electricity generation by a novel two-stroke biogas engine. *Journal of Cleaner Production*, *280*, 124473. https://doi.org/10.1016/j.jclepro.2020.124473

Nurdiyansah, I., Suherman, D., & Putranto, H. D. 2020. Relationship between farmer characteristics and scale of ownership of dairy cows in Kabawetan District, Kepahiang Regency. *Tropical Livestock Bulletin*, *1* (2), 64–74. https://doi.org/10.31186/bpt.1.2.64-74

Omelia, P., Suharyati, S., Dakhlan, A., & Hartono, M. 2023. Quantitative performance of male saburai goats in the saburai goat livestock development group in Sumberejo District, *Tanggamus Regency. Journal of Livestock Research and Innovation*, *7*(2), 261–270. https://doi.org/10.23960/jrip.2023.7.2.261-270

Putra, T. G., & Simanjuntak, M. C. 2023. System and management of bali cattle breeding in Kamuu East District, Dogiya Regency. *Para-Para Journal*, *4*(1), 36–47.

Sani, L. O. A., Ba'a, L. O., Abadi, M., & Ali, T. 2018. Financial analysis of bali cattle, plantation and horticultural business combination in Tinanggea District, South Konawe Regency. *Proceedings of the National Seminar on Animal Husbandry Technology*. Fpt UHO., 393–400.

Talakua, E. W., Kakisina, L. O., & Timisela, N. R. 2022. Lakor goat development strategy: A production, income, and SWOT analysis approach. *JSEP (Journal of Social and Agricultural Economics)*, *15*(1), 59. https://doi.org/10.19184/jsep.v15i1.26474

Technological Innovations in Tropical Livestock Development for Environmental Sustainability and Food Security – P. Dhian Isnaeni et al. (eds)
© 2025 The Author(s), ISBN 978-1-032-74373-8
Open Access: www.taylorfrancis.com, CC BY-NC-ND 4.0 license

Comprehensive marketing analysis of goat livestock enterprises in the North Poleang district, Bombana regency

H.A. Hadini*, M. Rusdin, M. Abadi, A.S. Aku, L.O.M. Munadi & Ardiansyah
Faculty of Animal Science, Universitas Halu Oleo, Kendari, Southeast Sulawesi, Indonesia

A. Tawai
Faculty of Social Science and Political Science, Universitas Halu Oleo, Kendari, Southeast Sulawesi, Indonesia

ABSTRACT: Bombana Regency, situated in Southeast Sulawesi Province, stands out as a favorable location for the development of goat farming businesses, boasting a population of 7,267 goats distributed across various sub-districts, including North Poleang Sub-district. This study aims to examine the marketing channels, margins, and efficiency within goat farming businesses in North Poleang District, Bombana Regency. Using the snowball sampling technique, all marketing institutions involved in goat marketing were selected as samples for this research, utilizing both primary and secondary data. The research delves into the analysis of marketing channel patterns, marketing margins, and marketing efficiency. The findings reveal the existence of three distinct marketing channels: 1) Direct transactions from breeders to final consumers, 2) Transactions involving breeders, collecting traders, and final consumers, and 3) Transactions involving breeders, collecting traders, retailers, and final consumers. Channel III exhibits the highest marketing margin for goat livestock at IDR 1,109,722/head, whereas the lowest margin is observed in Channel II at IDR 376,944/head. Channel I emerges as the most efficient marketing channel, while marketing channel II is identified as the most efficient when considering marketing institutions.

Keywords: Goat, Marketing Channels, Margin, Efficiency

1 INTRODUCTION

Efforts to increase global trade in goat livestock in the future era of free trade opportunities for export are still open. Approaching this era of free trade, countries must open their doors to imported products, with a minimum requirement of around 5% of consumption needs. Ultimately, the final decision rests with the consumer, who can choose between local and imported products. Therefore, local products must have strong competitiveness in quality, quantity, and sustainability to compete with imported products. Within the framework of the various livestock and livestock products, goat farming and its products have become the focus of continuous development to meet existing market demand (McDermott *et al.* 2010). The development of goat farming requires serious attention, considering the existence of domestic and international market opportunities, which aligns with changes in the political order in Indonesia towards the era of democratization and globalization (Kocho *et al.* 2011). Therefore, the agricultural sector in the future will face two main challenges simultaneously.

*Corresponding Author: hairil_hadini@uho.ac.id

 DOI: 10.1201/9781003468943-43

Countries are required to open the door to imported products with a minimum amount of around 5% of consumption needs. In this context, to successfully compete in the livestock industry in Indonesia, it is important to have stronger competitiveness. In particular, when dealing with similar products from abroad, competitiveness will vary depending on the type of livestock (Boogaard *et al.* 2015), such as ruminants (both large and small), beef cattle, dairy cattle, buffalo, horses, goats, and sheep, as well as non-ruminant livestock, such as pigs and poultry (Rehman *et al.* 2017). It provides views on the development of production structures and livestock businesses, prospects for livestock agribusiness, and the challenges and opportunities of global trade (Aldosari 2018). It shows the direction of development policies that need to be taken to increase the competitiveness of livestock businesses in Indonesia.

Livestock commodities, including the goat farming business, have a strategic role in providing animal protein for society. The goat farming business in Indonesia is generally still carried out traditionally with poor management of care and feeding. The livestock business is still part-time for farmers, so the resulting production is not optimal (Aku *et al.* 2021; Pagala, 2023). The existence of a goat farming business is a business that has a broad impact both socially and economically on society (Aku *et al.* 2022; Sandiah *et al.* 2021). Goats are a ruminant that is quite easy to maintain and breed because they have good adaptability to the tropical climate in Indonesia. Goats, classified as small ruminants, have great meaning for small people. This is indicated by the large spread of goat livestock throughout Indonesia, especially in Southeast Sulawesi Province, where their farming is still traditional.

Bombana Regency, located in Southeast Sulawesi Province, stands out as a promising hub for the development of goat farming enterprises. According to the 2022 Statistics Agency for Bombana Regency, the goat population in that year totaled 7,267 heads, distributed across various sub-districts. Notably, North Poleang District alone accounted for 457 heads. To establish a successful goat farming business, various factors must be taken into account, with marketing being a critical aspect. Marketing, as defined by Akash *et al.* (2022); Serra *et al.* (2020) is a social and managerial process that involves interactions among individuals and groups. In the context of livestock farming, marketing holds significant importance within the agribusiness system. It serves as a vital link, playing a crucial role in the overall development of livestock enterprises.

Marketing costs are greatly influenced by the various functions managed by each marketing agency. The more functions that are managed, the greater the costs required, which impacts the size of the marketing margin. Marketing margins will be higher when the prices received by consumers also increase. In addition, the longer the marketing channel chain, the more profits are taken and costs incurred by marketers, which ultimately contributes to increasing prices received by consumers) Nagpure *et al.* 2023. Marketing activities in the goat farming business will occur if components are involved, namely producers, traders, collectors, and consumers, where the producers set the selling price quite high, but the collectors want high profits. In contrast, consumers want relatively low livestock prices. Marketing activities are carried out using how to make a product, determine the price, determine the place of sale, and promote the product to consumers.

2 RESEARCH METHODS

This research was conducted in March 2023 in North Poleang District, Bombana Regency, Southeast Sulawesi Province. The research samples were breeders and traders involved in marketing goats using snowball sampling. The data collected in this research consists of primary data and secondary data. Data collection was carried out by observation and interviews using questionnaires. The data analysis used in this research is as follows:

Marketing channels are analyzed directly following the flow of producers, marketing institutions, and final consumers and then explained descriptively.

The marketing margin at each marketing institution can be calculated using the following formula:

$$MP = Pr - Pf$$

Information:

MP = Goat marketing margin (IDR/Head)
Pr = Price of goats the consumer level (IDR/Head)
Pf = price of goats at producer level (IDR/Head)

The marketing margin percentage is calculated using the following formula:

$$\%M = (M/HE) \times 100\%$$

Information:

%M = Margin percentage of all distribution channels
M = Margins
HE = Sales Price

Goat marketing efficiency is analyzed by comparing total marketing costs with total product value (turnover), which is calculated using the following formula:

$$Ep = (TC/TNP) \times 100\%$$

Information:

Ep = Marketing efficiency (100%)
TC = Total marketing costs (IDR/Head)
TNP = Total value of products marketed (IDR/Head)

Provision: Ep, the one with the smallest value, is the most efficient.

3 RESULTS AND DISCUSSION

3.1 *Characteristics of goat farmers and traders*

The characteristics of breeders and traders are characteristics of a person. There were 45 respondents in this study, namely 40 goat breeders and 5 traders. The characteristics of goat breeders and traders in North Poleang District, Bombana Regency, can be seen in Table 1.

Table 1 shows that the dominant ages of breeders and traders are 15–55 years, amounting to 36 people (80%), while 9 people aged 55 years and over (20%) are categorized as unproductive. Generally, breeders of productive age have high enthusiasm, including the enthusiasm to develop businesses in the agricultural sector (Zulkiram 2021). The gender of breeders and traders in this study was dominated by 42 men (93%) and 3 women (7%). Gender is an important factor that determines work productivity.

It is hoped that the educational factor can help the community increase the production and productivity of the livestock they raise. An adequate level of education will improve the performance and management capabilities of the livestock business being run. Table 1 shows that the education level of breeders and traders in marketing goat farming varies widely, from elementary school to university. The number of breeders and traders with elementary school education was 27 people (60%), 8 people at junior high school level (18%), 8 people at high school level (18%) and 2 people at tertiary level (4%). Based on this data, it can be said that the education of breeders and traders is still relatively low. This will affect the quality of breeders both in terms of skills and insight.

Table 1. Characteristics of Goat Breeders and Traders in North Poleang district, Bombana regency.

Description	Number of People	Percentage (%)
	Age of Farmers and Traders (years)	
15–55	36	80
>55	9	20
	Gender of Breeders and Traders	
Male	42	93
Female	3	7
	Breeder and Trader Education	
Elementary School	27	60
Junior High School	8	18
Senior High School	8	18
College	2	4
	Length of Business for Breeders and Traders (years)	
<5	15	33
5–10	21	47
10–20	9	20
	Number of Family Dependents	
1–2	13	29
3–4	24	53
5–6	5	11
>6	3	7

Source: Processed Primary Data, 2023.

Breeding experience is the length of time the farmer has been involved in the goat farming business independently. Table 1 shows that the length of business of goat breeders and traders in North Poleang District is less than 5 years, amounting to 15 people (33%), 15–0 years totaling 21 people (47%), and 10–20 years totaling 3 people (20%). This research shows that raising livestock for a long time indicates that the breeder's knowledge and skills regarding livestock rearing management have better abilities.

The large number of responsibilities of the farmer's family influences the increase in welfare to meet living needs. The greater the number of dependents in a family will influence the expenses. Table 1 shows that the number of household members of breeders and traders who have 1–2 family dependents is 13 people (29%), 3–4 is 24 people (53%), 4–6 is 5 people (11%) and more than 6 people totaling 3 people (7%). These results show that most breeders and traders have family members of less than 3–4 people. Apart from burdening the family, the farmer's family is also a source of labor for the family in managing their farming business, including their livestock business.

3.2 *Marketing*

3.2.1 *Goat farming marketing channels*

Marketing channels are the distribution of goat livestock from producers to final consumers. Marketing channels are sales tracking through existing marketing channels (Awaliyah and Saefudin 2020). The research results show that there are three goat marketing channels in the North Poleang District, as in the following Figure 1.

Marketing channel I is the process of marketing goats directly to final consumers and does not involve marketing institutions. The number of breeders involved in this channel is 17 people, and the number of goats traded is 25 goats, with an average price of male goats of IDR. 2,470,833/head and female goat IDR. 1,875,000/head. The breeder determines the price on this channel based on the livestock's age and body size. Then, a bargaining process occurs between the breeder and the buyer until an agreement is reached on the price.

Marketing channel II involves one marketing institution, namely collecting traders. The number of breeders in this channel is 20, and 1 collecting trader. The goats traded in this marketing channel are 56 heads with an average price of male goats of IDR. 3,636,111/head, while the average price of female goats amounting to IDR. 2,330,000/head. The farmer determines the price on this channel based on the age and body size of the livestock. Then, a bargaining process occurs until a price agreement is reached.

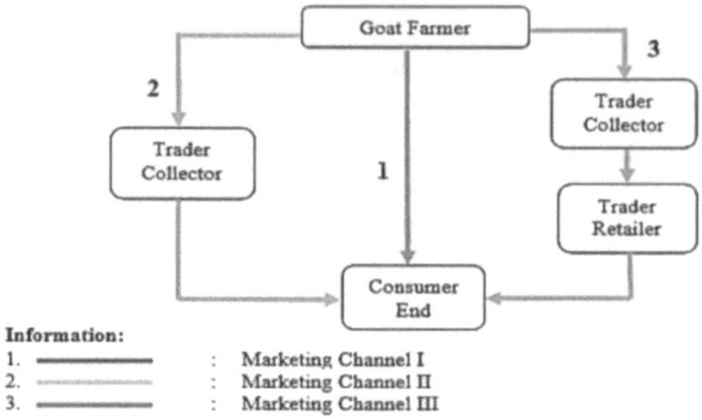

Figure 1. Marketing channel scheme I, II, and III for goat farming business in North Poleang district, Bombana regency.

Marketing channel III is a marketing channel that involves two marketing institutions, namely collectors and retailers. The number of breeders in this channel is 13, and 2 collecting traders. The number of goats traded is 49 heads, with an average price of male goats of IDR. 3,655,556/head and an average price of female goats of IDR. 2,625,000/head. Retail traders buy goats from collectors with an average price of male goats of IDR. 3,966,667/head and an average price of female goats of IDR. 3,016,667/head. The research findings indicate variations in prices among different traders.

3.2.2 *Margin, costs, profits and goat marketing efficiency*

The marketing margin for goat livestock is the difference between the selling and purchase price of goat livestock in North Poleang District, Bombana Regency. Goat marketing is carried out in two ways, namely, direct and indirect marketing. Direct marketing is in marketing channel I, where breeders directly market their goats to final consumers without going through intermediary traders, so there is no price difference or price margin between breeders and consumers.

Indirect marketing is marketing carried out by breeders through intermediary traders in channels II and III involving collectors and retailers. Marketing channel II involves 1 intermediary trader, namely the collector trader. The average price of goats at the farmer is IDR. 2,983,056, and the average price of goats at the collector level is IDR. 3,360,000, in this channel, there is a difference in prices at the farmer and the collecting trader level. The average price margin in channel II is IDR. 376,944/head. Marketing channel III involves 2 intermediary traders, namely collectors and retailers, with an average price of goats at breeders of IDR. 3,140,278, while the average selling price of goats at the collectors' level is IDR 3,601,667, and at retailers, the average is IDR. 3,601,667. Goat price is IDR. 4,250,000.

The price margin for collecting traders is IDR. 461,389/head and retail traders are IDR. 648,333/head, with a total price margin of IDR. 1,109,722/head. Based on this data, it is known that marketing channel III has a higher marketing margin when compared to channel II because channel III involves two intermediary traders, which causes costs and margins to be greater.

Marketing channel I breeders do not incur costs because consumers go directly to the breeder to buy the livestock, likewise for marketing channel II and III breeders. Marketing channel II, collecting traders, pay IDR. 35,714/head for buying and selling livestock, while in channel III, collecting traders and retail traders incur transportation costs for selling and buying goats in the amount of IDR. 227,584/head. The margins, costs, profits, and marketing efficiency for each marketing institution in the goat marketing channel can be seen in Table 2.

Table 2. Purchase price, selling price, cost margin, profit and marketing efficiency goat farming in North Poleang district, Bombana regency.

Trader	Marketing Channels II	Marketing Channels III
Collector Trader		
Purchase price (IDR/Head)	2,983,056	3,140,278
Selling price (IDR/Head)	3,360,000	3,601,667
Margins (IDR/Head)	376,944	461,389
Cost (IDR/Head)	35,714	100,441
Profit (IDR/Head)	341,230	360,948
Efficiency	1.06	
Retailer Trader		
Purchase price (IDR/Head)		3,601,667
Selling price (IDR/Head)		4,250,000
Margins (IDR/Head)		648,333
Cost (IDR/Head)		127,143
Profit (IDR/Head)		521,190
Efficiency		2.99

Source: Processed Primary Data, 2023

Table 2 shows that collecting traders in marketing channel II have a profit of IDR. 341,230/ head, and in marketing channel III, the marketing institution with the highest profit is the retailer IDR. 521,190/head, and the lowest is the collecting trader, amounting to IDR. 360,948/head. The marketing institution with the highest profits is marketing channel III, with total profits of IDR. 882,138/head, and the lowest is marketing channel II with total profits of IDR. 341,230/head. The high profits in Marketing Channel III are caused by the costs and number of marketing institutions being greater when compared to Marketing Channel II.

The most efficient marketing channel is channel I because marketing channel I do not involve marketing institutions, so there is no cost in marketing the livestock. Marketing channel II involves one marketing institution, namely collecting traders, which has an efficiency value of 1.06%, while marketing channel III involves two marketing institutions with an efficiency value of 2.99%. The results of this research state that the most efficient marketing channel involving marketing institutions is marketing channel II because it has the smallest efficiency value compared to marketing channel III.

4 CONCLUSION

The research findings can be summarized as follows: (1) In the North Poleang District of Bombana Regency, there exist three distinct marketing channels for goat livestock, namely: (a) Channel I, involving direct transactions from breeders to final consumers; (b) Channel II, which encompasses transactions from breeders to trader collectors and then to final consumers; and (c) Channel III, involving breeders, collectors, retailers, and final consumers. (2) Regarding the marketing margin for goat livestock in North Poleang District, Bombana Regency, Channel II exhibits a marketing margin of IDR 376,944/head for collectors, while Channel III shows marketing margins for collecting traders and retail traders at IDR

461,389/head and IDR 648,333/head, respectively, resulting in a total marketing margin of IDR 1,109,722/head. (3) The research concludes that the most efficient marketing channel for goat livestock in Poleang Utara District, Bombana Regency, is Channel I, while the most efficient channel through marketing institutions is Channel II.

ACKNOWLEDGMENTS

We thank the Rector and Dean of the Faculty of Animal Science, for holding the [4]th international seminar at the Faculty of Animal Science, Halu Oleo University. We hope that this seminar will run as expected and will certainly be an initial milestone for the institution's progress.

REFERENCES

Akash, M., Hoque, S., Mondal and Adusumilli, S. 2022. Chapter *Four–Sustainable livestock production and food security*. in *Emerging Issues in Climate Smart Livestock Production*, S. Mondal and R. L. Singh, Eds., Academic Press, 2022, pp. 71–90. doi: 10.1016/B978-0-12-822265-2.00011-9.

Aku, A. S., Hafid, H., Rusdin, M., Yaddi, Y., and Munadi, L., O. M. 2022. Sistem pemeliharaan dan pertambahan populasi ternak Kambing di Kabupaten Muna, Indonesia. *Jurnal Agribest*, vol. 6, no. 1, pp. 19–24, Mar. 2022, doi: 10.32528/agribest.v6i1.5828.

Aku, A., Takdir, S., Yaddi, Y., Abadi, M., and Munadi, L. O. M., 2021. Survey of disease incidence in goats in Muna Regency, Indonesia. *International Journal of Scientific Research in Science, Engineering and Technology*, vol. 8, no. 4, pp. 425–430, Aug. 2021, doi: 10.32628/IJSRSET218468.

Aldosari, F.O. 2018. Gender participation in sheep and goat farming in Najran, Southern Saudi Arabia. *Saudi Journal of Biological Sciences*, vol. 25, no. 1, pp. 144–148, Jan. 2018, doi: 10.1016/j.sjbs.2017.03.013.

Ayalew, W., King, J., Bruns, M. & Rischkowsky, B. 2003. Economic evaluation of smallholder subsistence livestock production: lessons from an Ethiopian goat development program. *Ecological Economics*, vol. 45, no. 3, pp. 473–485, Jul. 2003, doi: 10.1016/S0921-8009(03)00098-3.

Boogaard, B. K., Waithanji, E., Poole, E. J., and Cadilhon, J.-J., 2015. Smallholder goat production and marketing: a gendered baseline study from Inhassoro District Mozambique. *NJAS–Wageningen Journal of Life Sciences*, vol. 74–75, pp. 51–63, Dec. 2015, doi: 10.1016/j.njas.2015.09.002.

Kocho, T., Abebe, G., Tegegne, A., and Gebremedhin, B., 2011. Marketing value-chain of smallholder sheep and goats in crop-livestock mixed farming system of Alaba, Southern Ethiopia. *Small Ruminant Research*, vol. 96, no. 2, pp. 101–105, Apr. 2011, doi: 10.1016/j.smallrumres.2011.01.008.

McDermott, J. J., Staal, S. J., Freeman, H. A. Herrero, M., and Van de Steeg, J. A., 2010. Sustaining intensification of smallholder livestock systems in the tropics. *Livestock Science*, vol. 130, no. 1, pp. 95–109, May 2010, doi: 10.1016/j.livsci.2010.02.014.

Nagpure, G., Singh, K. R., Singh, J., Singh, A. P, and Singh, R. P., 2023. *Chapter 17–Livestock industry market trend and analysis. Nanobiotechnology for the Livestock Industry*, R. Pratap Singh, C. O. Adetunji, R. L. Singh, J. Singh, P. R. Solanki, and K. R. B. Singh, Eds., Elsevier, 2023, pp. 329–340. doi: 10.1016/B978-0-323-98387-7.00014-8.

Pagala, M. A., Rahim, A. Aku, A. S. Sani, L. O. A., Munadi, L. O. M., Melisa. Yaddi, Y., 2023. Characteristics of phenotypes of local goat quantitative properties in East Kolaka Regency, Indonesia. *International Journal on Advanced Science, Engineering and Information Technology*, vol. 13, no. 1, pp. 62–68, 2023.

Rehman, Jingdong, A., Chandio, A. A., and Hussain, I., 2017. Livestock production and population census in Pakistan: Determining their relationship with agricultural GDP using econometric analysis. *Information Processing in Agriculture*, vol. 4, no. 2, pp. 168–177, Jun. 2017, doi: 10.1016/j.inpa.2017.03.002.

Sandiah, N., Aku, A. S., Sani, L. O. A., Nafiu, L. O., and Munadi, L. O. M., 2021. Determination of base and non base sector of livestock commodity development in Southeast Sulawesi Province, Indonesia. *Technium Social Sciences Journal*, vol. 23, pp. 519–527, Sep. 2021.

Serra, R., Kiker, G. A., Minten, B., Valerio, V. C., Varijakshapanicker, P., and Wane, A. 2020. Filling knowledge gaps to strengthen livestock policies in low-income countries, *Global Food Security*, vol. 26, p. 100428, Sep. 2020, doi: 10.1016/j.gfs.2020.100428.

Zulkiram, Z. 2021. Sistem pemasaran domba di pasar hewan geurugok Kecamatan gandapura kabupaten bireuen. *Jurnal Sains Pertanian*, vol. 5, no. 3, pp. 99–106, Oct., doi: 10.51179/jsp.v5i3.1696.

Technological Innovations in Tropical Livestock Development for Environmental Sustainability and Food Security – P. Dhian Isnaeni et al. (eds)
© 2025 The Author(s), ISBN 978-1-032-74373-8
Open Access: www.taylorfrancis.com, CC BY-NC-ND 4.0 license

Social-economic study of Bali cattle farming: A case study in South Tiworo, West Muna

L.O.A. Sani*, H.A. Hadini & L.O.M. Munadi
Department of Animal Science, Faculty of Animal Science, Halu Oleo University, Indonesia

N. Rahayu
Student of Animal Science, Faculty of Animal Science, Halu Oleo University, Indonesia

A. Tawai
Faculty of Social Science and Political Science, Halu Oleo University, Indonesia

ABSTRACT: This research aims to identify the characteristics of Bali cattle farmers and analyze the influence of socio-economic factors on the community's interest in Bali cattle farming. The study was conducted from May to August 2023, involving a sample of 10 farmers from each village, totaling 50 respondents. Both quantitative and qualitative data were utilized, obtained from primary and secondary sources through observation, interviews, and documentation. The analytical tool employed was Multiple Linear Regression, with the goal of predicting the impact of socio-economic variables (income, family environment, community environment, social status) on the community's interest in Bali cattle farming, using SPSS 25.0 software for Windows. The research findings indicate that the farmers generally exhibit productive age (84%), relatively low educational attainment (38%), predominantly engaged in agriculture as their main occupation (66%), relatively low farming experience (1–5 years, 36%), and a relatively low level of livestock ownership (1–5 heads, 72%). Collectively, the independent variables (income/savings source, family environment, community environment, and social status) significantly influence the dependent variable (interest in Bali cattle farming). Partially, income/savings source, community environment, and social status each have a highly significant effect ($p < 0.01$) on the interest in cattle farming in South Tiworo District, West Muna Regency.

Keywords: Socioeconomic, Bali Cattle, West Muna

1 INTRODUCTION

The success of Bali cattle farming can be measured through its contribution to income and the fulfillment of daily needs for farmers. This evaluation can be conducted by considering the growth in the number of livestock owners and the increase in household income. The management and maintenance of Bali cattle are not only integral aspects of efforts to increase family income (Munadi *et al.* 2021) but also an effective strategy to improve economic conditions (Sandiah *et al.* 2021). One common approach adopted by communities to enhance household income is through Bali cattle farming (Sani *et al.* 2021). These beef cattle have become a popular choice among farmers due to their significant economic potential (Sani *et al.* 2021). Ownership and maintenance of Bali cattle encompass not only financial aspects (Asrika *et al.* 2023; Sani *et al.* 2021) but also take into account the growth in the weight of the livestock, indicating the health and quality of the cattle.

*Corresponding Author: arsadsani@uho.ac.id

DOI: 10.1201/9781003468943-44

The development of Bali cattle ownership enables farmers to optimize their efforts to achieve higher levels of productivity. The growth in the weight of cattle is a crucial parameter in evaluating the success of this livestock business, as it directly impacts the selling price and the potential for additional income (Sani *et al.* 2022, 2023). Furthermore, a significant increase in household income can serve as an indicator of the sustainability and competitiveness of Bali cattle farming amid market dynamics (Hadini *et al.* 2022). Bali cattle farming in South Tiworo District, West Muna Regency, plays a strategic role in the local economy. Bali cattle not only serve as the primary source of income for farmers but also make a significant contribution to meeting the animal protein needs of the population (Hadini *et al.* 2022; Sani *et al.* 2022). Therefore, a deeper understanding of the factors influencing community interest in Bali cattle farming is essential for optimizing the potential of this livestock sector.

In the socio-economic context, the South Tiworo District possesses distinctive characteristics. The dynamics of the community, patterns of social interaction, and the level of economic income can significantly contribute to the decision-making of the community regarding Bali cattle farming. This condition necessitates a further analysis of the impact of social and economic factors on the community's interest in engaging in Bali cattle farming activities. Additionally, West Muna Regency, as the research location, is facing economic and social changes that can influence the behavior of Bali cattle farmers. Regional economic transformations and government policies related to the agriculture and livestock sectors can also play a crucial role in shaping community interest in Bali cattle farming.

West Muna Regency is one of the centers for the development of Bali cattle farming in Southeast Sulawesi. In 2022, the population of Bali cattle reached 36,400 heads, contributing approximately 8.63% to the total cattle population in Southeast Sulawesi, which amounted to 421,454 heads (BPS Sultra 2023). Administratively, South Tiworo District comprises five villages: Barakkah Village, Sangia Tiworo Village, Kasimpa Jaya Village, Katangana Village, and Parura Jaya Village. Although the majority of the population in South Tiworo District relies on agricultural yields as their primary source of livelihood, Bali cattle farming also serves as a common side occupation among the local community.

The tradition of Bali cattle farming in the South Tiworo District has been passed down through generations, carried out in a traditional manner, or through extensive husbandry systems. The potential for developing cattle farming businesses in this area is still significant, given the extensive available vacant land, including plantation areas owned by residents used for grazing and as a source of feed for Bali cattle. According to data, the population of Bali cattle in South Tiworo District in 2021 reached 2,104 heads, experiencing an increase in 2022, with the number of livestock reaching 2,190 heads (BPS Muna Barat 2023). This increase is believed to be influenced by the annual rise in cattle prices and the ease of Bali cattle maintenance, which stimulates community interest in starting Bali cattle farming businesses.

Through this research, it is expected that suitable solutions or policy recommendations can be identified to enhance community interest in Bali cattle farming in the South Tiworo District. The conclusions and findings of this study are anticipated to provide valuable contributions to stakeholders, including local government, farmers, and other researchers interested in the development of the Bali cattle farming sector in this region.

2 RESEARCH METHODS

This research was conducted from May to August 2023 in South Tiworo District, West Muna Regency, Southeast Sulawesi Province. The selection of the research location was intentional (purposive) in South Tiworo District, involving five villages: Barakkah Village, Sangia Tiworo Village, Kasimpa Jaya Village, Katangana Village, and Parura Jaya Village. This decision was based on the consideration that the chosen location has a sufficient population of Bali cattle farms to be the focus of the research.

This research sampled a total of 50 respondents from the five villages, intentionally selecting 10 farmers from each village. The determination of this respondent court took into account that each respondent is a Bali cattle farmer. To analyze the obtained data, this research employs the Multiple Linear Regression method. The purpose of this analysis is to comprehend and predict the influence of socio-economic characteristics such as income, family environment, community environment, and social status on the community's interest in Bali cattle farming. The data analysis process is carried out using SPSS 22.0 software for Windows. The following is the Multiple Regression Equation used in this study:

$$\boldsymbol{Y = a + b1\ X_1 + b2\ X_2 + b3\ X_3 + b4\ X_4 + e}$$

In this equation:

Y = Public Interest in Bali Cattle Breeding (Score)
a = Konstant
X1 = Source of Income/Savings (Score)
X2 = Family Environment (Score)
X3 = Community Environment (Score)
X4 = Social Status (Score)
b1 b2 b3 and b4 = Variable Regression Coefficient X1, X2, X3, and X4
e = Standard Error

3 RESULTS AND DISCUSSION

3.1 *Respondent characteristics*

Table 1 illustrates the age distribution pattern of Bali cattle farmers in the South Tiworo District. From the data, it can be observed that 84% of farmers fall within the age range of 15–60 years, while the remaining 16% are above 60 years old. These results indicate that the majority of Bali cattle farmers in the region are still within the productive age range, demonstrating sufficient physical capability to carry out crucial tasks in farming activities. This forms a strong foundation for productivity in the context of Bali cattle farming in the area.

Table 1. Characteristics of respondents.

No	Description	Number of people)	Percentage (%)
1	Breeder Age		
	15–64	42	84
	> 64	8	16
2	Breeder Gender		
	Male	42	84
	Female	8	16
3	Breeder Education		
	Not completing primary school	7	14
	Primary School	13	26
	Junior High School	11	22
	Senior High School	14	28
	Bachelor	5	10
4.	The Main Job		
	Construction Laborers	1	2
	Fisherman	2	4
	Trader	1	2
	Private Employees	4	8
	Farmer	33	66
	Breeder	9	18

(*continued*)

Table 1. Continued

No	Description	Number of people)	Percentage (%)
5	Income Level (Rp)		
	1.000.000–2.000.000	40	80
	>2.000.000	10	20
6	Breeding Experience		
	1–5	28	56
	6–10	14	28
	>10	8	16
7	Livestock Ownership		
	1–5	36	72
	6–10	11	22
	>10	3	6

The gender distribution among Bali cattle farmers in the South Tiworo District is also noteworthy. Males dominate with a percentage of 82%, while female farmers constitute only about 16%. This fact indicates a gender disparity in cattle farming, which may be related to the perceived physical strength of males considered more capable in farming activities. Therefore, gender can influence interest and participation in cattle farming activities.

Education is also a significant factor in this context. Respondents fall into various levels of education, ranging from no elementary school completion (14%), elementary school (26%), lower secondary school (22%), upper secondary school (28%), to bachelor's degree (10%). This varied educational level reflects the educational challenges faced by farmers in the past related to limited school infrastructure and a lack of awareness of the importance of education.

The majority of respondents are employed as farmers, comprising 66%, while the lowest percentages are in occupations such as trading and construction labor, each at only 2%. Nevertheless, Bali cattle farming is still pursued as a side job. This indicates that cattle farming is seen as an opportunity to supplement their main income, even though their primary occupations differ. In terms of income, the majority of farmers (80%) earn monthly incomes ranging from Rp 1,000,000 to Rp 2,000,000. Conversely, only 20% earn more than Rp 2,000,000. Although these incomes are below the Provincial Minimum Wage (UMP), they are considered significant additional earnings. Income disparities can be attributed to variations in the types of occupations, as well as the number of cattle owned by each farmer.

Regarding the duration of cattle farming, the majority of respondents (56%) have been engaged in cattle farming for 1–5 years. Meanwhile, the ownership of Bali cattle in South Tiworo District varies significantly, with 72% owning 1–5 heads, 22% owning 6–10 heads, and 6% owning more than 10 heads. The average livestock ownership is 5 heads. This data reflects the diversity in cattle farming experience and ownership in the region.

3.2 *The influence of socio-economic factors on people's interest in breeding animals*

Based on the obtained primary data, further quantitative calculations were conducted to determine the influence between independent variables and their dependent variable. The data analysis model used is the multiple linear regression model. Through this model, the effects of independent variables, consisting of income/savings source (X1), family environment (X2), community environment (X3), and social status (X4), on the dependent variable, which is the interest in cattle farming (Y), can be easily evaluated. The results of the multiple linear regression analysis can be presented in Table 2.

Table 2. Results of multiple linear regression analysis of Socio-economic influence on interest in breeding Bali cattle.

Independent Variable	Regression Coefficients (B)	T_{hitung}	Sig	Information
Constant	0.981	0.565	0.575	
Source of Income (X1)	0.437	2.734	0.009	Significant
Family Environment (X2)	−0.014	−0.151	0.880	Not Significant
Community Environment (X3)	0.278	2.225	0.031	Significant
Social Status (X4)	0.250	2.600	0.013	Significant
Determinant coefficient (R^2)	0.350			
F_{Value}	6.059		0.001	Significant

Source: SPSS output results 2023.

The results of multiple linear regression analysis in Table 1 can be used to estimate the function in the regression equation model as follows:

$$Y = 0.098 + 0.437X_1 - 0.014X_2 + 0.278X_3 + 0.250X_4$$

The regression analysis results in the table indicate that independent variables (income/savings, family environment, community environment, and social status) have an impact on the dependent variable (interest in raising cattle). The analysis in Table 2 yielded an $F\text{-}_{value}$ of 6.059, and this value is greater than the critical $F\text{-}_{table}$ value of 2.578 ($p < 0.01$). This implies that the independent variables collectively have a significant influence on the interest in raising Bali cattle at a confidence level of 99%.

The regression analysis yielded a coefficient of determination (R^2) value of 0.350. This means that 35% of the variation in the dependent variable (interest in raising Bali cattle in the South Tiworo District) can be collectively explained by the examined independent variables. In comparison, the remaining 65% is explained by other variables not investigated in this study. The results of the test of independent variables against the related variable can be explained partially as follows:

3.2.1 *Source of income*

The coefficient of the variable representing the source of income/savings indicates a positive and statistically significant influence on the interest in raising Bali cattle. Specifically, the coefficient value for the income/savings source variable is 0.437, with a significance value of 0.009 ($p<0.01$). This implies a substantial and genuine impact, where an increase in the source of income/savings score by one unit is associated with a 0.437-unit increase in the interest in farming score.

The interpretation suggests that engaging in Bali cattle farming can offer a viable means of income to fulfill the financial needs of farmers. Given the high economic value associated with Bali cattle farming, it serves not only as a source of income but also as a form of savings. Farmers can sell their cattle whenever needed, providing a valuable asset that contributes to financial security. This economic aspect significantly influences people's interest in raising Bali cattle, as it aligns with their financial goals and needs.

The primary motivation for farmers to raise Bali cattle is driven by their aspirations to augment their income and accumulate savings. The livestock they possess, particularly Bali cattle, serves as a form of family savings that can be liquidated at any given time (Indrawirawan *et al.* 2021). The economic value attributed to beef cattle, including Bali cattle, lies in their role as a source of income and investment, effectively functioning as a form of savings (Lisson *et al.* 2010). This implies that farmers consider their cattle not only as a means of generating income but also as a valuable asset that can be sold whenever there is a need for financial resources.

The flexibility in selling cattle is highlighted, as farmers have the option to sell them through various channels, such as collectors, fellow breeders, or directly to consumers (Herlinae *et al.* 2012; Riszqina *et al.* 2014). This versatility in marketing provides farmers with the autonomy to choose the most suitable method based on their circumstances, contributing to the attractiveness of raising Bali cattle as a viable economic activity. The dual role of Bali cattle as both a source of income and a form of savings underscores its significance in meeting the economic aspirations of farmers.

3.2.2 *Family environment*

The coefficient of the family environment variable does not show a significant influence on the interest in raising Bali cattle. The family environment variable does not exhibit a substantial impact, as indicated by the coefficient value of −0.014 with a significance value of 0.880 ($p > 0.05$). A coefficient value of −0.014 implies that for every one-unit increase in the family environment score, there is a decrease in the interest in raising Bali cattle by 0.014 units.

In this context, it appears that the family environment variable, as measured in the study, does not play a significant role in influencing individuals' interest in raising Bali cattle. The negative coefficient suggests a minor negative relationship, but since the significance value is greater than 0.05, this relationship is not considered statistically significant. It's worth noting that the community's profession as farmers, engaging in sideline businesses to raise Bali cattle, and obtaining cattle seedlings through collaborative efforts or profit-sharing systems could be more influential factors compared to the family environment in shaping the interest of the community in raising Bali cattle.

Interest also typically arises from an individual's desire and the awareness that grows within them to engage in livestock farming. The emergence of interest from within a person is often initiated by the awareness that a particular activity has benefits for them and the satisfaction resulting from the positive impact that the activity brings to the individual (Baba *et al.* 2019; Roy *et al.* 2019). Additionally, interest can manifest as a result of internal motivations with specific goals occurring beyond an individual's conscious awareness.

3.2.3 *Community environment*

The coefficient of the community environment variable indicates a positive and significant influence on the interest in raising Bali cattle. The community environment variable has a substantial impact, with a coefficient value of 0.278 and a significance value of 0.031 ($p < 0.05$). A score value of 0.278 implies that for every one-unit increase in the community environment score, there is an increase in the interest in raising Bali cattle by 0.278 units.

The community environment factor is measured based on the encouragement from the surrounding environment, particularly individuals who have engaged in successful and experienced Bali cattle farming. The community environment, characterized by those who have succeeded in and gained experience in cattle farming, can influence individuals to cultivate beef cattle, especially in areas where there is a significant presence of livestock (Astaman *et al.* 2023; Firman & Nono 2021; Roy *et al.* 2019). External factors that influence an individual's desire include environmental factors (Sulfiar *et al.* 2022). Therefore, it can be concluded that the community environment plays a significant role in shaping character and interest.

3.2.4 *Social status*

The coefficient of the social status variable indicates a positive and significant influence on the interest in raising Bali cattle. The social status variable has a substantial impact, with a coefficient value of 0.250 and a significance value of 0.013 ($p<0.05$). A score value of 0.250 implies that for every one-unit increase in the social status score, there is an increase in the interest in raising Bali cattle by 0.250 units. The social status factor is measured based on the desire to be recognized, valued, and esteemed, as well as the ambition to be respected. This suggests that individuals with higher social status aspirations are more likely to show an increased interest in engaging in Bali cattle farming.

The influence of social status on the management of Bali cattle in the South Tiworo District indicates that the community perceives social status as important for livestock farmers. Social status occurs because some individuals strive for a higher purpose in the eyes of others compared to those who do not engage in any work at all. This aligns with the notion that a higher social status will also impact attitudes and garner high respect from the community.

4 CONCLUSION

Based on the research findings on the community's interest in raising Bali cattle in South Tiworo District, West Muna Regency, it can be concluded that the independent variables, namely income/savings (X1), family environment (X2), community environment (X3), and social status (X4), collectively have a significant influence on the dependent variable, which is the interest in raising Bali cattle (Y). Furthermore, income/savings (X1), community environment (X3), and social status (X4) individually and significantly ($p<0.01$) affect the interest in cattle farming in South Tiworo District, West Muna Regency.

REFERENCES

Asrika, R., Tawai, A., Sani, L. O. A., Pagala, M. A., Zulkarnain, D., Munadi, L. O. M., Aku, A. S., Abadi, M., & Jabuddin, L. O. (2023). Extension performance and satisfaction level of bali cattle farmers in South Konawe Regency, Indonesia. *Revista de Gestão Social e Ambiental*, 17(8), Article 8. https://doi.org/10.24857/rgsa.v17n8-004

Astaman, P., Siregar, A. R., Munizu, M., & Hastang. (2023). Identification of internal and external risk in Bali cattle business. *AIP Conference Proceedings*, 2628(1), 130027. https://doi.org/10.1063/5.0144044

Baba, S., Dagong, M. I. A., Sohrah, S., & Utamy, R. F. (2019). Factors affecting the adoption of agricultural by-products as feed by beef cattle farmers in Maros Regency of South Sulawesi, Indonesia. *Tropical Animal Science Journal*, 42(1), 76–80. https://doi.org/10.5398/tasj.2019.42.1.76

Firman, A., & Nono, O. H. (2021). A social-ecological system approach to Bali cattle raising in Timor Island, Indonesia. *Biodiversitas Journal of Biological Diversity*, 22(8), 3585–3593. https://doi.org/10.13057/biodiv/d220860

Hadini, H. A., Abadi, M., Sani, L. O. A., Munadi, L. O. M., Surahmanto, S., & Anggoro, W. S. (2022). Analysis of bali cattle business income on different scales in Tiworo Tengah District, Indonesia. *International Journal of Research in Business and Social Science*, 11(3), 168–174. https://doi.org/10.20525/ijrbs.v11i3.1735

Hadini, H. A., Karya, S., & Tawai, A. (2022). Factors affecting beef demand in Kendari City Southeast Sulawesi. *Indonesian Journal of Animal Agricultural Science*, 4(3), 24–29. http://dx.doi.org/10.33772/ijaas.v4i3.35537

Herlinae, H., Yemima, Y., & Jaya, D. A. (2012). Analisis sosial ekonomi peternakan sapi bali gaduhan terhadap perkembangan tinggi gumba ternak setelah dua tahun pemeliharaan, *Journal Of Tropical Animal Science*, 1(2), 83–88.

Indrawirawan, Suwignyo, B., & Kusumastuti, T. A. (2021). Analysis of factors affecting to the income of Bali cattle farmers in Barru Regency, South Sulawesi Province, Indonesia. *IOP Conference Series: Earth and Environmental Science*, 788, 012201. https://doi.org/10.1088/1755-1315/788/1/012201

Lisson, S., MacLeod, N., McDonald, C., Corfield, J., Pengelly, B., Wirajaswadi, L., Rahman, R., Bahar, S., Padjung, R., Razak, N., Puspadi, K., Dahlanuddin, Sutaryono, Y., Saenong, S., Panjaitan, T., Hadiawati, L., Ash, A., & Brennan, L. (2010). A participatory, farming systems approach to improving Bali cattle production in the smallholder crop-livestock systems of Eastern Indonesia. *Agricultural Systems*, 103(7), 486–497.

Munadi, L. O. M., Hidayat, H., Sahaba, L. O., & Inal, I. (2021). Pola dan sistem pemeliharaan ternak sapi bali di kabupaten muna. *Jurnal Ilmiah Penyuluhan Dan Pengembangan Masyarakat*, 1(3), 131–136. https://doi.org/10.56189/jippm.v1i2.19968

Riszqina, R., Isbandi, I., Rianto, E., & Santoso, S. I. (2014). The analysis of factors affecting the performance and benefit of karapan (Racing) cattle business in Madura Island, East Java, Indonesia. *Journal of the Indonesian Tropical Animal Agriculture*, 39(1), 65–72. https://doi.org/10.14710/jitaa.39.1.65-72

Roy, N. D., Charles, K., & Lika, B. (2019). The market structure of the Bali cattle in east nusa tenggara, Indonesia. *Russian Journal of Agricultural and Socio-Economic Sciences*, 95(11), 183–189.

Sandiah, N., Sani, L. O. A., Munadi, L. O. M., & Ernia, E. (2021). Analisis pemasaran sapi bali di kecamatan barangka kabupaten muna barat. *Jurnal Bisnis Tani*, 7(1), 44–53. https://doi.org/10.35308/jbt.v7i1.3309

Sani, L. O. A., Aka, R., Munadi, L. O. M., Ali, R., Pagala, M. A., & Syamsuddin. (2021). Marketing analysis of beef cattle in landono and mowila subdistricts of South Konawe Regency. *International Journal of Science, Technology & Management*, 2(3), 747–754. https://doi.org/10.46729/ijstm.v2i3.194

Sani, L. O. A., Hafid, H., Munadi, L. O. M., & Doni, A. (2022). Comparative income combination of farming and cattle bali in Palangga Subdistrict South Konawe Regency. *Jurnal Ilmu-Ilmu Peternakan (Indonesian Journal of Animal Science)*, 32(1), 35–41. https://doi.org/10.21776/ub.jiip.2022.032.01.04

Sani, L. O. A., Hafid, H., Munadi, L. O. M., Zulkarnain, D., & Pujian, S. R. R. (2021). Motivation of bali cattle farmers tinanggea and Palangga Subdistrict South Konawe Regency. *International Journal of Science, Technology & Management*, 2(3), 737–746. https://doi.org/10.46729/ijstm.v2i3.195

Sani, L. O. A., Sandiah, N., Ernia, E., Tawai, A., Zulkarnain, D., Astarika, R., & Munadi, L. O. M. (2023). Marketing channels for bali cattle in Barangka District, Regency West Muna, Southeast Sulawesi. *Indonesian Journal Of Animal Agricultural Science (IJAAS)*, 5(1), 01–11. https://doi.org/10.33772/ijaas.v5i1.40018

Sani, L. O. A., Sandiah, N., Munadi, L. O. M., & Darmin, D. (2021). Analisis pendapatan peternak dari kombinasi usaha ternak sapi bali dan perkebunan di Kabupaten buton utara. *Agrilan: Jurnal Agribisnis Kepulauan*, 9(2), 115–124. https://doi.org/10.30598/agrilan.v9i2.1176

Sani, L. O. A., Sutiana, S., Zulkarnain, D., Aku, A. S., Munadi, L. O. M., & Syamsuddin, S. (2022). Identification of livestock development inhibiting factors bali cattle transmigration and local community in Konawe District. *Budapest International Research and Critics Institute-Journal (BIRCI-Journal)*, 5(1), 674–685. https://doi.org/10.33258/birci.v5i1.3665

Sulfiar, A. E. T., Guntoro, B., Atmoko, B. A., & Budisatria, I. G. S. (2022). Sustainability of beef cattle farming production system in South Konawe Regency, Southeast Sulawesi. *Journal of the Indonesian Tropical Animal Agriculture*, 47(2), 155–165. https://doi.org/10.14710/jitaa.47.2.155-165

Technological Innovations in Tropical Livestock Development for Environmental Sustainability and Food Security – P. Dhian Isnaeni et al. (eds)
© 2025 The Editor(s), ISBN 978-1-032-74373-8

Author index